Reproductive Medicine for Clinical Practice

Reproductive Medicine for Clinical Practice

Editor: Cameron Baker

AMERICAN
MEDICAL PUBLISHERS
www.americanmedicalpublishers.com

AMERICAN
MEDICAL PUBLISHERS
www.americanmedicalpublishers.com

Cataloging-in-Publication Data

Reproductive medicine for clinical practice / edited by Cameron Baker.
p. cm.
Includes bibliographical references and index.
ISBN 979-8-88740-433-2
1. Reproductive health. 2. Human reproduction. 3. Fertility, Human.
4. Embryology, Human. 5. Birth control. I. Baker, Cameron.
RG133 .R47 2023
613.9--dc23

American Medical Publishers,
41 Flatbush Avenue,
1st Floor, New York,
NY 11217, USA

ISBN 979-8-88740-433-2 (Hardback)

Contents

Preface

Reproductive medicine refers to a branch of medicine that studies the female and male reproductive systems. Family planning, infertility, sexual education, diseases of the reproductive system, puberty, sexual dysfunction and birth control are the issues addressed by this branch of medicine. It deals with the diagnosis, prevention and treatment of diseases, such as cancer, endocrine disorders, infectious diseases and congenital abnormalities. It also deals with ovulation, menopause, menstruation and pregnancy in females, along with the gynecological conditions that affect fertility. Reproductive medicine has enabled the development of artificial reproductive techniques (ARTs), which have provided a solution to human infertility and are now being utilized in wildlife conservation and agriculture. These involve therapeutic approaches and novel technologies for enhancing IVF outcomes and preventing ovarian hyper stimulation syndrome. This book strives to provide a fair idea about reproductive medicine and to help develop a better understanding of the latest advances and clinical practices in this field. It covers in detail some existent and innovative concepts revolving around this domain. This book is appropriate for students seeking detailed information in this area as well as for experts.

This book has been the outcome of endless efforts put in by authors and researchers on various issues and topics within the field. The book is a comprehensive collection of significant researches that are addressed in a variety of chapters. It will surely enhance the knowledge of the field among readers across the globe.

It gives us an immense pleasure to thank our researchers and authors for their efforts to submit their piece of writing before the deadlines. Finally in the end, I would like to thank my family and colleagues who have been a great source of inspiration and support.

Editor

Effect of *Origanum vulgare* Essential Oil Supplementation on the Advanced Parameters of Mobility and on the Integrity of Human Sperm DNA

Modou M. Mbaye,[1,2] Bouchra El Khalfi,[1] Saida Ouzamode,[1] Brahim Saadani,[3] Noureddine Louanjli,[2] and Abdelaziz Soukri[1]

[1]*Laboratory of Physiopathology, Genetics Molecular and Biotechnology (PGMB), Faculty of Sciences Ain Chock, Research Center Health and Biotechnology, University Hassan II of Casablanca, Morocco*
[2]*In Vitro Fertilization Center IRIFIV, IRIS Clinic, Casablanca, Morocco*
[3]*Laboratory of Medical Analyses, Reproductive Biology, Labomac, Casablanca, Morocco*

Correspondence should be addressed to Abdelaziz Soukri; ab.soukri@gmail.com

Academic Editor: Yuksel Agca

The reduced sperm mobility is one of the most important causes of male infertility. Several reports have indicated that the treatment of subnormal sperm samples with certain agents prior to artificial insemination significantly improves the fertilizing potential of sperm. We have among others some stimulants such as pentoxifylline, relaxin, prostaglandin E, and diltiazem. In our precedent work, we had tested the effect of supplementation with three essential oils, namely, sage (*Salvia officinalis*), oregano (*Origanum vulgare*), and eucalyptus (*Eucalyptus globulus*), on sperm cell mobility and vitality. Oregano oil had shown interesting biological properties by giving the best values of progressive mobility and vitality. In this study, we aim to verify the effect of oregano oil supplementation on the advanced parameters of mobility and on the integrity of the sperm DNA of 25 male infertile volunteers. Our results showed that oregano oil over an incubation period of 5 to 10 min of exposure significantly improves the advanced parameters of mobility, namely, curvilinear velocity (VCL), linear velocity (VSL), the mean velocity of the path (VAP), and the amplitude of the displacement (ALH). The effect of the increase in the VCL decreased the linearity (LIN), the mean line (STR), and the mean wobble (WOB). Oregano oil at 5 min had no significant effect on the DNA fragmentation index (DFI) and sperm decondensation index (SDI). However, at 10 min, it had a significant effect on both DFI and SDI. The analysis of our results showed that this plant oil rich in terpenoids and phenolic antioxidants could be a quite good in vitro additive with high potential for the world of medically assisted reproduction.

1. Introduction

Asthenozoospermia characterized by a sperm cell mobility deficit is one of the major causes of male infertility [1]. This is due to a decrease in energy levels that can be caused by a failure of the main pathway of ATP hydrolysis, damage to sperm cell structures (flagella), or infections [2]. To overcome this energy deficiency, experts in reproductive biology propose many solutions, often of a chemical nature, thus encountering toxicity problems.

Finding natural biomolecules capable of improving sperm mobility and vitality in vitro is a promising, attractive, and very decisive path for a significant improvement in the low results of in vitro fertilization, which are stagnating at less than 20%.

Our previous work had shown that the in vitro supplementation of the essential oil of oregano during 5 and 10 min of incubation at 37°C under 5% of CO_2 significantly improved the mobility and the vitality of the spermatozoa [3].

Advanced mobility parameters, especially the different speeds, are positively correlated with sperm/oocyte interaction [4].

The rate of sperm DNA fragmentation and the level of sperm decondensation have a significant impact on embryo development and survival.

In order to show that oregano could be a potential beneficial additive for the preparation of sperm in vitro for the world of medically assisted reproduction, we considered necessary to study the effect of oregano oil supplementation on the advanced parameters of sperm cell mobility, namely, curvilinear velocity (VCL), linear velocity (VSL), mean path velocity (VAP), range of motion (ALH), linearity (LIN), mean straight line (STR), and mean wobble (WOB), as well as its impact on sperm DNA integrity through evaluation of the DNA fragmentation index (DFI) and the sperm decondensation index (SDI).

2. Materials and Methods

2.1. Chemical Products. All chemicals used in this study were obtained from Sigma-Aldrich (St. Louis, MO, USA).

2.2. Plant Material. Essential oil (EO) was obtained directly from the leaves of *Origanum vulgare L.* plants (Fliyou) collected at the Fez region (central Morocco). The plant material was randomly collected, washed, and dried in a well-ventilated place at room temperature for ten days before being used according to the method of Sabir et al. [5]. The sample was then isolated and stored for extraction.

2.3. Essential Oil. The essential oil was obtained by hydrodistillation 3.5 h using the Clevenger apparatus according to the method of Sabir et al. [5]. The oil was extracted from the distillate with hexane and dehydrated by passing through anhydrous sodium sulphate. After filtration, the solvent was removed by reduced pressure distillation in a rotary evaporator at 35°C, and the pure oil was stored in an amber bottle stored in the refrigerator (4°C), until use [5]. The nonlethal concentrations of the essential oil were determined by the dilution technique in series according to the method of Mar et al. [6].

2.4. Sample Collection. This study was carried out at the Laboratory of Medical Analysis and Reproductive Biology, "Labomac," Casablanca, Morocco. We have established a study group of 25 samples of men diagnosed with Asthenozoospermia ($\geq 20 \times$ concentrations $\times$ 106 ml; progressive motility is <32%). Informed consent was obtained from all patients included before using their sperm in this study. Then, samples were collected after 3 to 4 days of abstinence in sterile and labelled containers [3]. For liquefaction, the samples were stored at 37°C under 5% CO_2 until use. We checked at a time interval of 10 min until the liquefaction was done. The microscopic analysis was performed in accordance with World Health Organization (WHO) standards and guidelines [3].

2.5. Semen Treatment. After one hour of sperm production, a routine sperm analysis was performed to determine sperm count, motility, and vitality. To make it, a sample of 20 μl of sperm was deposited in a Makler room. The sperm pretreatment was performed using the density gradient optimization technique. Thus, 1 ml of PureSperm® 70%, 1 ml of PureSperm® 45%, and 1 ml of semen sample were added, respectively, in a 10 ml Falcon tube and centrifuged at 500 rpm for 20 min. The pellet (approx. 0.5 ml) was fortified with 10 to 20 μl of BM1, then divided into 2 equal aliquots in 10 ml Falcon tubes; the first tube containing the pellet and BM1 was incubated as a control; the second was also incubated with 1.5 μl of oregano oil at a final concentration of [10^{-3}]. Incubations were performed at 37°C under 5% CO_2 (Figure 1) [3].

2.6. Mobility Analysis. The effect of oregano oil on advanced parameters of human sperm cell mobility has been evaluated at different incubation periods: 0, 5, and 10 min at 37°C under 5% CO_2. The protocol consists of depositing an aliquot of 20 μl of the mixture (sperm/oil, control) in a preheated Makler chamber and analyzing by CASA (Hamilton-Thorne Semen Computer-Assisted Analysis version 10 HTM IVOS Analyzer (Hamilton-Thorne Biosciences, Beverly, MA, USA)). The parameters used for the analysis are as follows: number of images, 8; frame rate, 20 Hz; layer thickness 10 μl; temperature, 37°C; minimum contrast, 6; minimum size, 6; small size grid, 0.4; large size grid, 2.0; low intensity grid, 2.5; and high intensity grid, 4.3 [1]. Eight representative fields containing at least 100 mobile sperm cells were examined. Throughout the analysis, an integrated heated stage maintained the sample temperature at 37°C [1]. The parameters recorded for each sample were percentage viability, percentage progressive motility, and movement characteristics such as curvilinear velocity (VCL), linear velocity (VSL), mean path velocity (VAP), lateral displacement amplitude (ALH), mean linearity (LIN: VSL/VCL), mean straight line (STR: VSL/VAP), and mean wobble (WOB: VAP/VCL) [1].

2.7. Vitality Analysis. The assessment of sperm viability was performed with 2% eosin staining [3]. To do this, semen samples were mixed with an equal volume of eosin solution. A smear on a glass slide was made from the mixture and was allowed to air dry. Immediately after drying, each slide was examined under an optical microscope. The test is performed immediately after contact between the sperm cells and different concentrations of EO ($t = 0$ min), at exposure times ranging from 5 to 10 min, and the preparation was incubated at 37°C under 5% CO_2 [3].

2.8. Measurement of the DNA Fragmentation Index by TUNEL Test. The integrity of the sperm DNA was assessed by the TUNEL test using a commercial kit (Roche Diagnostics, Lewes, United Kingdom) according to the manufacturer's recommendations. The principle of the TUNEL technique is to use an enzyme, the Terminal Deoxynucleotidyl Transferase (TdT), capable of adding nucleotides to the 3′-OH ends of free DNA.

The sperm sample was washed twice in phosphate-buffered saline (PBS, Sigma-Aldrich, Gillingham, UK) and adjusted to a concentration of 2×10^7 cells/ml in PBS. The cell suspension was then fixed in PBS containing 2%

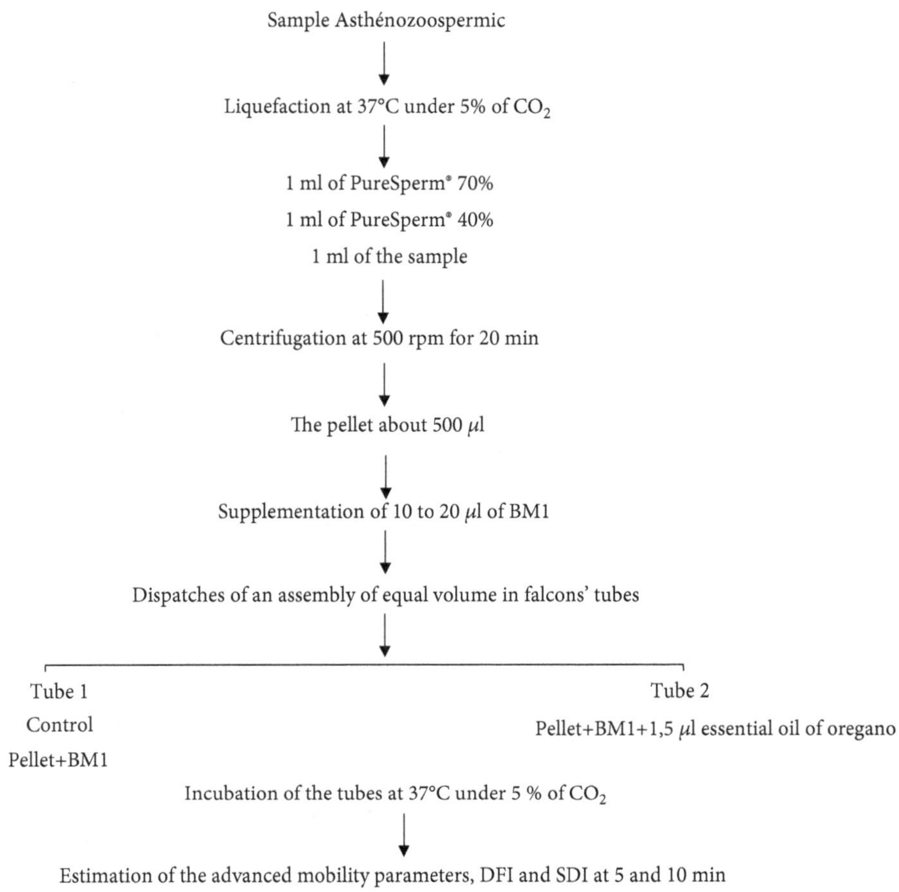

FIGURE 1: Sample processing method.

formaldehyde (Sigma-Aldrich) for 60 min at room temperature. Following a double wash with PBS, the sample is centrifuged at 1200 rpm. This step is repeated twice. Slides prepared were immediately analyzed using a fluorescence microscope (Nikon Eclipse 80i) equipped with appropriate filters. The images were captured using a CCD camera and XytoGen software (Excilone, version 3.8.46, France) (Figure 2) [7].

2.9. Measurement of the Index of Sperm Decondensation to Aniline Blue. The slides of the prepared sperm samples were rinsed twice with distilled water and then stained with 5% aniline blue bath pH 3.5 for five min. They are then quickly rinsed with distilled water and then dehydrated in alcohol baths (70, 90, and 100°, one minute each). The reading is done under white light at magnification ×1000 and immersion (Figure 2).

A total of 500 spermatozoa were counted on the slides made from the whole sperm. Positive for aniline blue (a poorly condensed chromatin spermatozoon) is any sperm for which the blue color occupies more than 50% of the surface of the head [7].

2.10. Statistical Test. The data obtained during our experiments were the subject of a statistical study. The results of the oregano oil supplementation on the characteristic parameters of mobility and nuclear quality were obtained by the Student t-test (t-test). All the graphs and histograms represented in this article have been created with the software GraphPad Prism 7.

3. Results

3.1. Effects of Origanum vulgare Oil on Mobility and Vitality. In vitro supplementation of oregano essential oil (*Origanum vulgare*) has significantly improved the percentage of progressive mobility as well as the vitality of human sperm cells (Figure 3) ($P < 0.001$).

3.2. Advice Effects of Origanum vulgare on Advanced Mobility Parameters. In vitro supplementation of oregano essential oil (*Origanum vulgare*) has shown a significant stimulating effect on advanced mobility parameters curvilinear velocity (VCL) ($P < 0.01$) (Figure 4), linear velocity (VSL) ($P < 0.01$) (Figure 5), mean path velocity (VAP) ($P < 0.01$) (Figure 6), and amplitude of displacement (ALH) ($P < 0.01$) (Figure 7).

The effect of the increased VCL decreased very substantially the linearity (LIN) ($P < 0.05$) (Figure 8), the mean line (STR) (Figure 9), and the mean wobble (WOB) (Figure 10).

3.3. Effect of Origanum vulgare on DNA Fragmentation Index. Supplementation of oregano in Asthenozoospermic sperm after 5 and 10 min of incubation at 37°C under 5% CO_2 does not alter the level of sperm with DNA fragmentation.

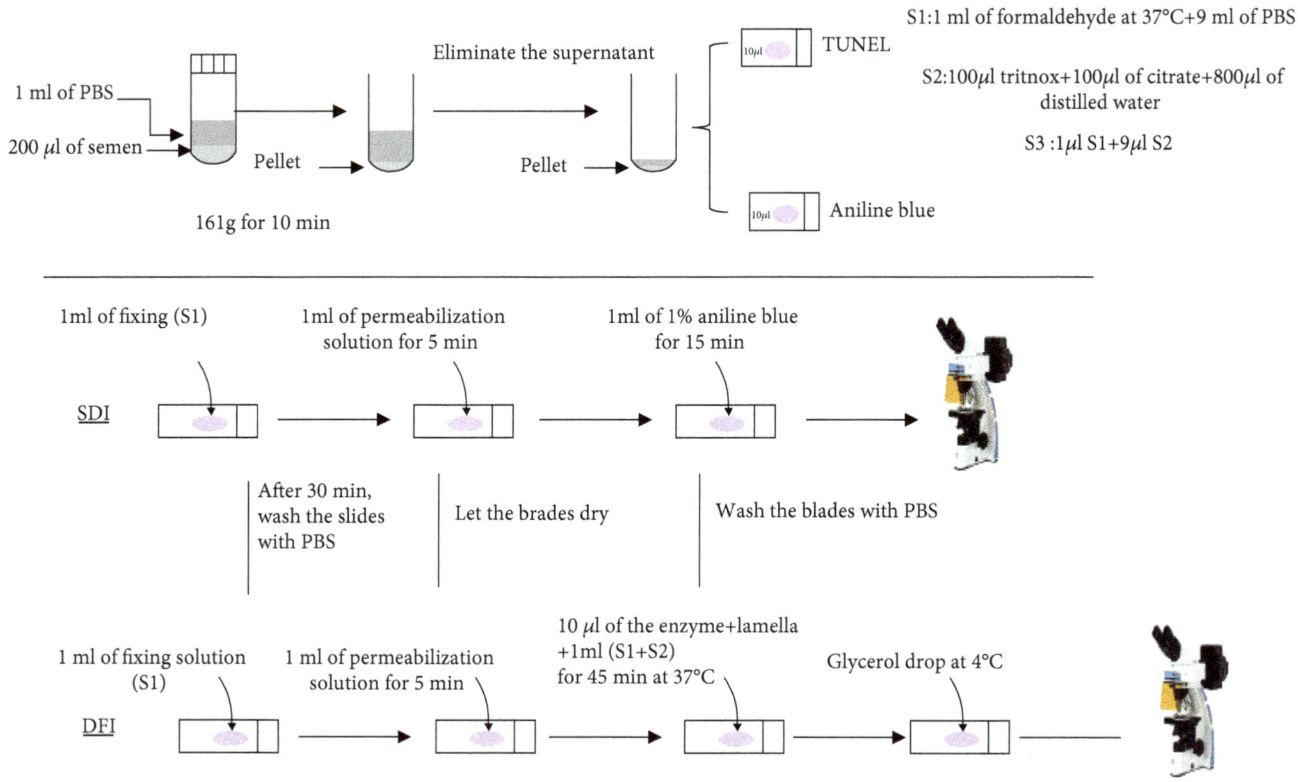

Figure 2: Processing method used for evaluating the sperm decondensation index (SDI) and the DNA fragmentation index (DFI).

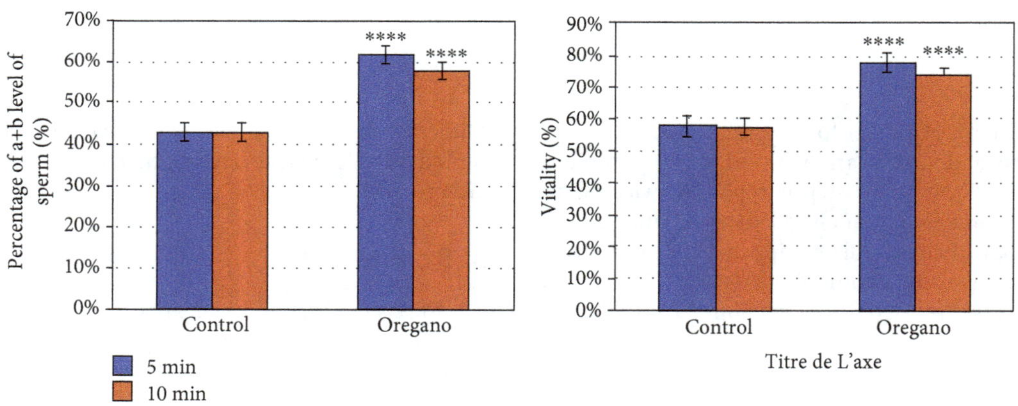

Figure 3: In vitro effect of oregano oil on the proportion of mobile sperm. The dilution of EO was done in a 0.2% (w/v) sterile agar solution. The percentage motility and vitality of each aliquot was measured after the addition of the EO and 5 min and 10 min treatment. Oregano oil could significantly increase the number of progressive mobile sperm cells and viability over a period of 5 to 10 min (****$P < 0.001$; $n = 25$).

Because the rate of sperm with DNA fragmentation is as high in the fortified sample as in the control, difference is not significant ($P = 0.53$) at 5 min. However, on the other hand, we noted a significant difference at 10 min ($P < 0.05$) (Figure 11).

3.4. Effect of Origanum vulgare on Sperm Decondensation Index. The level of spermatozoa with a condensation defect of DNA after 5 to 10 min of incubation at 37°C under 5% of CO_2 shows that the in vitro supplementation of oregano oil in human sperm has no deleterious effect on the normal condensation of sperm chromatin since mean values of supplemented and control samples do not show any significant difference ($P = 0.48$) at 5 min. However, we noted a significant difference at 10 min ($P < 0.05$) (Figure 12).

4. Discussion

Sperm transfer in the procedures of in vitro fertilization, intrauterine insemination, and intrafallopian gamete is done with washed sperm [1]. Finding methods to optimize sperm for all these procedures is utmost important for professionals in reproductive biology [8].

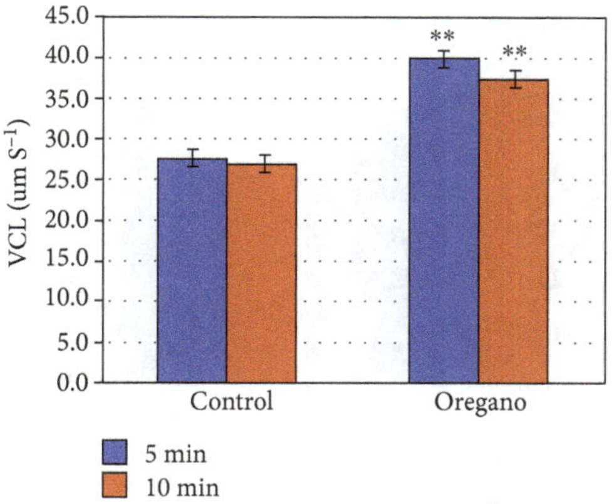

FIGURE 4: In vitro effects of oregano oil on the curvilinear velocity (VCL). The dilution of the EO was performed in 0.2% (*w*/*v*) sterile agar solution. The percentage of VCL of each aliquot was measured after the addition of the EO and 5 min and 10 min treatment. Oregano oil significantly improves the VCL over a period of 5 to 10 min (**$P < 0.01$; $n = 25$).

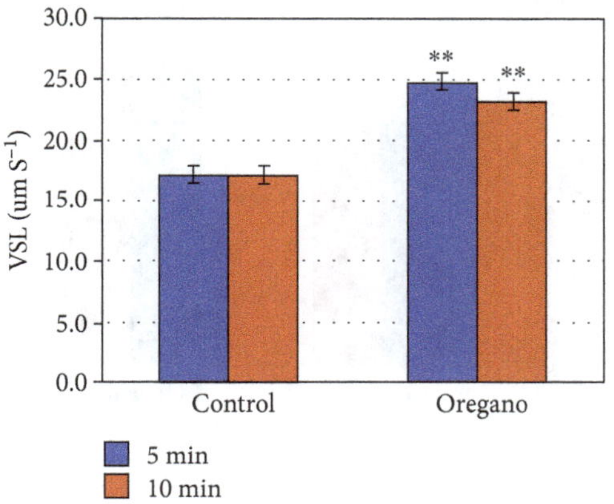

FIGURE 5: In vitro effect of oregano oil on the linear velocity (VSL). The dilution of EO was done in a 0.2% (*w*/*v*) sterile agar solution. The percentage of VSL of each aliquot was measured after the addition of the EO and 5 min and 10 min treatment. Oregano oil could significantly improve the VSL over a period of 5 to 10 min (**$P < 0.01$; $n = 25$).

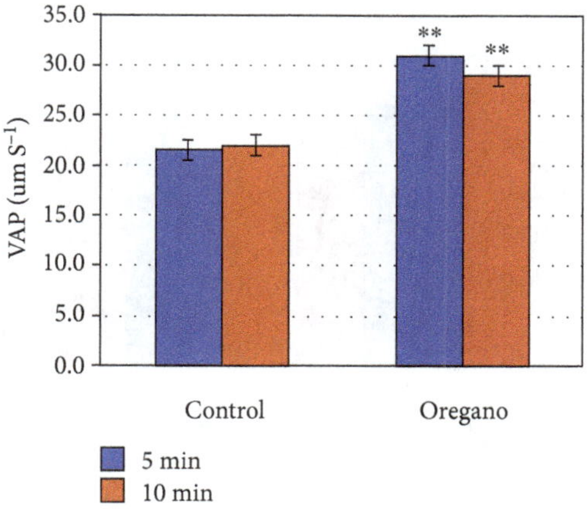

FIGURE 6: In vitro effect of oregano oil on the mean velocity of the path (VAP). The dilution of EO was done in a 0.2% (*w*/*v*) sterile agar solution. The percentage of VAP of each aliquot was measured after the addition of the EO and 5 min and 10 min treatment. Oregano oil could significantly improve the VAP over a period of 5 to 10 min (**$P < 0.01$; $n = 25$).

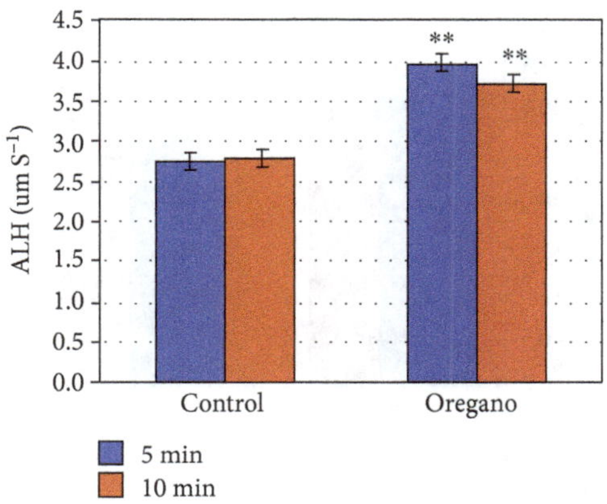

FIGURE 7: In vitro effect of oregano oil on the amplitude of displacement (ALH). The dilution of EO was done in a 0.2% (*w*/*v*) sterile agar solution. The percentage of ALH of each aliquot was measured after the addition of the EO and 5 min and 10 min treatment. Oregano oil could significantly improve ALH over a period of 5 to 10 min (**$P < 0.01$; $n = 25$).

Oregano essential oil could be included among the many plants reported in the literature with improving effects on human sperm mobility [9].

In our previous work, it has been shown that oregano at 5 min exposure at 37°C under 5% CO_2 significantly improves the progressive mobility and vitality of human sperm cells ($P < 0.001$) (Figure 3) [3].

Our experiments with oregano oil supplementation on advanced mobility parameters have shown that 5 and 10 min EO exposure at 37°C under 5% CO_2 significantly improves curvilinear velocity (VCL) (Figure 4), linear velocity (VSL) (Figure 5), mean path velocity (VAP) (Figure 6), and displacement amplitude (ALH) (Figure 7) of sperm cells.

On the other hand, sperm cell linearity (LIN) (Figure 8) as well as the average line (STR) (Figure 9) and the average wobble (WOB) (Figure 10) decreased substantially due to the increase in the VCL and VAP. Our results are in good agreement with those of Barlow and Liu groups [1, 10]. Our ALH values are also in agreement with the work of Liu et al., Aitken and Clarkson, and Bongo et al., by showing that ALH is higher in sperm cells of fertile men than those of infertile men; they show also a positive correlation of the effectiveness of penetration into the cervical mucus of sperm with increased ALH [1, 11, 12].

Several studies have shown that oregano essential oil contains phenolic compounds and flavonoids, in particular, rosmarinic acid, quercetin, kaempferol, apigenin, rutin, and oregano which can cleanse free radicals such as the superoxide anion and hydroxyl [13, 14]. Thus, the improvement in mobility, the advanced parameters of mobility, and the vitality of spermatozoa by the essential oil of oregano can be explained by its antioxidant activity against lipid peroxidation [14]. Moreover, Daghigh Kia et al. have shown that the

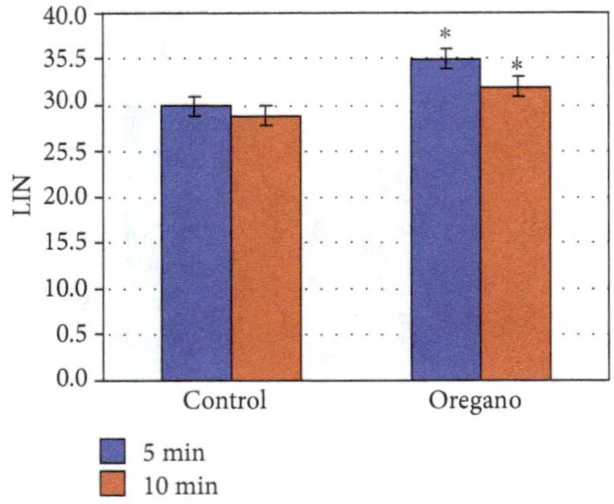

Figure 8: In vitro effect of oregano on the linearity (LIN). The dilution of EO was done in a 0.2% (w/v) sterile agar solution. The percentage of LIN of each aliquot was measured after the addition of the EO and 5 min and 10 min treatment. Oregano oil could significantly improve LIN over a period of 5 to 10 min ($^*P < 0.05$; $n = 25$).

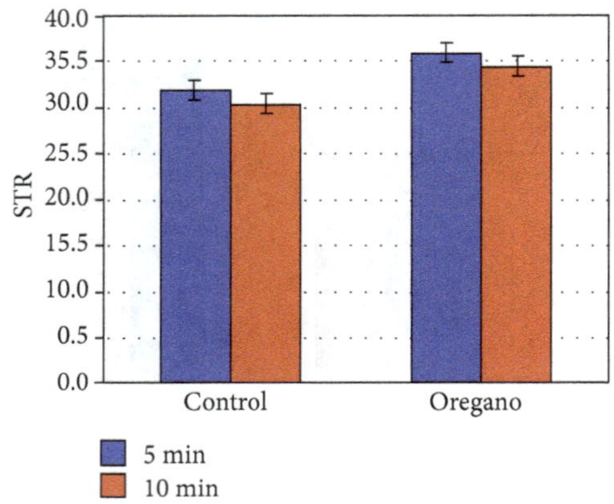

Figure 9: In vitro effect of oregano oil on the mean line (STR). The dilution of EO was done in a 0.2% (w/v) sterile agar solution. The percentage of STR of each aliquot was measured after the addition of the EO and 5 min and 10 min treatment. The effect of such an increase in VCL has resulted in a substantial reduction in STR, LIN, and WOB.

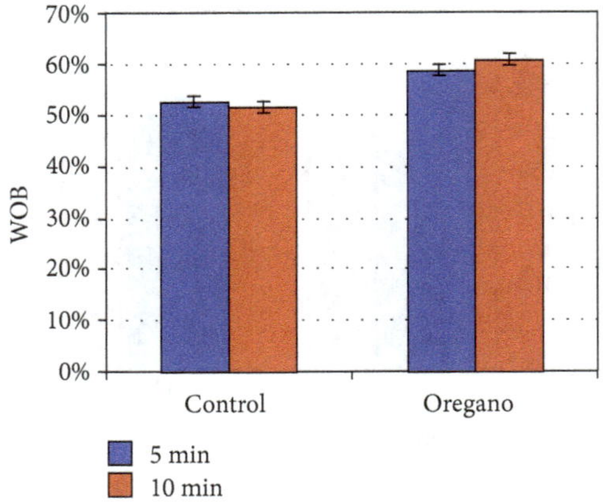

Figure 10: In vitro effect of oregano oil on the mean wobble (WOB). The dilution of EO was done in a 0.2% (w/v) sterile agar solution. The percentage of WOB of each aliquot was measured after the addition of the EO and 5 min and 10 min treatment ($P = 0.52$; $n = 25$).

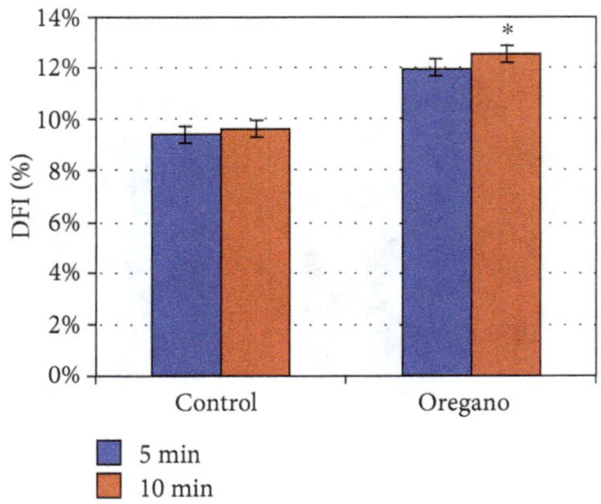

Figure 11: In vitro effect of oregano oil on DNA fragmentation index. DFI was measured after the addition of the EO and 5 min and 10 min treatment. The dilution of EO was done in a 0.2% (w/v) sterile agar solution. The percentage of DFI of each aliquot was measured immediately after the addition of the EO ($t = 5$ min) ($P = 0.53$; $n = 25$) and 10 minutes later ($t = 10$ min) ($^*P < 0.05$; $n = 25$).

peroxidation of lipids in sperm damages the structure of the lipid matrix in the membranes of sperm and that it is linked to a rapid loss of intracellular ATP which can lead to axonemal damage and reduced sperm viability [15]. It is in this same endeavor that Aitken determined that the peroxide radical (H_2O_2) could be distributed across the membranes of the spermatozoa and thus inhibit the activity of key enzymes such as glucose-6-phosphate dehydrogenase (enzyme which plays a major role in ATP production and sperm motility) [16].

Our ALH values agree well with the work of Liu et al., Aitken and Clarkson, and Bongo et al., by showing that ALH is higher in sperm of fertile men and also show a positive correlation of the effectiveness of penetration into the cervical mucus of sperm with an increase in ALH [1, 11, 12].

The evaluation of the effect of oregano oil supplementation on DNA integrity at 5 min incubation at 37°C under 5% CO_2 did not yield a significant difference for both DFI (Figure 11) and SDI (Figure 12) values. However, after 10 min of incubation, a significant difference was noted for both DFI ($P < 0.05$) and SDI ($P < 0.05$) with respect to the controls (Figures 11 and 12). The absence of a convention on the threshold values of the DFI and the SDI makes it difficult to interpret them. We can say that oregano essential oil does not impact the index of DNA fragmentation and sperm decondensation index because we have recorded lower values than the positive threshold value for DFI (4%) and for SDI (15%) [17]. Sperm abnormalities can cause not only embryonic development problems [4] but also spontaneous miscarriages [1]. The low DFI and SDI values can result from various factors in addition to the supplementation of oregano

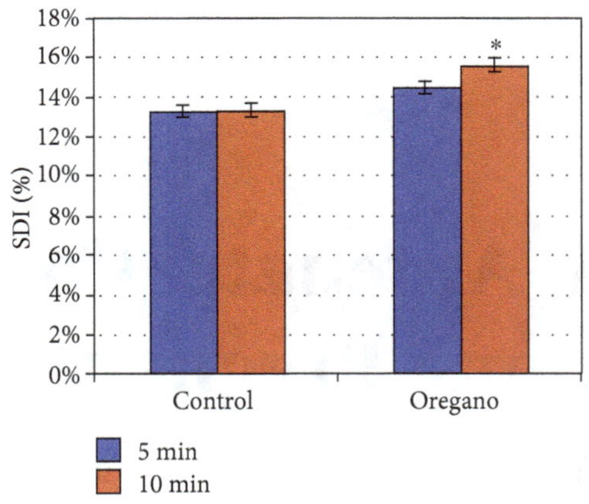

FIGURE 12: In vitro effect of oregano oil on the sperm decondensation index. SDI was measured immediately after the addition of the EO and 5 min and 10 min treatment. The dilution of EO was done in a 0.2% (*w/v*) sterile agar solution. The percentage of SDI of each aliquot was measured after 5 min ($P = 0.48$; $n = 25$) and 10 min ($^*P < 0.05$; $n = 25$).

oil because even in the control, we noted low DFI and SDI values. Moreover, numerous studies have shown that alteration of sperm DNA can result from various phenomena such as apoptosis, oxidative stress, production of endogenous Reactive Oxygen Species (ROS), and spontaneous and/or exogenous alterations (ionizing radiation, toxic components of the environment), which act on DNA elements by producing a very wide range of damage such as deletions or breaks in free nitrogenous bases [18].

The results of oregano oil supplementation on the advanced parameters of mobility and DNA quality of the sperm show that *Origanum vulgare* essential oil could be a promising alternative for better male infertility management especially in patients with Asthenozoospermia.

5. Conclusion

This study highlights the improving effects of in vitro supplementation with oregano essential oil on advanced sperm mobility parameters and its impact on sperm DNA quality. The results allowed us to observe an improvement in the advanced parameters of mobility, DFI and SDI, after 5 min of incubation. Based on the results, we can conclude that oregano oil could be a safe therapeutic alternative for the management of motility dysfunction in Asthenozoospermic patients.

References

[1] J. Liu, M. A. Carmell, F. V. Rivas et al., "Argonaute2 is the catalytic engine of mammalian RNAi," *Science*, vol. 305, no. 5689, pp. 1437–1441, 2004.

[2] M. Jodar, A. Soler-Ventura, R. Oliva, and Molecular Biology of Reproduction and Development Research Group, "Semen proteomics and male infertility," *Journal of proteomics*, vol. 162, pp. 125–134, 2017.

[3] M. M. Mbaye, B. El Khalfi, B. Addoum et al., "The effect of supplementation with some essential oils on the mobility and the vitality of human sperm," *The Scientific World Journal*, vol. 2019, Article ID 4878912, 6 pages, 2019.

[4] M. A. Jawad, A. A. W. Mohammed, H. B. Sahib, M. S. Abbood, and W. Shakir, "Effect of alcohol extract of Prunus avium on in vitro sperm activation of human semen samples," *Int J Pharm Science*, vol. 25, no. 1, pp. 65–68, 2014.

[5] A. Sabir, B. El Khalfi, F. Errachidi, I. Chemsi, A. Serrano, and A. Soukri, "Evaluation of the potential of some essential oils in biological control against phytopathogenic agent Pseudomonas syringae pv. tomato DC3000 responsible for the tomatoes speck," *J Plant Pathol Microbiol*, vol. 8, no. 9, 2017.

[6] P. D. Mar, B. El Khalfi, and A. Soukri, "Protective effect of oregano and sage essentials oils against the effect of extracellular H2O2 and SNP in Tetrahymena thermophila and Tetrahymena pyriformis," *Journal of King Saud University-Science*, vol. 32, no. 1, pp. 279–287, 2020.

[7] I. Kaarouch, N. Bouamoud, A. Madkour et al., "Paternal age: negative impact on sperm genome decays and IVF outcomes after 40 years," *Molecular Reproduction and Development*, vol. 85, no. 3, pp. 271–280, 2018.

[8] T. Bączkowski, R. Kurzawa, and W. Głąbowski, "Methods of embryo scoring in in vitro fertilization," *Reproduction biology*, vol. 4, no. 1, pp. 5–22, 2004.

[9] Y.-S. Yang, S. Melinda, H.-N. Ho et al., "Effect of the number and depth of embryos transferred and unilateral or bilateral transfer in tubal embryo transfer (TET)," *Journal of assisted reproduction and genetics*, vol. 9, no. 6, pp. 534–538, 1992.

[10] P. Barlow, A. Delvigne, J. Van Dromme, J. Van Hoeck, K. Vandenbosch, and F. Leroy, "Predictive value of classical and automated sperm analysis for in-vitro fertilization," *Human Reproduction*, vol. 6, no. 8, pp. 1119–1124, 1991.

[11] R. J. Aitken and J. S. Clarkson, "Cellular basis of defective sperm function and its association with the genesis of reactive oxygen species by human spermatozoa," *Reproduction*, vol. 81, no. 2, pp. 459–469, 1987.

[12] A. Bongso, S.-C. Ng, H. Mok et al., "Improved sperm concentration, motility, and fertilization rates following Ficoll treatment of sperm in a human in vitro fertilization program," *Fertility and Sterility*, vol. 51, no. 5, pp. 850–854, 1989.

[13] H. Kikuzaki and N. Nakatani, "Structure of a new antioxidative phenolic acid from oregano (Origanum vulgare L.)," *Agricultural and Biological Chemistry*, vol. 53, no. 2, pp. 519–524, 1989.

[14] C. B. Hollenbach, R. S. Bing, R. Stedile et al., "Reproductive toxicity assessment of Origanum vulgare essential oil on male Wistar rats," *Acta Scientiae Veterinariae*, vol. 43, p. 1295, 2015.

[15] H. Daghigh Kia, R. Farhadi, I. Ashrafi, and M. Mehdipour, "Anti-oxidative effects of ethanol extract of Origanum vulgare on kinetics, microscopic and oxidative parameters of cryopreserved Holstein bull spermatozoa," *Iranian Journal of Applied Animal Science*, vol. 6, no. 4, pp. 783–789, 2016.

[16] R. Aitken, "Molecular mechanisms regulating human sperm function," *Molecular human reproduction*, vol. 3, no. 3, pp. 169–173, 1997.

[17] C. Roux, C. Tripogney, C. Joanne, and J. Bresson, "Qualité nucléaire du spermatozoïde : tests d'exploration de la chromatine des spermatozoïdes humains (protéines nucléaires)," *Gynécologie Obstétrique & Fertilité*, vol. 32, no. 9, pp. 792–798, 2004.

[18] R. J. Aitken and C. Krausz, "Oxidative stress, DNA damage and the Y chromosome," *Reproduction*, vol. 122, no. 4, pp. 497–506, 2001.

2

Maternal Satisfaction with Antenatal Care and Associated Factors among Pregnant Women in Hossana Town

Dagmawit Birhanu Kebede, Yeshitila Belay Belachew, Desta Workneh Selbana, and Admasu Belay Gizaw

Jimma University School of Nursing and Midwifery, P.O. Box 378, Ethiopia

Correspondence should be addressed to Admasu Belay Gizaw; admasu2004@gmail.com

Academic Editor: Samir Hamamah

Background. A woman's satisfaction with antenatal care service has immediate and long-term impacts on maternal and her baby's health. It also ensures further use of service. However, it is not well studied in Ethiopia in general and at the southern region in particular. *Objective*. The main objective of this study is to assess the level of a maternal satisfaction with antenatal care services and associated factors. *Methods*. An institution-based cross-sectional study that involves both quantitative and qualitative methods of data collection was employed. A systematic sampling technique was used to obtain study participants, and quantitative data were collected using an interviewer-administered questionnaire. For qualitative data, Focus Group Discussions were done among clients that have a repeated visit by taking educational status as homogeneity criteria. EpiData version 3.1 and SPSS version 21 were used for analysis. Descriptive statistics, bivariate and multivariable logistic regression analyses were employed to describe and identify factors associated with maternal satisfaction on antenatal care. The qualitative data were analyzed thematically and manually. *Results*. Overall, 74% of mothers were satisfied with antenatal care services rendered in public health institutions of Hossana town. Most of the respondents were satisfied with privacy, cleanness, physical facility, and approaches of care. Age, educational status, privacy, cleanness, distance, and respect were significantly associated with a client's satisfaction. *Conclusion*. Three-fourths of the respondents were satisfied with the service. Age, education, living distance, maintenance of privacy, cleanness of the facility, and respect from providers were the significant predictors of the satisfaction level.

1. Introduction

Antenatal care can be broadly defined as encompassing pregnancy-related services provided between conception and the onset of labor with the aim of improving the pregnancy outcome and the heath of the mother or child and providing women and their families/partners with appropriate information and advice for a healthy pregnancy, childbirth, and postnatal recovery [1]. The measurement of patients' satisfaction is a common component of evaluations in quality care. Clients' reported levels of satisfaction reflect professionals' technical competence as judged by independent assessors and are an important indicator of the quality of care. It is known that a satisfied client is more likely to comply with treatment and advice she receives from health care professionals [2]. Client satisfaction was a function of patients' subjective responses to experienced care mediated by personal preferences and expectations. Also, it is a measurement designed to obtain reports or ratings from patients about services received from an organization, hospital, or health care provider. On a practical level, client satisfaction is equivalent to the actual measure [3].

Many maternal and prenatal deaths occur in women with low utilization of antenatal care (ANC), but utilization of ANC service is affected by a client's satisfaction. Nevertheless, true progress has been made globally in terms of increasing access. Worldwide, 70% of women ever receive any antenatal care, whereas in industrialized countries, more than 95% of pregnant women receive ANC [4]. Globally, an estimated 295,000 maternal deaths occurred in 2017, yielding an overall 211 maternal deaths per 100,000 live births [5]. Ninety-nine percent of this death occurs in developing countries, and the sub-Saharan African region alone accounts for 66% (19600) of maternal death. Maternal mortality is higher in women without skilled care before, during, and after childbirth. Ethiopia is one of the countries in sub-Saharan Africa with a markedly high maternal mortality ratio (401 deaths per 100,000 live births) [5].

ANC can reduce maternal mortality by 20% given good quality and regular attendance. ANC attendance during pregnancy has a positive impact on the use of postnatal healthcare services and an important entry point to convince expectant mothers about the health benefits of attended delivery [6–8]. However, the use of ANC service by pregnant women could be affected by the level of their satisfaction with the service provided at the health care facility. In southwestern Nigeria, only 44% of respondents utilized health care facilities. This was attributed to various factors causing dissatisfaction with services rendered at these centers [9–16].

Patients' use of health care is affected by the quality of care; those who are not satisfied with their providers may be less likely to continue with treatment or seek further services. According to the U.S. Agency for Healthcare Research and Quality, National Consumer Assessment of Healthcare Providers and Systems (CAHPS) Benchmarking Database in Africa, a maternal satisfaction survey was conducted at different times in different counties (for instance, in 2012 and 2018 and in Egypt and Nigeria, the level of maternal satisfaction with ANC was greater than 90% and 90%, respectively, whereas in Ethiopia, the levels of maternal satisfaction with antenatal care in 2008, 2013, 2014, 2018, and 2019 were 35%, 47.7%, 60.4%, 90%, and 90.8%, respectively [17–23].

The degree of patient satisfaction can be used as a means of assessing the quality of health care and personnel. It reflects the ability of the provider to meet the patients' needs. Satisfied patients are more likely than the unsatisfied ones to continue using health care services, maintain their relationships with specific health care providers, and comply with the care regimens [24–26]. Sociodemographic background of the patient, expectations of care, organizational factors (facility-related factors), and provider-related factors (communication and information, participation and involvement, and interpersonal relationships) are very important aspects or factors on which patient satisfaction depends [14, 18, 20, 27, 28].

Different studies in different parts of the world revealed that maternal satisfaction with antenatal care was affected by examination room cleanness, health care provider attitude, quality of antenatal care service provided, adequacy of information provided by the health care professionals, waiting time, supervision of antenatal care, adequacy of water supply, adequacy of waiting area, educational status of the mother, monthly income, type of pregnancy and history of stillbirth, patient's previous experiences, social and cultural norms, physical environment, availability of adequate resources (human, medicines, drugs, equipment, and supplies), adequacy of clinical care, and access to treatment in healthcare facilities [14, 29–38].

Despite these facts, client satisfaction on antenatal care service is one of the measures of quality care and is essential for further improvement of maternal and child health, and it is not well studied in the southern region of Ethiopia. Therefore, this study is aimed at assessing the level of maternal satisfaction with antenatal services and its associated factors in public health facilities of Hossana town.

2. Materials and Methods

2.1. Study Setting. The study was conducted in Southern Nations, Nationality, and People's Region (SNNPR) state, Hadiya zone, Hossana town, in Ethiopia. It is one of the political and administrative towns and lies 230 km southwest of the capital city, Addis Ababa. The town is divided into three subcities and eight kebeles. The total population size of the town projected to the year 2013 according to the 2007 population and housing census was 102,238 of which 50,094 are male and 52,144 are female with an annual growth rate of 5%. The census revealed that the town has a sex ratio of 51 : 49 females to males. The population of women in the reproductive age (WIRA) was 23,821, and the proportion of pregnant women constitutes 3.9% of the total population. Currently, in 2019, the town has one hospital, three health centers, and sixteen private clinics.

2.2. Study Design. A facility-based cross-sectional study that involves both qualitative and quantitative methods was conducted.

2.3. Sample Size Determination. The sample size for the quantitative study was determined using a single population proportion formula, and a total of 325 pregnant women are recruited:

$$n = \frac{(Z\alpha/2)2xp(1-p)}{d^2}, \quad (1)$$

where n is the sample size; $Z\alpha/2$ is the confidence level at $95\% = 1.96$; P is the proportion of satisfaction of women which is unknown, assumption of 50% ($P = 0.5$); and d is the margin of error of 4.5%:

$$n = \frac{(Z\alpha/2)^2 * P(1-P)}{d^2},$$
$$n = \frac{(1.96)^2 * 0.5(1-0.5)}{(0.05)^2}, \quad (2)$$
$$n = 384.$$

Since the source population is less than 10,000, the correction formula was used to get the final sample size as follows:

$$\text{nf} = \frac{n}{1 + n/N}, \quad (3)$$

where 'N' is the source population-all estimated pregnant women, 'nf' is the required sample size, and n is the calculated sample size. Hence, the sample size will be calculated at a total of source population $N = 1280$, $n = 384$, and $nf = 295$. Considering the nonresponse rate of 10%, the total sample size will be 325 pregnant women.

For the qualitative study, 32 pregnant women on an ANC follow-up were recruited out of the quantitative study area and categorized into 4 focus group discussions (FGDs) of equal size.

2.4. Sampling Technique. The entire four public health facilities in the town were included in the sampling process. The calculated sample size was proportionately allocated for each health facility, and the selection was performed using a systematic sampling technique. The number of clients in each health facility was determined by reviewing the annual document of each health facility and the number of subjects to be included in the study from each health facility. The first participant was randomly selected using a lottery method on the first date, and then, every fourth ANC client was selected.

2.5. Data Collection Instrument and Data Collection Procedure. Data was collected by a structured questionnaire. The questionnaire was adapted by reviewing relevant literatures on measures of satisfaction and modified to the local context (PSQ 18, PSQ-46, PSQ II SERVQUAL). The questionnaire consists of 27 items which measure the level of satisfaction with the different factors that contribute to client satisfaction of ANC services, i.e., provider-related factors and facility-related factors, sociodemographic variables, and clients' degree of knowledge, and service expectation of the respondents before utilizing the institution service was also included in the questionnaire. The questionnaire was first developed in English for the interview with pregnant women then translated first into Amharic and Hadiyesa and back-translated to English by someone who was native to those local languages to ensure its consistency and to make it simple during administration. The questionnaire was pretested on 5% of the sample in Balesa town before the data collection period to ensure clarity of the questionnaires, and then, necessary modifications and correction were made to ensure its validity. The reliability (internal consistency of the instrument) was cheeked by Cronbach's alpha. It measures the reliability of the instrument between each domain and the whole of the instrument. All domains had Cronbach's alpha greater than 0.7. The questionnaire consisted of five-point Likert scale items, with 1 and 5 indicating the lowest and highest levels of satisfaction, respectively. The level of satisfaction was indicated by selecting responses ranging from 5 = strongly agree, 4 = agree, 3 = uncertain, and 2 = disagree to 1 = strongly disagree. Five clinical nurse data collectors were selected from the health institution with two supervisors.

They were oriented for a day by the principal investigator about the study instrument, consent form, how to interview, and data collection procedure. Qualitative data focus group discussion (FGD) was conducted among clients that did not participate in the quantitative study in the same time period. Four FGDs were carried out, in the selected two public health facilities by taking educational status as homogeneity criteria. Each group had 6-10 members, an average of 8 female ANC users. The FGD was mediated by the principal investigator; the discussion of the participants was both audiotaped and manually written by two other note-takers and analyzed thematically and manually.

2.6. Data Quality Control. Data were collected by trained data collectors, and pretesting of the instrument was made out of the study site before the actual data collection. Every day, questionnaires were reviewed and checked for its completeness by the selected and trained supervisors and principal investigator; then, the necessary feedback was offered to data collectors in the next morning before data collection. Data were checked on the spot, errors were rectified, and missing data were incorporated into a form. The researcher with the supervisor checked the data collection procedure and counterchecked the entries at random to ensure the quality of data collection.

2.7. Ethical Consideration. Ethical clearance was obtained from the Institutional Review Board of Jimma University. A formal letter from the Institute of Health Science was given to the Hadiya zone health bureau and other concerned bodies to obtain their cooperation. An explanatory letter was added to each questionnaire to maintain participant rights; also, all patients were asked to participate in the study and received full explanations about the research purposes; respect, anonymity, and confidentiality were given and maintained by a consent form for each participant; they have the liberty to withdraw at any stage of the interview; and their participation will not undergo any pressure.

3. Data Processing and Analysis

Data were analyzed by using SPSS version 21.0 statistical software. The normality of data was tested using the Kolmogorov-Smirnov test. All the quantitative data were found to be not normally distributed if ($p \leq .0001$). Descriptive statistics was used for determining the frequency, percentage, mean, and standard deviation. Multivariable logistic regression analyses were used to understand the significance of the association between dependent and independent variables. All independent variables with P value < 0.05 were considered as statistically significant in this study.

4. Results

4.1. Sociodemographic Characteristics of Respondents. Among 325 pregnant women attenuating ANC, 303 participated in the study which makes a 93% response rate and four FGDs consisting of 6-8 members. Of the 303 women, 40.3% were below 24 years of age, 37.3% were between 24 and 29 years, and the rest are above 30 years of age (22.5%), and the mean age of the exit interview was 25 years. Around two-thirds of the study subjects (64.7%) were protestant followed by orthodox 21.8%, and the majority (98%) of the women were currently married. Regarding educational status, only 35 (11.6%) were illiterate, 28% were primary school level, and the rest 64.4% were secondary school and above. Regarding respondent ethnicity, more than two-thirds (69%) of them were Hadiya followed by 8.6% Amhara and 7.3% Kembata. Concerning the employment status of the study participants,

TABLE 1: Sociodemographic characteristics of respondents in Hossana town public health centers, Southern Ethiopia ($n = 303$).

Sociodemographic characteristics	f	%
Age ($N = 303$)		
<24	122	40.3
25-29	113	37.3
30-34	46	15.2
≥35	22	7.3
Median	25	
Marital status		
Currently married	297	98.0
Currently unmarried	6	2
Educational status		
Illiterate	35	11.6
Primary school	85	28.1
Secondary school	104	34.3
Tertiary school	79	26.1
Religion		
Orthodox	66	21.8
Protestant	196	64.7
Muslim	28	9.2
Catholic	13	4.3
Ethnicity		
Hadiya	209	69.0
Amhara	26	8.6
Silte	23	7.6
Gurage	19	6.3
Kembata	22	7.3
Oromo	4	1.3
Occupation		
Currently unemployed	170	56.1
Currently employed	133	43.9
Residence		
Urban	268	88.4
Rural	35	11.6
Health facility		
NEMH	79	26.1
Hossana HC	116	38.3
Lichamba HC	39	12.9
Bobuco HC	69	22.8

more than half of the study subjects (56.1%) were unemployed. More than eighty-eight percent of the respondents live in urban whereas the rest (about 12%) live in rural (Table 1).

4.2. Level of Client Satisfaction with Different Domains of Satisfaction. Most of the study subjects were satisfied by privacy (91.4%), cleanness of the center (87.5%), facility-related factors (82.8%), approaches of care by the care provider (80.2%), interpersonal and technical aspects (79.9%), and communication and information (75.2%). Overall, more than 74% of the study subjects were satisfied with the service that they received while the others (25.4%) are not satisfied (Table 2).

TABLE 2: Level of client satisfaction with different domains of satisfaction in Hossana town, public health centers, Southern Ethiopia ($n = 303$).

Components	Level of satisfaction ($n = 303$)	
	Satisfied N (%)	Not satisfied N
Approaches of care	243 (80.2)	60 (19.8)
Interpersonal and technical aspects	242 (79.9)	61 (20.1)
Communication and information	228 (75.2)	75 (24.8)
Privacy	277 (91.4)	26 (8.6)
Physical facility	251 (82.8)	52 (17.2)
Cleanness	265 (87.5)	38 (12.5)
Overall satisfaction	226 (74.6)	77 (25.4)

4.3. Factors Associated with Antenatal Care Satisfaction. Age is statistically significantly related to the level of satisfaction ($AOR = 5.584$; 95% CI: 1.76, 17.7). Younger mothers were more likely to be satisfied than their counterparts. Those study participants who are illiterate were four times more likely to be satisfied than those who were in primary school and above ($AOR = 4.53$; 95% CI: 1.228, 16.751). Study subjects whose privacies were maintained were more likely to be satisfied than those whose privacy was not maintained ($AOR = 8$; 95% CI: 3.375, 19.263). Cleanness of the institution is also an independent predictor of satisfaction; those who feel that the institution is clean were more likely to be satisfied than those who said that the institution is not clean ($AOR = 3.596$; 95% CI: 1.424, 9.079).

Distance from home to facility is significantly associated with satisfaction; those who travel less than 30 minutes to reach facilities were two times more likely to be satisfied than those who travel greater than 30 minutes ($AOR = 2.804$; 95% CI: 1.423, 5.522); also, one woman supports this idea from the qualitative finding by saying that ".... In the previous time I did not come to hospital when I need care because I travel long distance to reach health institution, but now the institution is near to my home so that I always came whenever I am in need." Respect has also a statistically significant association with satisfaction; those who reported that care providers were respectful were more satisfied than those who reported that care providers were not respectful ($AOR = 2.578$; 95% CI: 1.249, 5.325) (Table 3); also, one participant illustrates from qualitative findings: ".... I would say that she (the care provider) is a positive one because she greets me with a smile, and again, warm greets, even if she is exhausted too many clients, but she doesn't show any bored facial expression for me" (Table 3).

Table 3: Multivariate analysis showing factors associated with maternal satisfaction with antenatal care in public health centers, Hosanna town, Southern Ethiopia ($n = 303$).

Variables	Satisfied N (%)	COR (95% CI)	AOR (95% CI)
Age			
≤24	94 (77%)	3.3 (1, 8.5)	5.584 (1.76, 17.7)
25-29	89 (78%)	3.7 (1.4, 9.5)	8.6 (2.5, 28)
30-34	32 (69.5%)	2.2 (0.8, 6.5)	2.6 (0.757, 9.287)
≥35	11 (50%)	1	1
Educational status			
Illiterate	30 (85.7%)	2.4 (0.8, 7.1)	4.53 (1.228, 16.751)
Primary school	75 (88%)	3.1 (1.4, 7.0)	3.082 (1.169, 8.124)
Secondary school	65 (64.3%)	0.6 (0.3, 1.2)	0.538 (0.247, 1.17)
Tertiary school	56 (73.6%)	1	1
Residence			
Urban	205 (76.5%)	2.2 (1.0, 4.5)	1.987 (0.785, 5.0)
Rural	1 (0.4%)	1	1
Wanted status of pregnancy			
Yes	209 (76%)	2.05 (0.914, 4.59)	1.977 (0.671, 5.823)
No	17 (60.7%)	1	1
Parity			
Primipara	81 (78.6%)	1.397 (0.79, 2.45)	1.112 (0.511, 2.422)
Multipara	145 (72.5%)	1	1
Privacy respected			
Yes	214 (80.4%)	8.5 (4, 18)	8 (3.375, 19.263)
No	12 (32%)	1	1
Care provider was respectful			
Yes	207 (77.8%)	3.3 (1.6, 6.7)	2.578 (1.249, 5.325)
No	19 (51%)	1	1
Institution clean			
Yes	182 (77%)	1.87 (1, 3.35)	3.596 (1.424, 9.079)
No	44 (64.7%)	1	1
Distance from home			
≤30 minutes	166 (79.8%)	2.306 (1.348, 3.945)	2.804 (1.423, 5.522)
>30 minutes	60 (63.2%)	1	1
Waiting time			
≤30 minutes	198 (77.6%)	2.481 (1.302, 4.729)	2.17 (0.967, 4.878)
>30 minutes	28 (58%)	1	1
Expectation		1.067 (0.98, 1.161)	1.118 (0.986, 1.269)
Knowledge		1.130 (1.021, 1.25)	1.07 (0.956, 1.198)

5. Discussion

Antenatal care (ANC) is the key entry point of a pregnant woman to receive a broad range of health promotion and preventive services which provide the health of the mother and the baby [9]. Quality of ANC is an important determinant of the pregnancy outcome along with clean and safe delivery, essential obstetric care, and family planning which could contribute to the reduction of maternal mortality [10]. The majority of respondents (87.8%) reported that care providers were respectful. This finding is supported by a qualitative finding as one participant said that "I could say that she (the care provider) is a positive one because she greets me with a smile, warm greets, even if she's really tired of too many clients she doesn't act like she was tired."

Around 70% of the respondents took less than 30 minutes to reach the health facility. This was supported by the qualitative finding as one participant said that "it only took me around ten minutes to reach to the health institution it is very important that facilities were near to my home if I get seek or in need of immediate care it will be easy to reach." This finding is lower than that of a study conducted in Pakistan and Nepal which declared that it was easily accessible (within 30 minutes) [38]. A possible explanation for this might be the difference in infrastructure and economical difference in the countries [11]. Overall, in this study, almost 75% of women were satisfied with the antenatal care service rendered in the health institutions and 25.4% were dissatisfied. This finding is similar to a study conducted in Jimma University Specialized Hospital where 77% of respondents were satisfied [28]. This finding is not consistent with a study conducted in Belgium, at the University Hospital of Ghent (Belgium), Australia, Sweden, Nigeria, Shire North West Tigray, Bahir Dar, and Jimma town mothers in which majority of the study participants were satisfied by antenatal care services [13–20]. The difference might be due to competency, attitude, and skills of maternal care providers and overall service delivery structure differences between Ethiopia and European countries. Also, the study finding was not consistent with the study conducted in Malaysia which found that more than half of the respondents were satisfied with the service that they received 56.7% [32]. This variation may be due to thedifference in the level of health facilities.

In this study, it was found that younger age groups (below 34 years) tend to get high satisfaction than older ages; this is also true after adjusting for the other variables included in the model (multivariate analysis). Also, a significant association was shown in the finding which is in congruence with a study done in Addis Ababa; the study revealed that age is negatively and significantly associated with satisfaction [30]. Because the elders were more experienced than their younger counterparts, they may compare the service with the previous one they encountered.

It was determined that clients who belonged to "illiterate and primary" education levels were more satisfied than the secondary and higher groups, and the association was also significant in multivariate analysis; the finding is similar to several studies, for example, a study conducted by Javed and Hasen [11, 18] and Elsaba [19]. In this study, respondents who travel more than 30 minutes were two times more satisfied than those whose travel time is less than 30 minutes. This is a similar study conducted in Pakistan, and another study in Adama revealed that those who live far (30 minutes of travel time) from the health facility were highly dissatisfied than those who live near [35, 36]. It might be that those who live near the health institution had the chance to use the facility any time they want which makes them more satisfied.

Also, the findings of this study revealed that clients respected by health care providers were significantly associated with satisfaction. Those who reported that they were respected by the care provider were two times more likely satisfied than those not respected by care providers. This finding is similar to a previous study conducted in Addis Ababa in which the study revealed a significant relationship between the level of satisfaction and client respect, and clients who were respected by the health care service provider were more satisfied compared to those not respected [21].

In this study, client satisfaction with the ANC services was significantly related to privacy during the ANC session. Study subjects who feel secured regarding their privacy were more satisfied than their referents. This finding is in congruence with a study done in Bahir Dar in which respondents whose privacy was maintained were about two times more likely to be satisfied than those whose privacy was not maintained [22]. Findings of this study also showed that cleanness of the facility had a significant association with satisfaction. This is in line with a study conducted in Wolaita where respondents who reported that the institution was clean were seven times as high to be satisfied than those who reported that the institution was not clean [23]. It is obvious that a clean and attractive environment will enhance someone's satisfaction with the existing service.

6. Conclusions

Generally, around three-fourths of the respondents were satisfied with the service that they received. Most of the clients were satisfied with privacy, approaches of care from the care provider, interpersonal and technical aspects, facility-related factors, and cleanness of the center. Relatively low satisfaction was reported on the communication and information domain. Age, education status, distance from the facility, respect of privacy, cleanness of the facility, and provider respectfulness were the significant predictors of the satisfaction level. The authors of this study kindly request any additional support from governmental and nongovernmental organizations at the national and international levels including family doctor's practice to improve maternal care quality more specifically antenatal care services.

Acknowledgments

We would like thank the Jimma University Institute of Health for permitting us to conduct this study and covering the survey cost and Hadiya zone health bureau administrators and Hossana town public health center staffs for all the help and support given to us during the data collection period. Last but not least, we would like to acknowledge and thank study participants and data collectors.

References

[1] J. Hollowell, J. J. Kurinczuk, L. Oakley, P. Brocklehurst, and R. Gray, *A Systematic Review of the Effectiveness of Antenatal Care Programs to Reduce Infant Mortality and Its Major Causes in Socially Disadvantaged and Vulnerable Women Final Report*, BMC Pregnancy and Childbirth, 2009.

[2] F. S. Chawani, *Patient Satifaction with Nursing Care a Meta Synthesis*, University of the Witwatersrand, Johannesburg, 2009.

[3] O. O. Chirdan, L. A. Lar, T. O. Afolaranmi, E. O. Inalegwu, C. S. Igoh, and G. U. Adah, "Client satisfaction with maternal health services comparim between public and private hospitals in JOS nigeria," *Journal of Medicine*, vol. 7, no. 1, pp. 1–9, 2009.

[4] WHO, *Provision of effective antenatal care, integrated management of pregnancy and childbirth (IMPAC). Mak pregnancy safer*, World Health Organization, 2006.

[5] WHO, *Trends in Maternal Mortality 2000 to 2017: Estimates by WHO, UNICEF, UNFPA, World Bank Group and the United Nations Population Division*, World Health Organization, Geneva, 2019.

[6] *World Data Atlas Ethiopia - Maternal mortality ratio*, 2017, https://knoema.com/atlas/Ethiopia/Maternal-mortality-ratio.

[7] T. Nimi, S. Fraga, D. Costa, P. Campos, and H. Barros, "Prenatal care and pregnancy outcomes: a cross-sectional study in Luanda, Angola," *International Journal of Gynaecology and Obstetrics*, vol. 135, Suppl 1, pp. S72–S78, 2016.

[8] P. A. Afulani, "Determinants of stillbirths in Ghana: does quality of antenatal care matter?," *BMC Pregnancy and Childbirth*, vol. 16, no. 1, p. 132, 2016.

[9] J. Kuhnt and S. Vollmer, "Antenatal care services and its implications for vital and health outcomes of children: evidence from 193 surveys in 69 low-income and middle- income countries," *BMJ Open*, vol. 7, no. 11, article e017122, 2017.

[10] WHO and UNICEF U, *Trends in Maternal Mortality : 1990 to 2013*, World Health Organization, 2013.

[11] Ethiopian Public Health Institute (EPHI) [Ethiopia] and ICF, *Ethiopia Mini Demographic and Health Survey 2019: Key Indicators*, EPHI and ICF P12-22, Rockville, MD, USA, 2019.

[12] I. S. Abdulraheem, A. R. Olapipo, and M. O. Amodu, "Primary health care services in Nigeria : critical issues and strategies for enhancing the use by the rural communities," *Journal of Public Health and Epidemiology*, vol. 4, no. 1, pp. 5–13, 2012.

[13] S. Kumar Acharya, S. Kumar Sharma, B. Dulal, and A. K. Kumar, *Nepal Health Sector Support Program, Ministry of Health and Population*, 2018, http://www.newera.com.np/.

[14] A. Galle, A. S. Van Parys, K. Roelens, and I. Keygnaert, "Expectations and satisfaction with antenatal care among pregnant women with a focus on vulnerable groups: a descriptive study in Ghent," *BMC Womens Health*, vol. 15, no. 1, pp. 1–12, 2015.

[15] N. A. E. Montasser, R. M. Helal, W. M. Megahed et al., "Egyptian women's satisfaction and perception of antenatal care," *International Journal of TROPICAL DISEASE & Health*, vol. 2, no. 2, pp. 145–156, 2012.

[16] A. Srivastava, B. I. Avan, P. Rajbangshi, and S. Bhattacharyya, "Determinants of women's satisfaction with maternal health care: a review of literature from developing countries," *BMC Pregnancy and Childbirth*, vol. 15, no. 1, pp. 1–12, 2015.

[17] P. H. Fulpagare, A. Saraswat, K. Dinachandra et al., "Antenatal care service utilization among adolescent pregnant women–evidence from Swabhimaan programme in India," *Frontiers in Public Health*, vol. 7, 2019.

[18] D. J. Onyeajam, S. Xirasagar, M. M. Khan, J. W. Hardin, and O. Odutolu, "Antenatal care satisfaction in a developing country: a cross-sectional study from Nigeria," *BMC Public Health*, vol. 18, no. 1, pp. 1–9, 2018.

[19] F. Chemir, F. Alemseged, and D. Workneh, "Satisfaction with focused antenatal care service and associated factors among pregnant women attending focused antenatal care at health centers in Jimma town, Jimma zone, South West Ethiopia; a facility based cross-sectional study triangulated with qualitative study," *BMC Research Notes*, vol. 7, no. 1, pp. 1–8, 2014.

[20] B. Fseha, "Assessment of mothers level of satisfaction with antenatal care services provided at Alganesh Health Center Shire, North West Tigray, Ethiopia," *Biomedical Journal of Scientific & Technical Research*, vol. 16, no. 1, pp. 11798–11802, 2019.

[21] A. N. Terefe and A. B. Gelaw, "Determinants of antenatal care visit utilization of child-bearing mothers in Kaffa, Sheka, and Bench Maji Zones of SNNPR, Southwestern Ethiopia," *Health Services Research and Managerial Epidemiology*, vol. 6, no. 1, article 233339281986662, 2019.

[22] T. Ejigu, M. Woldie, and Y. Kifle, "Quality of antenatal care services at public health facilities of Bahir-Dar special zone, Northwest Ethiopia," *BMC Health Services Research*, vol. 13, no. 1, p. 1, 2013.

[23] Wikipedia, the free encyclopedia, *Health Services Utilization in United States of America*, pp. 3–10, 2020, https://en.wikipedia.org/wiki/Health_care_in_the_United_States.

[24] M. I. A. Yousef Hamoud Aldebasi, "Patients' satisfaction with medical services in the Qassim Area," *Journal of Clinical and Diagnostic Research*, vol. 5, no. 4, pp. 813–817, 2011.

[25] F. M. Mgawadere, *Assessing the Quality of Antenatal Care at Lungwena Health Centre in Rural Malawi*, UNIVERSITY OF MALAŴI College of Medicine Assessing, 2009.

[26] J. M. Turan, H. Nalbant, N. Ortaylı, and A. A. Kolog, "The quality of hospital-based antenatal care in Istanbul," *Studies in Family Planning*, vol. 37, no. 1, pp. 49–60, 2006.

[27] F. Assefa, A. Mosse, and Y. H. Michael, "Assessment of clients' satisfaction with health service deliveries At Jimma University Specialized Hospital," *Ethiopian Journal of Health Sciences*, vol. 21, no. 2, pp. 101–109, 2011.

[28] I. Hildingsson and I. Rådestad, "Swedish women's satisfaction with medical and emotional aspects of antenatal care," *Journal of Advanced Nursing*, vol. 52, no. 3, pp. 239–249, 2005.

[29] I. Hildingsson, H. Haines, M. Cross, J. F. Pallant, and C. Rubertsson, "Women's satisfaction with antenatal care: comparing women in Sweden and Australia," *Women and Birth*, vol. 26, no. 1, pp. e9–14, 2013.

[30] S. Clement, J. Sikorski, J. Wilson, S. Das, and N. Smeeton, "Women's satisfaction with traditional and reduced antenatal visit schedules," *Midwifery*, vol. 12, no. 3, article 10.1016/s0266-6138(96)90055-8, pp. 120–128, 1996.

[31] S. Dyah Pitaloka and A. M. Rizal, "Patients' satisfaction in antenatal clinic hospital University Kebanggaan Malaysia," *Jurnal Kesihatan Masyarakat (Malaysia)*, vol. 12, no. 1, article 91737825, p. 1, 2005.

[32] W. Sinishaw, *Assessment of Quality of Antenatal Care in Public Health Center of Addis Ababa Health Centers*, Addis Ababa university school of graduate studies, 2009.

[33] A. Hasan, *Patient satisfaction with maternal and child health services among mothers attending the maternal and child health training institute in Dhaka Bangladesh*, Mahidol University, 2007.

[34] S. M. Lamadah and H. A. Elsaba, "Women's satisfaction with the quality of antenatal care at the primary health care centers in Al-Madinah Al-Menawarh, KSA," *Life Science Journal*, vol. 9, no. 4, pp. 4291–4299, 2012.

[35] S. Yousuf, *Assessment of Quality of Care in Antenatal Services in Adama Special Zone of Oromia Region*, Addis Ababa University, Ethiopia, 2009.

[36] Y. Melkamu, "Quality of reproductive health services at private for-profit institutions in Addis Ababa," *Ethiopian Journal of Reproductive Health*, vol. 2, no. 1, pp. 35–51, 2008.

[37] B. Yohannes, M. Tarekegn, and W. Paulos, "Mothers' utilization of antenatal care and their satisfaction with delivery services in selected public health facilities of Wolaita zone, Southern Ethiopia," *International Journal of Scientific & Technology Research*, vol. 2, no. 2, pp. 74–85, 2013.

[38] R. Adhikari, "Effect of Women's autonomy on maternal health service utilization in Nepal: a cross sectional study," *BMC Women's Health*, vol. 16, no. 1, p. 1, 2016.

3

Prevalence and Associated Factors of Self-Medication among Pregnant Women on Antenatal Care Follow-Up at University of Gondar Comprehensive Specialized Hospital in Gondar, Northwest Ethiopia

Faisel Dula Sema,[1] **Deres Gezahegn Addis**,[2] **Eshetie Azezew Melese**,[2] **Demeke Dana Nassa**,[2] **and Zemene Demelash Kifle**[3]

[1]*Department of Clinical Pharmacy, School of Pharmacy, College of Medicine and Health Sciences, University of Gondar, Ethiopia*
[2]*School of Pharmacy, College of Medicine and Health Sciences, University of Gondar, Ethiopia*
[3]*Department of Pharmacology, School of Pharmacy, College of Medicine and Health Sciences, University of Gondar, Ethiopia*

Correspondence should be addressed to Faisel Dula Sema; faiselye1203@gmail.com

Academic Editor: Robert Gaspar

Background. Self-medication is being prevalent throughout the globe. Although pregnant women are among the most vulnerable group of the population for drug-induced adverse effects on their fetus and themselves, many pregnant women use self-medication without adequate safety precautions. *Objective.* This study was aimed at assessing the prevalence and associated factors of self-medication among pregnant women on antenatal care follow-up at University of Gondar Comprehensive Specialized Hospital. *Methods.* A cross-sectional study was employed among 400 pregnant women attending antenatal care clinic at the University of Gondar Comprehensive Specialized Hospital between February 01 and May 30, 2019. A structured interviewer-administered questionnaire was used for data collection. Data were analyzed using SPSS® (IBM Corporation) version 22. Descriptive statistics were presented using frequency and proportion. Binary logistic regression was used to identify factors associated with self-medication with a 95% confidence level and p value of 0.05. *Results.* Among 400 respondents, the prevalence of self-medication during the current pregnancy was 44.8% (95% CI = 40.5-50). Among all respondents (400), 38.0% (95% CI = 33.3-42.8) and 12.5% (95% CI = 9.5-15) used herbal and conventional medicine, respectively. Self-medication showed a significant association with a previous history of self-medication and monthly income. *Conclusions.* The prevalence of self-medication among pregnant women is considerably high. The previous history of self-medication and monthly income showed a significant association with self-medication. Awareness creation should be done for reproductive-age women on the potential risks of self-medication.

1. Introduction

"Self-medication can be broadly defined as a decision made by a patient to consume a drug with or without the approval of a health professional" [1]. Traditionally, it has been defined as "the taking of drugs, herbs or home remedies on one's own initiative, or on the advice of another person, without consulting a doctor" [2]. "It involves the use of medicinal products by the consumer to treat self-recognized disorders or symptoms, or the intermittent or continued use of a medication prescribed by a physician for chronic or recurring diseases or symptoms. In practice, it also includes use of the medication of family members, especially where the treatment of children or the elderly is involved" [3]. Self-medication can be practiced by using both conventional/modern and herbal medicines ("Herbal medicine include herbs and/or herbal materials and/or herbal preparations and/or finished herbal products in a form suitable for administration to patients") [4].

The prevalence of self-medication is alarmingly high throughout the globe. It ranges from 8.5 to 98%, showing variation with different subgroups of the population (e.g., male vs. female) and between a developed versus developing region [5].

Even though self-medication may have a considerable benefit as a part of self-care, it also poses many potential risks at both the individual and the community levels, as well as at the health care system [3]. It commonly associates with risks such as misdiagnosis, use of excessive drug dosage, prolonged duration of use, drug interactions, and polypharmacy [6]. Moreover, it is one of the major reasons for antibiotic resistance [7]. It may also cause skin problem, hypersensitivity, and allergy, especially in the case of those patients that do not follow the instructions given by the label of package insert [8].

Previous studies reported that the most frequent reasons for self-medications are having a minor illness, health care costs, lack of adequate time to visit a physician, prior experience in using a drug, and long waiting time to visit a qualified practitioner [5, 9]. In the developing world like sub-Saharan African countries where health care resource is very limited, people live with extreme poverty, and illiteracy rate is very high; the practice of self-medication could have a greater negative impacts, especially when practiced by very fragile population like pregnant women.

Since pregnant women are among the most vulnerable group of the population for drug-induced adverse effects on their fetus and themselves, the harmful effect of medication use is expected to be high if they are not used after prescription, supervision, and follow-up of authorized health care providers [10, 11], because the pharmacokinetic profile of the drug may be altered due to maternal physiologic changes during pregnancy. As a result, unexpected adverse drug reactions may occur. Moreover, medications may pass through the placenta and cause harm to the fetus [12].

Despite the occurrence of an adverse outcome that depends not only on the physical and chemical nature of the drug but also on the dose, duration, frequency, route of exposure, and gestational timing involved [11, 13], many pregnant women use self-medication without adequate safety precautions. The prevalence of self-medication among pregnant women was reported to be high throughout the world. It is estimated to be 22%-44% [14]. Furthermore, a relatively higher magnitude, up to 85%, is being reported from a resource-limited setting, particularly in Africa [15–20].

Pregnant women may use both over-the-counter and prescription medications like vitamins, analgesics, antibiotics, antimalaria, and herbal medicines for self-medication [15–22]. However, it is difficult to conclude that any drug is absolutely risk-free for pregnant women; even the most familiar and easily accessed drugs like nonsteroidal anti-inflammatory drugs are reported to have a risk of pregnancy adverse outcomes [23].

The low awareness of the potential risks of medication use during pregnancy [13, 24] and the relative difference in the knowledge, attitude, and sociocultural condition of pregnant women [19, 25–27] may cause the prevalence of self-medication in different settings to fluctuate. Unlike relatively resource-rich settings, self-medication may be highly widespread among illiterate, unemployed, women with low socioeconomic status, and women on their first trimester of pregnancy [18, 28–30].

In Ethiopia, the situation of self-medication among pregnant women could be worst due to limited access to health facilities, low socioeconomic status, relatively high illiteracy, and lack of awareness on the adverse effects of self-medication [9, 31–33]. Therefore, this study was aimed at assessing the prevalence and associated factors of self-medication among pregnant women on antenatal care follow-up at University of Gondar Comprehensive Specialized Hospital (UoGCSH), northwest Ethiopia. So, all possible necessary measures can be taken by a policymaker, health care providers, and all concerned stake holders of the area based on the findings of this study.

2. Methods

2.1. Study Design and Settings. An institution-based cross-sectional study was conducted among pregnant women attending the ANC (antenatal care) clinic at UoGCSH in Gondar town, northwest Ethiopia, from February 01 to May 30, 2019.

The study was conducted at UoGCSH, Gondar town, northwest Ethiopia, which is found at 738 km from Addis Ababa (capital city of Ethiopia). The hospital is the only referral hospital in the area of Gondar with multiple specialty clinics including an ANC follow-up clinic. It serves around 7 million people both rural and urban inhabitants. Currently, around 16,000 pregnant women visit the hospital for ANC services per year. At the ANC clinic, gynecologists, residents, interns, and midwife nurses participate in the delivery of ANC to pregnant women.

2.2. Population. All pregnant women who attended to the ANC clinic at UoGCSH were the source population. All pregnant women who were attending the antenatal care clinic at UoGCSH during the study period were the study population.

2.3. Inclusion and Exclusion Criteria. All pregnant women who visited the ANC clinic of the UoGCSH within the study period were included. Pregnant women who were critically ill, on labor pain, and unable to communicate at the time of data collection were excluded.

2.4. Sample Size Determination and Sampling Procedure. The sample size was determined by using a single-population proportion formula: $n = (Z^2(P)(1 - P))/W^2$, where n is the sample size required, W is the marginal error of 5% ($W = 0.05$), Z is the degree of accuracy required (95% level of significance = 1.96). $p = 0.5$ (50%) was used to increase the study precision by getting the maximum possible sample size. $n = ((1.96)^2(0.5)(1 - 0.5))/(0.05)^2 = 384$. With an addition of 5% nonresponse rate, the final sample size was 400.

By using simple random sampling, 400 patients were identified for data collection. According to the UoGCSH statistic and information office record, around 25 pregnant women visit the ANC clinic every day for ANC service. Thus, by calculating the number for the data collection period (60 days), we estimated the number of pregnant women (1500) who would visit the ANC clinic for ANC service. We have labeled 1500 lotteries, "label 1" for 400 pregnant women and "label 0" for 1100 pregnant women, and mixed them within a bag. Then, all pregnant women were asked to take out the lottery from the bag when they came for ANC service. Only pregnant women (400) who took out the lottery labeled as 1 were incorporated in the study.

2.5. Operational Definitions. Self-medication is the use of conventional/modern or herbal medicine by pregnant women without the prescription of authorized health care provider for the treatment of self-recognized disorders or symptoms or the intermittent or continued use of a medication prescribed by an authorized health care provider for chronic or recurring diseases or symptoms.

Illiterate is those who cannot read and write.

2.6. Data Collection Method and Procedures. Three clinical pharmacists were employed for the data collection. The data was collected by using a structured interviewer-administered questionnaire (Supplementary Materials Annex2). Although, the questionnaire was prepared in the English language after a thorough literature review of previously validated published studies [15, 16, 17, 18, 20–22], it was sent to one faculty member and two physicians to assess the face validity, because it was subject to slight modification. For internal consistency, we have used the alpha Cronbach test which had an index of 0.75. Then, the questionnaire was translated to the Amharic language by experts at the area and translated back to the English language to minimize translation error. It was pretested by 5% (20 pregnant women) of the sample size before the commencement of the actual data collection. The data collected for the purpose of the pretest was not included in the final analysis. Also, data was not recollected on individuals who had participated for the purpose of pretesting the questionnaire. The questionnaire has 33 questions categorized into 5 sections. The first section encompasses the sociodemographic information of the participants like age (in years), marital status, occupation, monthly income (in ETB), education level, religion, place of residence, and distance from health facility (hospital or health center). The second section, the obstetrics information of the participants, consists of the number of gravida, number of parity, number of children, history and reason of abortion, and stage of pregnancy. The third section contains pregnant women's attitude towards self-medication. In this part, pregnant women were asked whether they believe self-medication is important for maternal and fetal health and unusual health problem can occur on the infant(s) due to self-medication during pregnancy. They were also asked at which trimester of pregnancy the negative effect of self-medication can occur. The fourth and fifth sections comprise self-medication by conventional and herbal medicine, respectively. Under these parts, pregnant women were asked whether they have used conventional and/or herbal medicine during the current pregnancy for the purpose of self-medication. They were also asked for history of self-medication, reason for self-medication, and types of ailments treated by self-medication by both conventional and herbal medicines. The name, source of information, and source of medicine were asked for both the conventional and herbal medicines.

2.7. Data Quality Control. One-day training was given to the data collectors and supervisors on the objectives of the study, the contents of the questionnaire, and issues related to confidentiality before starting data collection. Data collection was supervised frequently. The questionnaire was pretested on 5% of the sample size.

2.8. Data Processing. The collected data were checked for completeness and consistency and then entered into SPSS® (IBM Corporation) version 22 for analysis. Also, the data was cleaned for possible errors. When there was an error, data were corrected by crosschecking with the data on the data abstraction format using the original ID variable on the SPSS immediately.

2.9. Data Analysis and Interpretation. At the end of data collection, data were coded, entered, and analyzed by using IBM SPSS version 22 software. Descriptive statistics were used to describe the result of the study in frequency, proportion, mean, and standard deviation. Independent variables were tested for association with self-medication (conventional and herbal medicine). Independent variables were also tested for association with conventional and herbal medicine separately. The association between dependent and independent variables was determined by using the chi-squared test (the results of the chi-squared test is submitted separately as Supplementary Materials Supporting information) and binary logistic regression. The chi-squared test was used to apply Fisher's exact test for identifying variables which could not fulfill the assumption for the Pearson chi-squared test and logistic regression. The score was dichotomized as yes = pregnant women with self-medication practice and no = pregnant women with no self-medication practice. The Pearson chi-squared test and Fisher exact test of independence were used to determine the association between the independent and dependent variables. Then, we have checked the magnitude of the association by using binary logistic regression for those variables that fulfill the assumption for model fitting. Statistical significance was considered when a p value was less than 0.05. Although we had perform analysis by both chi-squared test and binary logistic regression, we preferred to report our finding from the binary logistic regression, since it is a more stronger analysis method. The independent variables were checked for multicollinearity (with variance inflation factors for all models 1 = 1.079) and the presence of outliers (with a probability of Mahalanobis distances = 0.06). The bivariable logistic regression analysis was done to identify an association between the dependent and each independent variable. The model was tested by using Hosmer–Lemeshow goodness of fit (model 1: chi-squared test = 1.615, df = 7, sig. = 0.978; model 2: chi-squared test = 18.209, df = 7, sig. = 0.011; and model 3: chi-squared test = 5.397, df = 7, sig. = 0.612). All independent variables with $p < 0.2$ in the bivariable logistic regression analysis were entered for multivariable analysis using the enter method. Finally, the result of the study was presented in tables and pie chart.

2.10. Ethical Consideration. To conduct the study, ethical clearance and approval were obtained from the Ethical Review Committee Department of School of Pharmacy, College of Medicine and Health Sciences, and then, formal permission was obtained from the medical director of UoGCSH. Then, written informed consent (Supplementary Materials AnnexI) was obtained from the study participants after the objective of the study was made clear and permission for cooperation was asked politely.

3. Results

3.1. Sociodemographic Information of the Respondents. A total of 400 pregnant women participated in this study with a response rate of 100%. From the entire participant, 199 (49.8%) women were at the age of 28–37 years, with a mean and standard deviation of 27.83 ± 4.27 years. Most of them ($N = 364$, 91.0%) were married. Concerning their occupation, 126 (31.5%) women were a housewife. According to the WHO income scale level, 159 (39.8%) women had a low monthly income (<3000 ETB (Ethiopian birr)). Less than half of the pregnant women had a diploma/degree ($N = 162$, 40.5%). The commonest religion of the participant was orthodox ($N = 305$, 76.3%). For most pregnant women, place of residence was urban ($N = 337$, 84.3%) with a distance from health facility less than 5 km ($N = 237$, 59.3%) (Table 1).

3.2. Obstetrics Information of the Respondents. One hundred fifty (67.5%) pregnant women were gravida II. Most of the respondents ($N = 159$, 39.8%) had one child with parity one. The previous history of abortion was recorded on 26 (6.5%) pregnant women. The major reason for their abortion was a health problem ($N = 14$, 3.5%). Most of the respondents ($N = 300$, 75%) were in the third trimester of pregnancy (Table 2).

3.3. Pregnant Women's Attitude towards Self-Medication. Among 400 pregnant women, 35 (8.8%) of them believed that self-medication is important for maternal health and 8 (2.0%) of them believed that self-medication is important for the health of the unborn child. Around one-third of the pregnant women thought that the negative effect of self-medication occurs during the first trimester ($N = 261$, 65.3%). Also, 289 (72.3%) of 400 pregnant women had a belief that unusual health problem can occur on the infant(s) due to self-medication use during pregnancy (Table 3).

3.4. Prevalence of Self-Medication. Among 400 pregnant women, 179 (44.8%) (95% CI = 40.5-50) of them used self-medication during the current pregnancy (Figure 1). It includes the prevalence of both conventional 50 (12.5%) (95% CI = 9.5-15) and HM 152 (38.0%) (95% CI = 33.3 -42.8) (Tables 4 and 5). Around one-third of the participants, 146 (36.5%), had a previous history of self-medication (Table 4).

3.5. Self-Medication with Conventional Medication. In this study, around half of the CM users ($N = 26$, 52.0%) had prior experience of the drug. Headache was the main ailment sated for CM use ($N = 30$, 60%). The commonly used drug was paracetamol ($N = 29$, 58.0%). Pharmacists/druggists were the most used source of information about the drug ($N = 37$, 74.0%). Private community pharmacies/drug stores ($N = 46$, 92.0%) were the major sources of the drugs. However, most of the users have no information on the dose and side effects of the drugs they used ($N = 28$, 56.0%). Around 149 (37.3%) of the study participants had previous history of self-medication by conventional medicine (Table 4).

3.6. Self-Medication with Herbal Medicine. The study showed that 152 (38.0%) pregnant women used HM. The most frequent disease for HM use was common cold ($N = 69$, 44.08%). Ginger was a commonly used HM ($N = 87$, 55.92%). The users mainly got information about HM from neighbors ($N = 77$, 48.68%). In most cases, pregnant women prepare HM by themselves ($N = 146$, 94.73%). However, 107 (70.39%) of them could not state the specific reason for HM use for self-medication. Half of the participants, 200 (50%) of them, had previous history of self-medication by herbal medicine (Table 5).

3.7. Factors Associated with Self-Medication. The only variables which fulfill the assumption for model fitting were age, monthly income, and previous history of self-medication. Pregnant women having previous history of self-medication associated with self-medication 26.816 (13.064, 15.064; p value = 0.001) times more likely than pregnant women with no previous history of self-medication. Pregnant women who had monthly income greater than 6000 Ethiopian birr associated 2.441 (1.197, 4.977) times more likely than pregnant women with monthly income less than 3000 Ethiopian birr with an overall p value of 0.022 (Table 6).

3.8. Factors Associated with Self-Medication with Conventional Medication. By binary logistic regression, the only variable associated with self-medication with CM was previous history of self-medication. Pregnant women who had previous history of self-medication associated with self-medication with CM 5.223 (2.007, 13.592; p value = 0.001) times more likely than pregnant women with no previous history of self-medication (Table 6).

3.9. Factors Associated with Self-Medication with Herbal Medicine. The previous history of self-medication and monthly income significantly associated with self-medication with HM. The previous history of self-medication associated with self-medication of pregnant women with HM around 27.164 (11.913, 61.935; p value = 0.001) times more likely than pregnant women with no previous history of self-medication. Similarly, pregnant women with monthly income greater than 6000 Ethiopian birr associated with self-medication with HM

Table 1: Sociodemographic information of the respondents at UoGCSH, June 2019.

Characteristics		*N* (400)	%
Age group in years	18-27	193	48.2
	28-37	199	49.8
	>38	8	2.0
Marital status	Single	12	3.0
	Married	364	91.0
	Divorced	40	5.0
	Widowed	4	1.0
Occupation	Governmental employed	125	31.3
	Self-employee	106	26.5
	Housewife	126	31.5
	Farmer	23	5.8
	Student	9	2.3
	Unemployed	11	2.8
Monthly income in ETB*	<3000	159	39.8
	3000-6000	135	33.8
	>6000	106	26.5
Education level	Illiterate	23	5.8
	Primary school [1–8]	57	14.3
	Secondary school [9–12]	151	37.8
	College/university student	7	1.8
	Diploma/degree	162	40.5
Religion	Orthodox	305	76.3
	Muslim	80	20.0
	Protestant	14	3.5
	Jehovah witness	1	0.3
Place of residence	Urban	337	84.3
	Rural	63	15.8
Distance from a health facility	<5 km	237	59.3
	5-10 km	102	25.5
	>10 km	61	15.3

*ETB: Ethiopian birr.

2.739 (1.376, 5.452; p value = 0.004) times more likely than pregnant women with monthly income of less than 3000 Ethiopian birr with overall p value = 0.005 (Table 6).

4. Discussion

This study assessed the prevalence and associated factors of self-medication among pregnant women who were attending to the ANC clinic of UoGCSH. In this study, we have reported the prevalence and associated factors of self-medication as a whole to have the overall picture of it. In addition, we are also convinced to report the prevalence, reasons, ailments, type of medicine, source of information, source of the medicine, and associated factors for both conventional and herbal medicines separately, because some of the previous studies reported self-medication by considering only either conventional or herbal medicine.

The prevalence of self-medication during the current pregnancy was high, 44.8% (95% CI = 40.5-50). This is a composite of both conventional and herbal medicine use. This finding is consistent with the study done in Mwanza and Tanzania (46.24%) [29]. However, it is higher than the studies done in Addis Ababa, Ethiopia (26.6%) [20], Goba town, southeast Ethiopia (15.5%) [21], Iran (35%) [25], and Mexico (21.9%) [34]. On the contrary, it is lower than the study done in Harar town, Ethiopia (69%) [16]; Nigeria (85%) [18]; Bukavu in Eastern DR Congo (61.3%) [17]; and Central Region of Ghana (69%) [35]. When we look into its subparts, conventional and herbal medicines, the prevalence of CM practice was 12.5% (95% CI = 9.5-15). It is higher than the study done in Mexico (6.11%) [34]. Conversely, it is lower than the studies done in Harar town, Ethiopia (29.1%) [16], and Addis Ababa, Ethiopia (18.2%) [20]. The prevalence of HM practice was 38.0% (95% CI = 33.3-42.8). It is higher than the study done in Addis Ababa, Ethiopia (10.9%) [20];

TABLE 2: Obstetrics information of the respondents at UoGCSH, June 2019.

Characteristics		N (400)	%
Number of gravidae	One	120	30.0
	Two	150	37.5
	Three	93	23.3
	≥Four	37	9.4
Number of parity	No child	125	31.3
	One child	159	39.8
	Two children	84	21.0
	More than two children	32	8.2
Previous abortion	Yes	26	6.5
	No	374	93.5
Reason for abortion ($N = 26$)	Health problem	14	3.5
	Low economic level	1	0.3
	Unwanted pregnancy	5	1.3
	Unspecified	6	1.5
Stage of pregnancy	First trimester	11	2.8
	Second trimester	89	22.3
	Third trimester	300	75.0

TABLE 3: Pregnant women's attitude towards self-medication at UoGCSH, June 2019.

Characteristics		N (400)	%
Self-medication is important for maternal health	Yes	35	8.8
	No	365	91.3
Self-medication is important for fetal health	Yes	8	2.0
	No	308	77.0
	I have no idea	84	21.0
I believe that the negative effect of self-medication occurs at the X[a] week of pregnancy	First trimester	261	65.3
	Second trimester	13	3.3
	Third trimester	4	1.0
	I have no idea	122	30.5
I believe that unusual health problem can occur on the infant(s) due to self-medication use during pregnancy	Yes	289	72.3
	No	13	3.3
	I have no idea	98	24.5

[a]X represents first trimester, second trimester, third trimester, and I have no idea.

Mexico (14.68%) [34], Gulu district in Northern Uganda (20%) [22]; and Mwanza in Tanzania (25.3%) [29]. In opposite, it is lower than the study done in Gondar, Ethiopia (48.6%) [15], and Harar town, Ethiopia (58.2%) [16]. The difference may be due to the diversity in the socioeconomic factors, geographic location, accessibility, and study settings.

The high prevalence of self-medication by pregnant women may be due to multiple reasons. From these, the lack of knowledge of pregnant women on the potential risks of self-medication during pregnancy could be among the major one. Like most of sub-Saharan African countries, because of the high work load on the health care workers and patient flow on the study setting, health care providers may not give adequate health education on the possible risks of self-medication on the pregnant women's health and their fetus adequately. In addition, the attitude of the pregnant women towards self-medication can have a significant impact on the prevalence. In this study, we have noticed that 35 (8.8%) of the pregnant women believed that self-medication is important for maternal health and 8 (2.0%) of them believed that self-medication is important for the health of the unborn child. Moreover, 21% of them had no idea

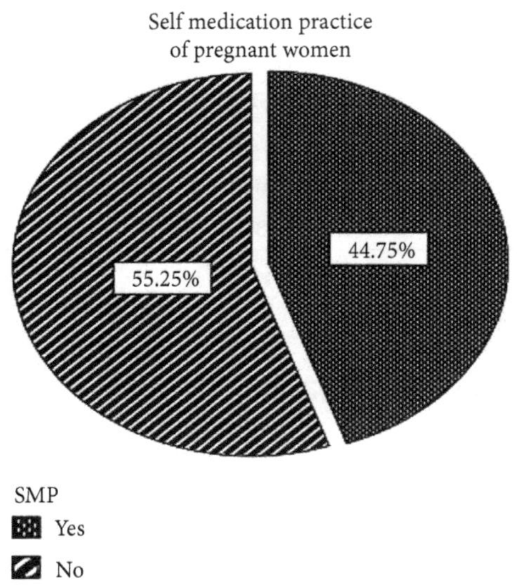

Figure 1: Self-medication of pregnant women at UoGCSH, June 2019.

whether self-medication during pregnancy is important or harmful for fetal health. Similarly, 30.5% of them had no idea at which trimester the negative effect of self-medication occurs and 24.5% of them also had no idea on whether unusual health problem can occur on the infant(s) due to self-medication use during pregnancy (Table 3). The awareness creation of pregnant mothers about self-medication to improve their knowledge and attitude of potentially childbearing aged women particularly pregnant women towards self-medication through different techniques like mass-media and inclusion of the issues of self-medication as a routine counseling point during ANC clinic follow-up may have a reasonable contribution to counteract the challenge.

However, despite having a good knowledge and attitude of self-medication, pregnant women may practice self-medication for other various reasons including sociocultural and economic reasons [16–18, 20, 21, 35, 36]. Thus, the pregnant women were asked the reasons for self-medication by both conventional and herbal medicines. The commonest reasons given for the conventional and herbal medicine use were having prior experience of the drug (52%) and easy accessibility (23.6%), respectively. This is supported by the study done in Harar town, Ethiopia [16]; Addis Ababa, Ethiopia [20]; Bukavu, Eastern DR Congo [17]; and Jos, Nigeria [18]. Additionally, knowing about the disease and treatment was the reason for self-medication by CM. Likewise, the less frequent reasons for HM use were better effectiveness, lower cost, and fewer side effects than CM (Harar town, Ethiopia) [16]. The other commonly mentioned reasons for self-medication in previous studies were time-saving [20, 21], the disease was not serious (61) (54.5) [20, 35, 36], lack of trust in drugs prescribed by health workers [21], cheaper treatment cost, positive outcomes [35], expensive drug prescription in the health facility, and availability of old prescription [36]. Even though pregnant women self-medicate due to prior experience of the medicine and knowing about the disease and treatment, it does not mean the medicine is free from any potential risk for the fetus. The risk may be overwhelming especially for herbal medicines in countries like Ethiopia where there is no standardization of the dose, frequency, and duration of herbal medicine. So, due to the various nature of the reason given for self-medication, interventions should be based on case-by-case scenario. In addition to well-planned awareness creation, improving health care accessibility, strengthening the legal restriction of the dispensing of medicine without prescription for pregnant women, and financial empowerment of pregnant women may be helpful.

Paracetamol (58.0%) and ginger (55.9%) were the most commonly used conventional and herbal medicines, respectively. This is consistent with many previous studies [15–17, 20, 21, 26, 34]. Due to the easy accessibility of paracetamol as over-the-counter (OTC) medicine and ginger on the free market, many pregnant women were motivated to self-medicate with these agents. Even though these medicines are reported to be relatively safe, there are also evidences on potential risk of paracetamol and ginger on the pregnancy adverse outcomes if they are not used under precaution [37–39]. In addition, due to lack of standardization of traditionally used medicine and inability of most pregnant women to understand the package insert prepared in the English language, many self-medicating women may use the medicines for the wrong indication, dose, and duration, which may result in adverse pregnancy outcome.

Headache (60.0%) and common cold (44.08%) were the most commonly mentioned ailments for the use of conventional and herbal medicine, respectively. In addition, self-medication was practiced for treating nausea/vomiting, typhoid, and cough. It is in line with many of the previous studies [15–18, 29, 34]. Because of physiologic disturbance during pregnancy, pregnant women may be prone to many illnesses; however, pregnant women should consult their doctors before taking any medication to minimize the potential risks of self-medication.

Pharmacist/druggist (74.0) for CM use and neighbors (48.68) followed by family and friends (46.05) for HM were the commonest source of information about self-medication. This is consistent with studies done in Harar town, Ethiopia [16]; Gondar, Ethiopia [15]; Mexico [34]; and Addis Ababa, Ethiopia) [20]. So, empowering pharmacists/druggists, consideration of families, close relatives, and friends in the health education of pregnant women may prevent potential risk and maximize the possible benefit of self-medication.

The conventional medicines used were mostly obtained from a community pharmacy or drug store (92.0). However, the HMs were mainly self-prepared (94.7%). It is consistent with the previous studies done in Harar town, Ethiopia [16], and Addis Ababa, Ethiopia [20]. However, HMs were purchased from the supermarket in the study done in Mexico [34]. This may be due to the presence of tradition of herbal remedy preparation at home in Ethiopia. However, most of the respondents (56.0%) in this study did not have adequate information about the drug. So the preparation of local standard guidelines and availability to the population for herbal medicine and capacity building of pharmacy professionals regarding commonly used medication by pregnant women,

TABLE 4: Self-medication among pregnant women by conventional medicine at UoGCSH, June 2019.

Characteristics		N	%
CM use during the current pregnancy($N = 400$)	Yes	50	12.5
	No	350	87.5
Reasons for CM ($N = 50$)	Easily available	8	16.0
	Better knowledge about the disease and the treatment	5	10.0
	Had prior experience on the drug	26	52.0
	Unable to specify the reason	11	22.0
Ailments for CM ($N = 50$)	Headache	30	60.0
	Nausea/vomiting	3	6.0
	Typhoid	4	8.0
	Common cold	4	8.0
	Cough	8	16.0
	Unspecified	1	2.0
Drugs for CM ($N = 50$)	Paracetamol	29	58.0
	Amoxicillin	8	16.0
	Cough syrup	2	4.0
	Hyoscine	2	4.0
	Metronidazole	4	8.0
	I do not know the name of the drug	5	10.0
Source of information about the drugs ($N = 50$)	From friends	4	8.0
	Internet	3	6.0
	Pharmacist/druggist	37	74.0
	Other health professionals	6	12.0
Where did you get the drugs ($N = 50$)	Neighbors	4	8.0
	Private community pharmacies/drug stores	46	92.0
What did you know about the drugs ($N = 50$)	Dose	14	28.0
	Side effect	8	16.0
	No information	28	56.0
Previous history of self-medication by conventional medicine	Yes	149	37.3
	No	251	62.7

*Some of the pregnant women use both conventional and herbal medications.

especially OTC medication, may prevent risks and encourage more safe self-medication.

In this study, self-medication significantly associated with a previous history of self-medication and monthly income. However, in the study done in Hosanna town, southern Ethiopia [28], it strongly associated with pregnant women who were unable to read and write followed by women who had health problems during pregnancy and those who can read and write and had primary education [28]. In the study done in Tanzania, it showed a significant association with illiteracy, being unemployed, and being in the first trimester of pregnancy [29]. In the study done in Mexico [34], it significantly associated with smoking followed by alcohol consumption and higher education [34]. The discrepancy in the predictors of self-medication in different studies may be due to difference in study setting. So, it is a good reflection that studies are very essential to identify the driving factors and better understand the nature of self-medication in different settings. In addition, since some of the previous studies only consider either conventional or herbal medicine as self-medication, it may be appropriate to identify factors for each of them independently.

In this study, CM use significantly associated with a previous history of self-medication. This may be due to the sense of perceived experience to the CM. Thus, pregnant women may believe that using drugs that were used out of pregnancy may not harm their pregnancy. The remaining medications that had been obtained before the current pregnancy at home may be used for the same symptoms or illnesses that they had had before they were getting pregnant. However, it could be a harmful practice because previously used medicines may not be safe for pregnant mothers.

Similarly, the use of HM significantly associated with previous history of self-medication and monthly income. Likewise, herbal medicine was highly practiced by pregnant women with relatively higher monthly income (greater than 6000 Ethiopian birr). This may be due to affordability issue of locally available herbal medicine. However, lower monthly

Table 5: Self-medication among pregnant women by using herbal medicine at UoGCSH, June 2019.

Characteristics		$N = 400$	%
HM during the current pregnancy	Yes	152	38.0
	No	248	62.0
Reason for HM use ($N = 152$)	Herbal medicines are effective than conventional medicines	5	3.28
	Herbal medicines have fewer side effects	3	1.97
	Herbal medicines have a lower cost	1	0.66
	Herbal medicines are accessible without a prescription	36	23.68
	Unable to specify	107	70.39
Ailments ($N = 152$)	Headache	65	42.76
	Nausea/vomiting	17	11.18
	Typhoid	1	0.66
	Common cold	67	44.08
	Unable to specify	2	1.32
Types of herb(s) ($N = 152$)	Ginger	85	55.92
	Garlic	2	1.31
	Ocimum lamiifolium	60	39.45
	Unable to specify	5	3.28
Source of information about HM ($N = 152$)	Traditional healers	2	1.32
	Health professionals	6	3.95
	Family and friends	70	46.05
	Neighbors	74	48.68
Where did you get the herbal medicine? ($N = 152$)	Self-preparation	144	94.73
	Traditional healers/herbalist	1	0.66
	Traditional birth attendants	1	0.66
	Neighbors	8	3.95
Previous history of self-medication by herbal medicine	Yes	200	50
	No	200	50

income (less than 3000 Ethiopian birr) was tending to associate with conventional medicine. It seems obvious that pregnant women with lower monthly income tend to practice self-medication by conventional medicine, because they may not afford the necessary health care cost to visit the nearby health care facility.

Considering the high prevalence of self-medication and variability in the magnitude, reasons, the types of illness, and medicines used for self-medication, all concerned bodies should pay due attention to the self-medication of pregnant women. Health care providers may contribute a lot through education, provision of adequate information, and counseling of pregnant women about self-medication depending on case-by-case circumstances.

5. Limitations

A recall bias among the participants and being shy to tell the truth because the study was institutional and the data were collected through interviewer-administered structured questionnaire may reduce the magnitude of self-medication.

6. Conclusions

The reported prevalence of self-medication among pregnant women is considerably high. Pregnant women use both herbal and conventional medicines for the purpose of self-medication.

However, a relatively higher prevalence of herbal than conventional medicine use is reported by pregnant women. Previous history of self-medication significantly associates with self-medication. It also significantly associates with herbal and conventional medicine use independently. Monthly income showed a significant association with self-medication in general and self-medication with herbal medicine.

Given that self-medication is common, awareness creation should be done for reproductive-age women about the risks of self-medication by both herbal and conventional medicines through different techniques. In addition, health care providers, especially those who are involved in ANC, should be aware of evidence regarding the prevalence, potential benefits, and harms of self-medication. A detailed study on self-medication is also recommended, particularly to establish the efficacy, safety, and standardization of commonly used herbs during pregnancy.

Table 6: Binary logistic regression analysis of factors associated with self-medication, self-medication with conventional medicine, and self-medication with herbal medicine among pregnant women at UoGCSH, 2018.

(a) Model 1: binary logistic regression analysis of factors associated with self-medication

Characteristics		Self-medication Yes	Self-medication No	COR with 95% CI	AOR with 95% CI	*p* value
Age group in years	18-27	74	119	0.604 (0.406, 0.899)	0.776 (0.474, 1.274)	0.315
	>28	105	102	1.655 (1.112, 2.465)		
Monthly income						0.022
	<3000	72	87	1	1	
	3000-6000	60	97	0.74 (0.477, 1.170)	0.934 (0.547, 1.593)	0.801
	>6000	47	37	1.535 (0.902, 2.613)	2.441 (1.197, 4.977)	0.014
Previous history of self-medication	Yes	169	91	24.123 (12.087, 48.223)	26.816 (13.064, 15,064)	0.001
	No	10	130	1		

(b) Model 2: binary logistic regression analysis of factors associated with self-medication with conventional medicine

Characteristics		SMCM Yes	SMCM No	COR with 95% CI	AOR with 95% CI	*p* value
Age group in years	18-27	19	174	0.620 (0.337, 1.139)	0.589 (0.311, 1.14)	0.103
	>28	31	176	1		
Monthly income						0.139
	<3000	25	134	2.425 (0.953, 6.170)	2.669 (1.013, 7.035)	0.047
	3000-6000	19	138	1.790 (0.686, 4.669)	2.154 (0.804, 5.771)	0.127
	>6000	6	78	1		
Previous history of self-medication	Yes	45	215	5.651 (2.188, 14.593)	5.223 (2.007, 13.592)	0.001
	No	5	135	1		

(c) Model 3: binary logistic regression analysis of factors associated self-medication with herbal medicine

Characteristics		SMHM Yes	SMHM No	COR with 95% CI	AOR with 95% CI	*p* value
Age group in years	18-27	63	130	0.643 (0.427, 0.966)	0.870 (0.534, 1.418)	0.576
	>28	89	118	1		
Monthly income						0.005
	<3000	60	99	1		
	3000-6000	49	108	0.749 (0.470, 1.193)	0.922 (0.543, 1.566)	0.763
	>6000	43	41	1.730 (1.014, 2.954)	2.739 (1.376, 5.452)	0.004
Previous history of self-medication	Yes	145	115	23.957 (10.781, 53.235)	27.164 (11.913, 61.935)	0.001
	No	7	133	1		

Abbreviations

CM: Conventional medicine
ETB: Ethiopian birr
HM: Herbal medicine
UoGCSH: University of Gondar Comprehensive Specialized Hospital.

Authors' Contributions

FDS was responsible for the conceptualization, data curation, formal analysis, investigation, methodology, project administration, resources, software, supervision, visualization, writing of the original draft preparation, reviewing, and editing. DGA was responsible for the conceptualization, data curation, supervision, investigation, writing, reviewing, and editing. EAM was responsible for the data curation, supervision, investigation, writing, reviewing, and editing. DDN was responsible for the supervision, writing, reviewing, and editing. ZDK was responsible for the supervision, writing, reviewing, and editing.

Acknowledgments

The authors express their appreciation to the University of Gondar Comprehensive Specialized Hospital, particularly the ANC clinic staff, for their kind cooperation during data collection. The authors are grateful to data collectors too.

References

[1] M. A. Chisholm-Burns, B. G. Wells, and T. L. Schwinghammer, *Pharmacotherapy Principles and Practice*, McGraw-Hill, 2016.

[2] M. Hernandez-Juyol and J. Job-Quesada, "Dentistry and self-medication: a current challenge," *Medicina Oral: organo oficial de la Sociedad Espanola de Medicina Oral y de la Academia Iberoamericana de Patologia y Medicina Bucal*, vol. 7, no. 5, pp. 344–347, 2002.

[3] World Health Organization, *Guidelines for the regulatory assessment of medicinal products for use in self-medication*, World Health Organization, Geneva, 2000.

[4] WHO, *WHO guidelines for selecting marker substances of herbal origin for quality control of herbal medicines*, WHO Expert Committee on Specifications for Pharmaceutical Preparations, 2017.

[5] A. Shaghaghi, M. Asadi, and H. Allahverdipour, "Predictors of self-medication behavior: a systematic review," *Iranian Journal of Public Health*, vol. 43, no. 2, pp. 136–146, 2014.

[6] C. M. Hughes, J. C. McElnay, and G. F. Fleming, "Benefits and risks of self medication," *Drug Safety*, vol. 24, no. 14, pp. 1027–1037, 2001.

[7] I. A. Rather, B.-C. Kim, V. K. Bajpai, and Y.-H. Park, "Self-medication and antibiotic resistance: crisis, current challenges, and prevention," *Saudi Journal of Biological Sciences*, vol. 24, no. 4, pp. 808–812, 2017.

[8] D. Bennadi, "Self-medication: a current challenge," *Journal of Basic and Clinical Pharmacy*, vol. 5, no. 1, pp. 19–23, 2013.

[9] M. Sisay, G. Mengistu, and D. Edessa, "Epidemiology of self-medication in Ethiopia: a systematic review and meta-analysis of observational studies," *BMC Pharmacology and Toxicology*, vol. 19, no. 1, p. 56, 2018.

[10] J. N. Trønnes, A. Lupattelli, and H. Nordeng, "Safety profile of medication used during pregnancy: results of a multinational European study," *Pharmacoepidemiology and Drug Safety*, vol. 26, no. 7, pp. 802–811, 2017.

[11] Food and Drug Administration, *Reviewer guidance: evaluating the risks of drug exposure in human pregnancies*, Center for Drug Evaluation and Research, Rockville, MD, 2005.

[12] A. I. Adanikin and J. O. Awoleke, "Antenatal drug consumption: the burden of self-medication in a developing world setting," *Tropical Doctor*, vol. 47, no. 3, pp. 193–197, 2017.

[13] K. D. L. da Silva, F. E. M. Fernandes, T. de Lima Pessoa, S. I. V. C. Lima, A. G. Oliveira, and R. R. Martins, "Prevalence and profile of adverse drug reactions in high-risk pregnancy: a cohort study," *BMC Pregnancy and Childbirth*, vol. 19, no. 1, p. 199, 2019.

[14] M. Mohseni, S. Azami-Aghdash, S. Gareh Sheyklo et al., "Prevalence and reasons of self-medication in pregnant women: a systematic review and meta-analysis," *International Journal of Community Based Nursing and Midwifery*, vol. 6, no. 4, pp. 272–284, 2018.

[15] A. B. Mekuria, D. A. Erku, B. M. Gebresillassie, E. M. Birru, B. Tizazu, and A. Ahmedin, "Prevalence and associated factors of herbal medicine use among pregnant women on antenatal care follow-up at University of Gondar referral and teaching hospital, Ethiopia: a cross-sectional study," *BMC Complementary and Alternative Medicine*, vol. 17, no. 1, p. 86, 2017.

[16] A. Jambo, G. Mengistu, M. Sisay, F. Amare, and D. Edessa, "Self-medication and contributing factors among pregnant women attending antenatal care at public hospitals of Harar town, Ethiopia," *Frontiers in pharmacology*, vol. 9, 2018.

[17] P. M. Mbarambara, P. B. Songa, L. M. Wansubi, P. M. Mututa, B. B. K. Minga, and C. K. Bisangamo, "Self-medication practice among pregnant women attending antenatal care at health centers in Bukavu, Eastern DR Congo," *International Journal of Innovation and Applied Studies*, vol. 16, no. 1, p. 38, 2016.

[18] A. Emmanuel, G. Achema, B. B. Afoi, and R. Maroof, "Self medicaltion practice among pregnant women attending antenatal clinic in selected hospitals in Jos, Nigeria," *International Journal of Nursing and Health Science*, vol. 1, no. 6, pp. 55–59, 2014.

[19] S. Adama, *Self-medication perception and practice among pregnant women in Wa Municipality*, University of Ghana, 2017.

[20] S. W. Beza, "Self-medication practice and associated factors among pregnant women in Addis Ababa, Ethiopia," *Tropical Medicine and Health*, vol. 46, no. 1, p. 10, 2018.

[21] T. Zewdie, T. Azale, A. Shimeka, and A. M. Lakew, "Self-medication during pregnancy and associated factors among pregnant women in Goba town, southeast Ethiopia: a community based cross sectional study," *BMC Research Notes*, vol. 11, no. 1, p. 713, 2018.

[22] R. Nyeko, N. M. Tumwesigye, and A. A. Halage, "Prevalence and factors associated with use of herbal medicines during pregnancy among women attending postnatal clinics in Gulu district, Northern Uganda," *BMC Pregnancy and Childbirth*, vol. 16, no. 1, p. 296, 2016.

[23] D.-K. Li, J. R. Ferber, R. Odouli, and C. Quesenberry, "Use of nonsteroidal antiinflammatory drugs during pregnancy and the risk of miscarriage," *American Journal of Obstetrics and Gynecology*, vol. 219, no. 3, pp. 275.e1–275.e8, 2018.

[24] D. Limaye, V. Limaye, G. Krause, and G. Fortwengel, "A systematic review of the literature to assess self-medication practices," *Annals of Medical and Health Sciences Research*, vol. 7, 2017.

[25] M. Baghianimoghadam, "Attitude and practice of pregnant women regarding self-medication in Yazd, Iran," *Archives of Iranian Medicine*, vol. 16, no. 10, pp. 580–583, 2013.

[26] N. M. Zaki and A. A. Albarraq, "Use, attitudes and knowledge of medications among pregnant women: a Saudi study," *Saudi Pharmaceutical Journal*, vol. 22, no. 5, pp. 419–428, 2014.

[27] R. Sharma, B. Kapoor, and U. Verma, "Drug utilization pattern during pregnancy in North India," *Indian Journal of Medical Sciences*, vol. 60, no. 7, pp. 277–287, 2006.

[28] T. Laelago, T. Yohannes, and F. Lemango, "Prevalence of herbal medicine use and associated factors among pregnant women attending antenatal care at public health facilities in Hossana town, Southern Ethiopia: facility based cross sectional study," *Archives of Public Health*, vol. 74, no. 1, 2016.

[29] K. J. Marwa, A. Njalika, D. Ruganuza, D. Katabalo, and E. Kamugisha, "Self-medication among pregnant women attending antenatal clinic at Makongoro health centre in Mwanza, Tanzania: a challenge to health systems," *BMC Pregnancy and Childbirth*, vol. 18, no. 1, p. 16, 2018.

[30] G. Abeje, C. Admasie, and B. Wasie, "Factors associated with self medication practice among pregnant mothers attending antenatal care at governmental health centers in Bahir Dar city administration, Northwest Ethiopia, a cross sectional study," *The Pan African Medical Journal*, vol. 20, 2015.

[31] E. Ernst, "Herbal medicinal products during pregnancy: are they safe?," *BJOG: An International Journal of Obstetrics and Gynaecology*, vol. 109, no. 3, pp. 227–235, 2002.

[32] P. Kulkarni, A. Garg, A. Ajmera, A. Mahajan, S. Gadekar, and P. K. (India), "Global scenario of self medication: a review of literature," *Indian Journal of Commerce and Management Studies*, vol. 9, no. 1, pp. 99–107, 2018.

[33] M. B. Ayalew, "Self-medication practice in Ethiopia: a systematic review," *Patient Preference and Adherence*, vol. 11, pp. 401–413, 2017.

[34] A. J. Alonso-Castro, A. J. Ruiz-Padilla, Y. Ruiz-Noa et al., "Self-medication practice in pregnant women from central Mexico," *Saudi Pharmaceutical Journal*, vol. 26, no. 6, pp. 886–890, 2018.

[35] F. Y. Gbagbo and J. Nkrumah, "Self-medication among pregnant women in two municipalities in the Central Region of Ghana," *Health Care for Women International*, pp. 1–16, 2020.

[36] I. C. Ojo, N. A. Okafor, O. E. Adeola, M. M. Adamolekun, and R. F. Adewoyin, "Factors influencing self-medication practice among pregnant women attending antenatal clinic in primary health facilities in Akure South Local Government, Ondo State," *IOSR Journal of Nursing and Health Science (IOSR-JNHS)*, vol. 9, no. 2, pp. 16–22, 2020.

[37] D.-K. Li, L. Liu, and R. Odouli, "Exposure to non-steroidal anti-inflammatory drugs during pregnancy and risk of miscarriage: population based cohort study," *BMJ*, vol. 327, no. 7411, p. 368, 2003.

[38] S. Daniel, G. Koren, E. Lunenfeld, N. Bilenko, R. Ratzon, and A. Levy, "Fetal exposure to nonsteroidal anti-inflammatory drugs and spontaneous abortions," *CMAJ*, vol. 186, no. 5, pp. E177–E182, 2014.

[39] J. Stanisiere, P.-Y. Mousset, and S. Lafay, "How safe is ginger rhizome for decreasing nausea and vomiting in women during early pregnancy?," *Food*, vol. 7, no. 4, p. 50, 2018.

4

Increased Vulnerability to Pregnancy and Sexual Violence in Adolescents with Precocious Menstruation

Giani Silvana Schwengber Cezimbra,[1] Dioclécio Campos Junior,[1] Edward Araujo Júnior,[2] Cristina Aparecida Falbo Guazzelli,[2] and Álvaro Nagib Atallah[3]

[1]*Department of Pediatrics, Faculty of Medical Sciences-University of Brasília (UnB), Brasília-DF 70.910-900, Brazil*
[2]*Department of Obstetrics, Paulista School of Medicine-Federal University of São Paulo (EPM-UNIFESP), São Paulo-SP 04021-001, Brazil*
[3]*Discipline of Evidence-Based Medicine, Paulista School of Medicine-Federal University of São Paulo (EPM-UNIFESP), São Paulo-SP 04024-002, Brazil*

Correspondence should be addressed to Edward Araujo Júnior; araujojred@terra.com.br

Academic Editor: Robert Gaspar

This cross-sectional, observational, and descriptive study was conducted to evaluate the association between age at menarche in the adolescent population and the age at sexual initiation, age at first pregnancy, and experience of sexual violence in the adolescent population visiting a primary health unit in Brazil. We recruited 201 female adolescents who visited the gynecology outpatient clinic of a Basic Health Unit in the Federal District of Brazil. These adolescents answered a questionnaire with regard to sexual and reproductive health during doctor's appointments. To calculate the association, we recorded data for age at menarche, age at first sexual intercourse, age at first pregnancy, and experience of sexual violence. Pearson and Mann–Whitney correlation coefficient statistical tests were performed to evaluate the association between these variables. Mean age at menarche was lower among adolescents who became pregnant ($p = 0.0004$) and those who experienced sexual violence ($p = 0.0008$). Further, there was a strong association between age at menarche and age at first sexual intercourse ($p < 0.0001$). This study also demonstrated that the earlier the age at menarche, the earlier was the age at sexual initiation and age at first unintended pregnancy and the greater was the risk of experiencing sexual violence. Early menarche may be considered a vulnerability factor during adolescence.

1. Introduction

Menarche, or the first menstrual bleeding, is a significant event in the reproductive life of a woman. The onset of menarche is preceded by a complex cascade of hormonal changes during puberty [1]. Hormonal regulation of sexual maturation is susceptible to several factors from the beginning of prenatal life. Early pubertal development induces medical and social problems and, eventually, results in increased morbidity and mortality in adulthood. Age at menarche is one of the most significant features commonly used for retrospective epidemiological studies on female sexual maturation in a population [1].

According to Karapanou and Papadimitriou [2], variability in the date of the first menstruation is due to complex interactions between genetic characteristics and environmental factors. Genetic factors contribute to age at menarche by approximately 57–82% [2, 3]. These factors include prenatal and postnatal determinants of menarcheal age, such as ethnic differences, maternal history, maternal weight gain during pregnancy, gestational diabetes, prematurity, and birth weight [4, 5].

Environmental factors have attracted increasing attention because many of them are potentially controllable and are related to climate, geographic location, nutritional status, socioeconomic level, education, ethnicity, number of children in the family, and other variables [2].

Other factors such as family disruption, childhood adversity, and ongoing stress may also accelerate a girl's sexual and reproductive development. Adverse childhood experience such as sexual abuse and presence of psychological disorders such as autistic spectrum, Down syndrome, and cerebral palsy may cause variation in the onset of menses [5–9].

Yermachenco and Dvornyk [1] state that general improvement in the socioeconomic and health conditions of populations has resulted in an earlier onset of puberty and the anticipated onset of menses. These conditions impact the nutritional and psychosocial state of girls during childhood and adolescence. In this way, early menarche may be considered a positive trend with regard to improvements in socioeconomic conditions and wellbeing in countries where hunger, drought, and local conflicts continue to be serious problems [10].

Studies conducted in developed countries suggest that early menarche (at the age of 11 years or below) increases the vulnerability of these adolescents to negative sexual and reproductive health outcomes including early sexual initiation, early pregnancy and delivery, and sexual violence [1, 11–13].

This study is aimed at evaluating the association between age at menarche and age at sexual initiation, age at pregnancy, and experience of sexual violence in the adolescent population visiting a primary health unit in the Federal District, Brazil. Establishing this relationship may help contribute to preventive strategies, protective health interventions, and the sexual and reproductive rights of adolescents.

2. Materials and Methods

This clinical cross-sectional, observational, descriptive study was conducted among low-income female adolescents who sought care by spontaneous demand and visited the gynecology outpatient clinic in a Basic Health Unit (BHU), Sobradinho, Federal District, Brazil. The sample consisted of 201 female adolescents, aged 10–19 years, who attended the BHU for adolescents for 12 months. The project was approved by the Research Ethics Committee of the Faculty of Medicine at the University of Brasília and registered under number 119/2007. In addition, a duly completed and signed consent form was received from the participants and their guardians for those under 18 years of age, to accept participation in the study and the delivery of the Terms of Free and Informed Consent.

Inclusion criteria were age between 10 and 19 years, female gender, previous menarche, and those who agreed to participate in the study. Exclusion criteria were presence of any disease or use of medications that could interfere with sexual maturation.

The questionnaire was composed of direct questions with yes or no answers or related numbers, such as in the case of the participants' age. A database was then constructed with the information of the following variables: age at menarche (independent variable), age at sexual initiation, age at first pregnancy, and experience of sexual violence in the adolescents' dependent variables. The answers in the questionnaire were exclusively filled by the researcher for questions directed to the adolescents, who answered freely and independently. Questions on sexual violence required direct, affirmative (yes) or negative (no) answers after clarifying the concept. In Brazil, sexual activity with girls under the age of 14 years is legally considered sexual violence [14, 15].

The database was constructed using Excel 2000 software (Microsoft Corp., Redmond, WA, USA). Statistical tests such as ANOVA and Mann–Whitney tests were performed using SAS software version 8.02 (SAS Institute Inc., Cary, NC, USA), and a mathematical model of linear regression was established.

Pearson correlation coefficients (r) were also used to quantify the degree of association between two variables. Initially, each variable was analyzed individually, and then statistical analysis was performed to access the association between the independent variable and the other dependent variables by crossing the data of age at menarche with the data of age at first sexual intercourse, age at first pregnancy, and occurrence of sexual violence. To verify this, frequencies, averages, standard deviations, and confidence intervals (CIs) were calculated. Statistical significance at $p < 0.05$ was used for all analyses.

3. Results

At the BHU, 768 adolescents sought services during the 12 months of evaluation, of them, 201 agreed to participate and answered the questionnaire. The mean age of the adolescents during care was 16.9 years. Of the 201 adolescents, 191 (95%) were aged 15 years or older at the time of the consultation. The mean age at menarche was 12.1 years, and of the 201 participants, 135 (67%) menstruated before 12 years of age and 66 (33%) after 13 years of age.

Of the 201 adolescents, 171 (85%) reported having initiated sexual activity at the time of visiting the BHU. The mean age at first sexual intercourse was 15 years. Of those 171 participants, 58 (34%) reported having started their sexual life at 14 years or younger and 21 (12%) began at the age of 15 years. For 92 (54%) of the adolescents interviewed, sexual initiation occurred at the age of 16 years.

During the evaluation of the findings, we observed that age at first sexual intercourse is usually after menarche and that the later the age at menarche, the later is the age at first sexual intercourse (Figure 1). These data show an association between age at menarche and age at first sexual intercourse. The Pearson correlation coefficient (r) was 0.38, and it indicated a moderate positive association between the two sets of information ($p < 0.0001$).

Among the 201 adolescents, 114 (56.7%) had already become pregnant, and the mean age was 16.2 ± 1.5 years for the first pregnancy. The CI was 15.9–16.5 years for the first pregnancy, ranging from 11 to 18 years (Table 1).

Among the adolescents, 30 (26.3%) became pregnant at the age of 15 years or younger. Age at menarche and age at first pregnancy showed a significant association ($p = 0.0004$). Thus, age at menarche also exerted influence on age at first pregnancy in this group (Figure 2).

The number of respondents who answered the questions on sexual violence was 103. Of these 103 participants, 51 (49%) experienced some form of sexual violence. There were 28 declared cases of sexual violence, and in 23 cases, there

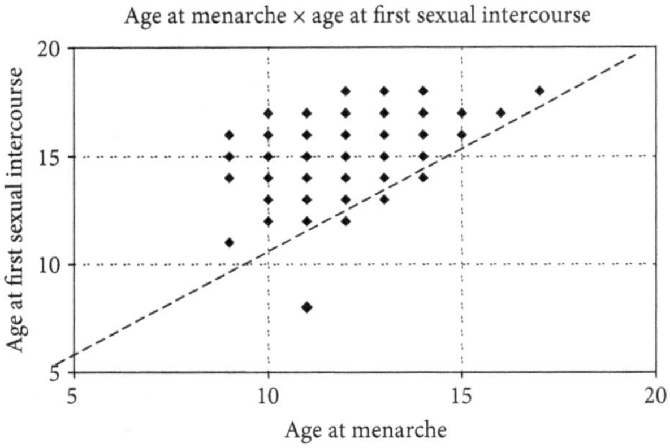

FIGURE 1: Correlation between the age at menarche and age at first sexual intercourse of adolescents attended at a Basic Health Unit (age at menarche × age at first intercourse).

TABLE 1: Distribution of the age at the first pregnancy of adolescents attended at a Basic Health Unit.

Age at first pregnancy	N	%
11	1	0.88
12	2	1.75
13	2	1.75
14	10	8.77
15	15	13.16
16	34	29.82
17	26	22.81
18	24	21.05
Total of respondents	114	100

*Nonrespondents: 87 (30 without sexual activity so far and 57 who never got pregnant).

was a presumption of violence, as these adolescents were under 14 years of age. Experience of sexual violence was also significantly associated with early menarche, with a mean age at menarche of 11.5 years. This age was different from that of participants with negative answers for this event, in which the mean age at menarche was 12.2 years. The age difference in the onset of menarche among adolescents who experienced sexual violence was statistically significant ($p < 0.05$) (Table 2).

The statistical model, as shown in Table 3, provided details on which factors were related to age at menarche. This model provided details on the association of age at first sexual intercourse and age at first pregnancy with age at menarche ($R^2 = 0.9865$).

4. Discussion

The results of this study corroborate the literature, confirming that there is a progressive tendency toward precocity of sexual maturation. This is an important medical and social problem, as it can result in increased morbidity and mortality in adult life [1–3]. According to the data obtained in the study, age at menarche predominated at approximately 12 years. It is estimated that during the twentieth century, age at menarche fell by approximately 3 months per decade [2, 16, 17]. This universal phenomenon can result in higher risks such as early sexual initiation, unplanned pregnancy, and sexual violence in girls and adolescents [1, 11–13]. Currently, age at menarche is considered a reliable marker among the other positive changes that occur in pubertal development [2, 18, 19].

The data obtained from the group showed that the earlier the menarche, the earlier the sexual life begins. Among all associations, the relationship between early menarche and the earliest onset of sexual activity has the greatest impact ($p < 0.0001$). The data in the literature are similar to ours', and because of psychoemotional immaturity, misinformation, and lack of access to contraceptives, there is a high risk of pregnancy and sexually transmitted diseases [13].

The precocity of age at menarche may be associated with other consequences such as health problems at a later age, presence of risk behaviors, early sexual initiation, smoking, breast cancer, diabetes, impaired fertility, cardiovascular diseases, obesity, and psychological disorders. Data from other studies corroborate the data of this study by identifying that early menarche (at the age of 11 years or less) increases the vulnerability of adolescents to negative sexual health outcomes and reproductive health in high-income countries. This includes early sexual initiation, early pregnancy and childbirth, and sexual violence [10–13].

A study conducted in New Zealand demonstrated findings similar to ours in girls who reached menarche at 10–11 years of age were significantly more likely to be pregnant at 18 years of age than those who reached menarche at a later age [11]. In studies conducted among young women in the United States, age at menarche was associated with the initiation of sexual life, which, in turn, correlated directly and positively with age at first pregnancy [10, 13].

In the population evaluated in this study, 114 (56.7%) adolescents had already become pregnant at least once, and 10% of them, two or more times. Mean age at first pregnancy was 16.2 years and our results showed an association between first pregnancy and early menarche. A major concern among teenagers is the risk of recurrence of pregnancy. A review of the American literature showed that 35% of low- and middle-income adolescents became pregnant again in less than 2 years [20]. The same trend was seen in another study [21].

An experience of sexual violence was confirmed by 61 (49%) adolescents in the evaluated group (considering the presumed violence). This study showed a significant association between experiencing sexual violence and early menarche, corroborating the findings in the literature [13, 15]. According to a study conducted by Wise et al., sexual violence was positively associated with early menarche, with an increase in the frequency of sexual abuse cases [15]. In this study, a weak but statistically significant association between physical violence and early menarche was observed. The association between sexual violence and early menarche was stronger when menarche occurred before the age of 11 years.

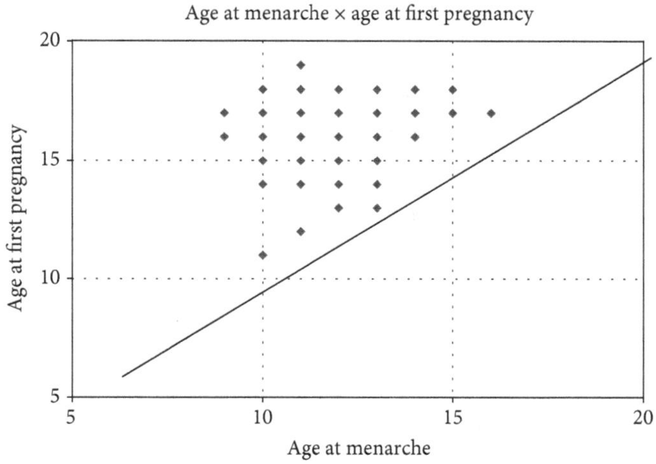

Figure 2: Correlation between the age at menarche and the age at first pregnancy of adolescents attended at a Basic Health Unit (age at menarche × age at first pregnancy).

Table 2: Correlation between age at menarche and the experience of sexual violence among adolescents attended at a Basic Health Unit.

Sexual violence	N	Mean	Standard deviation	Confidence interval	p^*
Yes	51	11.5	1.2	(11.1–11.8)	0,0008
No	62	12.2	1.3	(11.9–12.6)	

*Mann–Whitney test.

Table 3: Linear regression model between age at menarche and age at first pregnancy among adolescents attended at a Basic Health Unit.

Age at menarche = 0.3935 (age at first sexual intercourse) + 0.3825 (age at first pregnancy) − 0.0034

Variable	Parameter	p
Age at first intercourse	0.39346	0.0049
Age at first pregnancy	0.38254	0.003

*Linear regression model without intercept.

Although the data are consistent with the data reported in the literature, longitudinal studies with a larger number of participants are required to elucidate the association of these findings.

Early sexual maturation is not always accompanied by psychoemotional and social maturity, which hinders autonomy for self-care and protection as well as restricts access to resources for living in a healthy and safe manner. It can definitively compromise life projects in adolescence and adulthood. It is possible, therefore, to associate early menarche with a greater frequency of unprepared and unprotected sexual initiation in relation to various biopsychosocial aspects, unintended pregnancy in adolescence and experiencing sexual violence, and whether the violence is declared by the adolescent or not yet perceived by them but presumed by justice and pseudopermitted by society.

Investing in research on sexual and reproductive health is an effective strategy to identify the factors associated with the increased risks that adolescents face concerning sexual violence, unintended pregnancies, and other diseases and injuries to which they are vulnerable. The data obtained will allow the development of necessary and effective measures to protect and positively influence a new generation of children and adolescents. Thus, this research will assist them in achieving their goals, fulfilling their aspirations, guaranteeing their rights, and achieving an overall improved quality of life.

References

[1] A. Yermachenko and V. Dvornyk, "Nongenetic determinants of age at menarche: a systematic review," *BioMed Research International*, vol. 2014, Article ID 371583, 14 pages, 2014.

[2] O. Karapanou and A. Papadimitriou, "Determinants of menarche," *Reproductive Biology and Endocrinology*, vol. 8, no. 1, p. 115, 2010.

[3] J. Clarkson, W. C. Boon, E. R. Simpson, and A. E. Herbison, "Postnatal development of an estradiol-kisspeptin positive feedback mechanism implicated in puberty onset," *Endocrinology*, vol. 150, no. 7, pp. 3214–3220, 2009.

[4] M. G. Teles, S. D. C. Bianco, V. N. Brito et al., "AGPR54-Activating mutation in a patient with central precocious puberty," *The New England Journal of Medicine*, vol. 358, no. 7, pp. 709–715, 2008.

[5] M. S. Vitalle, C. Y. Tomioka, Y. Juliano, and O. M. Amancio, "Body mass index, pubertal development and their relationship with menarche," *Revista da Associação Médica Brasileira*, vol. 49, no. 4, pp. 429–433, 2003.

[6] J. Mendle, L. D. Leve, M. Van Ryzin, M. N. Natsuaki, and X. Ge, "Associations between early life stress, child maltreatment, and pubertal development among girls in foster care," *Journal of Research on Adolescence*, vol. 21, no. 4, pp. 871–880, 2011.

[7] A. J. O. Whitehouse, M. T. Maybery, M. Hickey, and D. Sloboda, "Brief report: autistic-like traits in childhood pre-

dict later age at menarche in girls," *Journal of Autism and Developmental Disorders*, vol. 41, no. 8, pp. 1125–1130, 2011.

[8] L. M. Burke, C. Z. Kalpakjian, Y. R. Smith, and E. H. Quint, "Gynecologic issues of adolescents with down syndrome, autism, and cerebral palsy," *Journal of Pediatric and Adolescent Gynecology*, vol. 23, no. 1, pp. 11–15, 2010.

[9] K. A. Tunau, M. A. Hassan, B. A. Ekele, A. N. Adamu, and Y. Ahmed, "Age at menarche among school girls in Sokoto, Northern Nigeria," *Annals of African Medicine*, vol. 11, no. 2, pp. 103–107, 2012.

[10] J. Deardorff, N. A. Gonzales, F. S. Christopher, M. W. Roosa, and R. E. Millsap, "Early puberty and adolescent pregnancy: the influence of alcohol use," *Pediatrics*, vol. 116, no. 6, pp. 1451–1456, 2005.

[11] J. M. Boden, D. M. Fergusson, and L. J. Horwood, "Age of menarche and psychosocial outcomes in a New Zealand birth cohort," *Journal of the American Academy of Child and Adolescent Psychiatry*, vol. 50, no. 2, pp. 132–140.e5, 2011.

[12] W. Copeland, L. Shanahan, S. Miller, E. J. Costello, A. Angold, and B. Maughan, "Outcomes of early pubertal timing in young women: a prospective population-based study," *American Journal of Psychiatry*, vol. 167, no. 10, pp. 1218–1225, 2010.

[13] M. Ibitoye, C. Choi, H. Tai, G. Lee, and M. Sommer, "Early menarche: a systematic review of its effect on sexual and reproductive health in low- and middle-income countries," *PLoS One*, vol. 12, no. 6, article e0178884, 2017.

[14] "Brasil, Lei n 12.015/09, 2009- Artigo 217-A," December 2019, http://www.planalto.gov.br/ccivil_03/_Ato2007-2010/2009/Lei/L12015.htm.

[15] L. A. Wise, J. R. Palmer, E. F. Rothman, and L. Rosenberg, "Childhood abuse and early menarche: findings from the Black Women's Health Study," *American Journal of Public Health*, vol. 99, no. S2, pp. S460–S466, 2009.

[16] T. C. Dann and D. F. Roberts, "Menarcheal age in University of Warwick young women," *Journal of Biosocial Science*, vol. 25, no. 4, pp. 531–538, 1993.

[17] G. W. Lindgren, I. L. Degerfors, A. Fredriksson et al., "Menarche 1990 in Stockholm schoolgirls," *Acta Paediatrica Scandinavica*, vol. 80, no. 10, pp. 953–955, 1991.

[18] I. Nakamura, M. Shimura, K. Nonaka, and T. Miura, "Changes of recollected menarcheal age and month among women in Tokyo over a period of 90 years," *Annals of Human Biology*, vol. 13, no. 6, pp. 547–554, 1986.

[19] F. Rigon, L. Bianchin, S. Bernasconi et al., "Update on age at menarche in Italy: toward the leveling off of the secular trend," *The Journal of Adolescent Health*, vol. 46, no. 3, pp. 238–244, 2010.

[20] M. K. Baldwin and A. B. Edelman, "The effect of long-acting reversible contraception on rapid repeat pregnancy in adolescents: a review," *The Journal of Adolescent Health*, vol. 52, 4 Suppl, pp. S47–S53, 2013.

[21] L. A. McDaid, J. Collier, and M. J. Platt, "Previous pregnancies among young women having an abortion in England and Wales," *The Journal of Adolescent Health*, vol. 57, no. 4, pp. 387–392, 2015.

5

Menstrual Hygiene Management and School Absenteeism among Adolescents in Ghana: Results from a School-Based Cross-Sectional Study in a Rural Community

Shamsudeen Mohammed,[1] **Roderick Emil Larsen-Reindorf**,[2] **and Issahaku Awal**[3]

[1]*Department of Population, Family and Reproductive Health, School of Public Health, Kwame Nkrumah University of Science and Technology, Kumasi, Ghana*
[2]*Department of Obstetrics & Gynaecology, School of Medical Science, Kwame Nkrumah University of Science and Technology, Kumasi, Ghana*
[3]*Department of Medicine, Renal Dialysis Unit, Tamale Teaching Hospital, Tamale, Ghana*

Correspondence should be addressed to Shamsudeen Mohammed; deen0233@gmail.com

Academic Editor: Hind A. Beydoun

The study aimed to deepen our understanding of the menstrual hygiene management (MHM) of adolescents and the influence of menstruation on school absenteeism. We employed a school-based cross-sectional design in five Junior High Schools combining both quantitative and qualitative data collection methods. A questionnaire was used to collect quantitative data from 250 schoolgirls, and key informant interviews were conducted with a teacher in each of the five schools. We performed logistic regression analysis to provide crude and adjusted effect estimates and 95% confidence intervals. About fifty percent of the girls were engaged in good MHM, and approximately forty percent of them reported menstrual-related school absenteeism. We did not find evidence ($p = 0.858$) of association between MHM and menstrual-related school absenteeism. However, after controlling for the effect of other factors, we found evidence that the age of the schoolgirls, their father's occupation, and the receipt of allowance for menstrual care products were associated with MHM. When compared to those aged 17 to 19, those aged 10 to 13 years had 0.72 (95% CI 0.21, 2.44) decreased odds of poor MHM while those aged 14 to 16 had almost 3-fold increased odds (95% CI 1.49, 4.55) of poor MHM. The adolescents whose fathers were farmers had 0.42 (95% CI 0.21, 0.82) decreased odds of poor MHM while those whose fathers were unemployed had 0.24 (95% CI 0.10, 0.61) decreased odds of poor MHM. We found that girls who did not receive regular allowance for menstrual care products had nearly 2-fold increased odds (95% CI 1.06, 3.09) of poor MHM compared to those who received allowance for menstrual care products. Menstrual pain (82.2%), fear of staining clothing (70.3%), fear of being teased (70.3%), nonavailability of sanitary pad (63.4%), and lack of private place to manage period at school (60.4%) were the common reasons cited for menstrual-related school absenteeism.

1. Introduction

Menstruation is a natural part of the reproductive cycle during which blood is lost through the vagina [1]. Most adolescents experience their first menstruation (menarche) between the ages of 11 and 14 years. However, some girls start as early as 8 and some at 17 or older [2, 3]. Hygiene during the period of menstruation is fundamental to the dignity and well-being of women and girls and an issue that every girl has to deal with once she enters adolescence around the age of 12 and until she reaches menopause [4, 5]. Menstrual hygiene products such as tampons, sanitary pads, menstrual cups, cloths, paper material, or plant material are used by women and girls to absorb menstrual blood and to maintain personal hygiene during the period of menstruation [6]. To prevent physical discomfort and leakages, adolescent girls need to know the types of menstrual care products that exist and how to appropriately use and dispose of them hygienically [7]. Knowledge of what product to use, how often to change it, and access to adequate water, sanitation, and hygiene facilities help women and girls to maintain good hygiene during menstruation [1, 8]. In the absence of suitable and affordable menstrual care products, some women and girls may resort to using unhygienic and inappropriate products such as newspaper, old rags, dried leaves, or socks to collect menstrual blood and manage their periods [1, 8]. For instance, a study in Mali reported the use of old cotton fabric (*pagnes*) to absorb menstrual blood among adolescent girls [9]. Also, findings from a study in Ethiopia showed that 35.4% of students used sanitary napkins, 55.6% used homemade cloth, and 9% used underwear as absorbent materials for menstrual blood [10]. Although research on the health risks of poor menstrual hygiene practices is inconclusive [3], it is believed that hygiene practices during menstruation have a health impact as the risk of reproductive and urinary tract infections is higher than normal during menstruation [1]. Poor, unhygienic, and unsafe sanitary materials to absorb menstrual blood, therefore, predispose adolescent girls to reproductive tract infections with potential long-term effects on their reproductive health [11]. UNICEF suggests that, during menstruation, girls and women need to change their sanitary napkins regularly, especially in the first two to three days [5]. Sommer and Connolly proposed that menstrual absorbent products should change three or four times a day and woman and girls should wash the area around the vagina at least twice a day with soap and water [2].

Globally, menstruation and menstrual hygiene insecurity contribute to school absenteeism of millions of girls and women and increase the likelihood of school dropout [12]. According to UNESCO, many adolescent girls stay home from school due to menstrual cramping, deficient menstrual hygiene materials, lack of water and sanitation facilities in schools, unsupportive environments, and fear of a menstrual accident [7]. Some adolescents also shun standing up to answer questions in class because of fear of leakage or smell and discomfort; others hesitate to write on the board for fear of menstrual accidents and others seeing blood on their clothes and the subsequent shame and embarrassment this causes [13–16]. Tegegne and Sisay found that girls sometimes miss exams in school when the date of the exam coincides with their menstruation days [10]. This limits the right of women and girls to get an education and contribute to maintaining gender inequalities between schoolgirls and their male peers [12]. In some cases, girls completely drop out of school because of the stress and embarrassment associated with managing menstruation in a school environment [1]. With accessible water and adequate sanitation facilities that are safe, socially and culturally acceptable within the school premises, women and girls are able to manage menstruation in privacy and with dignity and do not have to miss out on their studies when they menstruate [12]. This study was undertaken to deepen understanding of the menstrual hygiene management of adolescents and the impact of menstruation and menstrual hygiene practices on school absenteeism among adolescent schoolgirls in a rural community in Ghana.

2. Materials and Methods

This was a school-based cross-sectional study conducted in Kumbungu in the Northern Region of Ghana. Kumbungu is the capital of the Kumbungu District in the Northern Region of Ghana with an estimated population of 39,341 [17]. All the people in this district live in rural areas with the population equally distributed between males and females [17]. There are five main Junior High Schools in the district capital. Adolescent schoolgirls in all the five Junior High Schools in the district constituted the population for the study, and data were collected from Junior High Schoolgirls between the ages of 10 and 19 years who had attained menarche. Participants were selected from Junior High Schools because girls experience menarche between 11 and 14 years and during this period they are in Junior High School.

2.1. Sample Size and Sampling Procedure. The sample size for the study was determined using Cochran's correction formula for a finite population [18] based on 40% prevalence of menstrual hygiene practices from a previous study [19], 95% confidence interval, and 5% margin of error. With the population of 387 adolescent schoolgirls in the five Junior High Schools and the assumption of 30% nonresponse rate, the calculated sample size for the study was estimated to be approximately 250.

The estimated sample size was apportioned to each school using probability proportional to size sampling approach centred on the number of adolescent girls in each of the five schools. A sampling frame of eligible participants for each school was designed with the help of schoolteachers using class registers. A list of random numbers was then generated and compared to the sampling frame to select participants through simple random sampling method. Using the classroom registers, selected students were identified and approached in their respective classrooms in each of the five schools. They were then put together in one classroom for completion of the study questionnaire. A teacher was purposively selected in each of the five schools for key informant interview (KII) on the impact of menstruation on school attendance. We selected classroom teachers who taught in their school for at least a year and were willing to consent to participate in the study, and female teachers who met the criteria were selected over male teachers because adolescent girls are more likely to disclose their menstrual challenges to them.

The research team then generated a table of random numbers with OpenEpi version 3, which was compared to a sampling frame to sample participants for the study in each of the five schools using simple random sampling method.

2.2. Data Collection Procedure. Quantitative data were collected with a pretested self-administered questionnaire consisting of both opened-ended and closed questions on sociodemographic characteristics of the participants, menstrual hygiene management, and the influence of menstruation on school attendance of adolescent girls. The questionnaire was field-tested among 30 adolescent girls with similar characteristics as the study population. The field test offered an opportunity to assess the reliability of the instrument and the ability of the participants to understand and respond to the questions. Necessary changes were made to improve the questionnaire after the review and the field test. Three female research assistants were recruited and trained to administer the questionnaire. With the assistance of teachers in each of the schools, participants were positioned apart from each other in classrooms to prevent discussions between them during completion of the questionnaire. Due to the culturally sensitive nature of menstruation and its management, adolescent boys and male teachers were not allowed in classrooms where quantitative data collection took place. The female research assistants explained to the participants how to complete the questionnaires and offered help to those who required it.

In addition, key informant interviews were conducted with a teacher in each of the five schools on the impact of menstruation on the school attendance of the adolescent schoolgirls. Trained research assistants used an interview guide to facilitate the key informant interviews. The questions were open-ended with probes, to help facilitators ask for more details where necessary. All the interviews were conducted in English language and recorded with an audio tape recorder with notes taken. The participants were informed of the purpose of the study and their right to decline to answer any question or withdraw from participation at any time during the study.

2.3. Definition of Terms

2.3.1. Menstrual Hygiene Management. The study adopted the menstrual hygiene management definition proposed by the World Health Organization and UNICEF as the "use of clean menstrual management material to absorb or collect menstrual blood that can be changed in privacy as often as necessary for the duration of a menstrual period, using soap and water for washing the body as required, and having access to safe and convenient facilities to dispose of used menstrual management materials" [13].

2.3.2. Menstrual-Related School Absenteeism. This was defined as missing one or more days of school because of menstruation or its management.

2.3.3. Adolescent. Schoolgirls between the ages of 10 and 19 years were considered as adolescents in this study.

2.4. Data Management and Statistical Analysis. Data were checked for completeness, coded, and entered into Microsoft Excel Spreadsheet before imported into Stata version 16.0 for analysis. Background characteristics of the schoolgirls were summarised by whether they ever experienced menstrual-related school absenteeism. The adolescents' menstrual hygiene management was measured out of nine menstrual hygiene management questions and scored based on the scoring scheme of a previous study [19]. Each correct response scored one point while an incorrect response earned no score. The scores of participants were summed to determine their overall menstrual hygiene management score. Participants were classified as engaged in good menstrual hygiene management if they scored 6-9 points and poor menstrual hygiene management if they scored 0-5 points. We performed univariate and multivariable logistic regression analysis to provide crude and adjusted effect estimates and 95% confidence intervals for the association between sociodemographic factors and the menstrual hygiene management of the schoolgirls. Independent factors that showed strong or statistical significant ($p < 0.05$) effect in the initial univariate analysis were moved to the multivariable regression model where the effect of other factors was controlled to determine the factors that were independently associated with the menstrual hygiene management of the schoolgirls. Variables were only retained in the multivariable logistic regression model if they showed at least good evidence of association ($p < 0.05$). All p values presented are from the likelihood ratio test. Qualitative data from key informant interviews were transcribed verbatim. The transcripts were read several times to generate codes, which were then organised into one major theme, and narrated with quotations from the participants.

2.5. Ethical Consideration. The ethics committee of Kwame Nkrumah University of Science and Technology, School of Medical Sciences, and Komfo Anokye Teaching Hospital provided ethical clearance for the study, and permission was obtained from the Kumbungu District Director of Education. Participants indicated their consent by signing a consent form designed for the study after the purpose and significance of the study was explained to them. For participants under the age of consent, informed verbal consent was obtained from headteachers of their respective schools and signed informed assent from the participants. Parental consent was not obtained since headteachers act as guardians in school. The consent procedure was approved by the ethics committee and accepted by the headteachers. Confidentiality of the information collected was ensured.

3. Results

3.1. Sociodemographic Characteristics of Adolescent Schoolgirls. A little over half of the participants ($n = 137$, 54.8%) were 14 to 16 years old, and sixty-eight percent ($n = 171$) of them experienced menarche between 13 and 15 years (Table 1). Of the two hundred and fifty participants, 244 (97.6%) were Muslims, 132 (52.8%) lived in families that owned radio/television, and 66 (26.4%) of them were engaged in income-earning activities after school hours. More than half ($n = 145$, 58.2%) of the participants said they do not receive money for the purchase of menstrual care products.

3.2. Menstrual Hygiene Management of Adolescent Schoolgirls. Less than half ($n = 113$, 45.2%) of the schoolgirls changed their used absorbent materials three times or more in a day, and seventy-six percent ($n = 190$) of them reported that they wash their hands before changing their pads (Table 2). A little over half ($n = 104$, 54.74%) of the girls who washed their hands before changing their pads reported doing so always. The results showed that almost all ($n = 237$, 94.80%) the girls washed their hands after changing their

TABLE 1: Sociodemographic characteristics of adolescent schoolgirls.

Characteristics	Menstrual-related school absenteeism Yes (%)	No (%)	Total (%)
Age group (years)			
10-13	7 (6.93)	9 (6.04)	16 (6.40)
14-16	50 (49.50)	87 (58.39)	137 (54.80)
17-19	44 (43.56)	53 (35.57)	97 (38.80)
Age at menarche			
10-12	27 (26.73)	46 (30.87)	73 (29.20)
13-15	70 (69.31)	101 (67.79)	171 (68.40)
16-17	4 (3.96)	2 (1.34)	6 (2.40)
Have television/radio			
Yes	57 (56.44)	75 (50.34)	132 (52.80)
No	44 (43.56)	74 (49.66)	118 (47.20)
Earn money			
Yes	29 (28.71)	37 (24.83)	66 (26.40)
No	72 (71.29)	112 (75.17)	184 (73.60)
Father's occupation			
Trader	5 (4.95)	11 (7.38)	16 (6.40)
Farmer	71 (70.30)	87 (58.39)	158 (63.20)
Formal sector employee	1 (0.99)	14 (9.40)	15 (6.00)
Unemployed	14 (13.86)	24 (16.11)	38 (15.20)
Others[a]	10 (9.90)	13 (8.72)	23 (9.20)
Mother's occupation			
Trader	23 (22.77)	35 (23.49)	58 (23.20)
Farmer	33 (32.67)	37 (24.83)	70 (28.00)
Formal sector employee	6 (5.94)	15 (10.07)	21 (8.40)
Unemployed	28 (27.72)	51 (34.23)	79 (31.60)
Others[a]	11 (10.89)	11 (7.38)	22 (8.80)
Receive money for sanitary pad			
Yes	38 (38.00)	66 (44.30)	104 (41.77)
No	62 (62.00)	83 (55.70)	145 (58.23)
Summary of menstrual hygiene management[b]			
Good MHM	52 (40.9)	75 (59.06)	127 (50.8)
Poor MHM	49 (39.8)	74 (60.2)	123 (49.2)

[a]Others include tailor, daily labourer, butcher, imam, and mason. [b]Chi-squared test: $x^2 = 0.0318$, p value = 0.858. MHM: menstrual hygiene management.

used absorbent materials, and more than half ($n = 168$, 70.89%) of them do so always. Forty-five percent ($n = 113$) of the girls reported that they disposed of their used sanitary pads in latrine (pit latrine). One hundred and sixty-two (64.80%) of the girls cleaned their genitals with water and soap when menstruating, and almost all the girls ($n = 235$, 94.38%) bath during menstruation. Based on the overall menstrual hygiene management score, 127 (50.80%) of the participants were engaged in good menstrual hygiene management while 123 (49.20%) were engaged in poor menstrual hygiene management.

3.3. Factors Associated with Menstrual Hygiene Management of Adolescent Schoolgirls. In the bivariate analysis, independent factors that were associated with menstrual hygiene management (MHM) were the age of the schoolgirls, their father's occupation, and receipt of money for sanitary products (Table 3).

In the adjusted analysis, there was very strong evidence ($p < 0.001$) of association between age and poor menstrual hygiene management of the schoolgirls (Table 3). Compared to those aged 17 to 19, those aged 10 to 13 years had 0.72 (95% CI 0.21, 2.44) decreased odds of poor menstrual hygiene management while those aged 14 to 16 had almost 3-fold increased odds (95% CI 1.49, 4.55) of poor menstrual hygiene management. We found strong evidence ($p = 0.005$) that father's occupation was associated with the menstrual hygiene management of adolescents. Those whose fathers were farmers had 0.42 (95% CI 0.21, 0.82) decreased odds of poor menstrual hygiene management whereas those whose fathers were unemployed had 0.24 (95% CI 0.10, 0.61) decreased odds of poor menstrual hygiene management compared to those

TABLE 2: Menstrual hygiene management of adolescent schoolgirls.

Parameters of practice	Number	Percent
Absorbent material used during the last menstrual period		
Commercial sanitary pad	118	47.20
Reusable cloth pad	85	34.00
Disposable cloth	25	10.00
Cotton	7	2.80
Underwear/underpants	15	6.00
Change of absorbent material		
Once daily	28	11.20
Twice daily	101	40.40
Thrice or more daily	113	45.20
Do not change until the next day	8	3.20
Wash hands before changing pad		
Yes	190	76.00
No	60	24.00
How often do you wash your hands before changing your pad ($n = 190$)		
Always	104	54.74
Most of the time	54	28.42
Sometimes	32	16.84
Wash hands after changing pad		
Yes	237	94.80
No	13	5.20
How often do you wash your hands after changing your pad ($n = 237$)		
Always	168	70.89
Most of the time	38	16.03
Sometimes	31	13.08
Disposal of used absorbent materials		
Dustbin	38	15.20
Toilet	113	45.20
Open environment	2	0.80
Burnt	25	10.00
Buried	72	28.80
Materials for cleaning genitals when menstruating		
Water only	71	28.40
Water and soap	162	64.80
Tissue paper	8	3.20
Towel	3	1.20
I do not clean/wash	6	2.40
Bath during menstruation		
Yes	235	94.38
No	14	5.62
Overall menstrual hygiene practice		
Good practice	127	50.80
Poor practice	123	49.20

Note: all the menstrual hygiene practice questions were self-reported by the adolescents.

whose fathers had other forms of occupation. The results show good evidence ($p = 0.028$) of association between receipt of regular allowance for sanitary products and the menstrual hygiene management of the schoolgirls. Schoolgirls who did not receive regular allowance for sanitary products had nearly 2-fold increased odds (AOR 1.81, 95% CI 1.06, 3.09) of poor menstrual hygiene management compared to those who received an allowance for sanitary products.

3.4. Influence of Menstruation on the School Attendance of Adolescent Girls. Of the two hundred and fifty schoolgirls, 101 (40.4%) ever absented from school because of menstruation (self-reported); the rest ($n = 149$, 59.6%) of the girls said they have never missed school because of menstruation. Less than half of the girls who were engaged in good menstrual hygiene management ($n = 52$, 40.9%) and 49 (39.8%) of those engaged in poor menstrual hygiene management reported menstrual-related school absenteeism (Table 3). However, we did not find any evidence ($p = 0.858$) of association between menstrual hygiene management and menstrual-related school absenteeism. The most frequently reported reason for missing school among the one hundred and one respondents who experienced menstrual-related absenteeism was pain ($n = 83$, 82.2%) followed by fear of staining clothing ($n = 71$, 70.3%), fear of being teased ($n = 71$, 70.3%), nonavailability of sanitary pad ($n = 64$, 63.4%), and lack of private place to manage period at school ($n = 61$, 60.4%) (Table 4).

3.5. Schoolteachers' Perspective on Menstrual-Related Absenteeism. Almost all the teachers we interviewed said menstruation does not affect the school attendance of most of the girls in the schools. However, they disclosed that some girls occasionally ask for permission from teachers to go home and manage severe menstrual symptoms (e.g., menstrual pains). One teacher said some girls come to school late when they are menstruating. A teacher mentioned that they do not advise girls to absent from school when they are menstruating "because menstruation is not a disease and lessons will not be revisited when they resume school after their periods." The teachers, however, stated that menstruation negatively influences the participation of girls during lessons. Some of the teachers cited absenteeism, poor concentration in class, and loss of self-confidence during the period of menstruation as some of the factors that may impact negatively on the academic performance of girls.

It doesn't affect their attendance that much because most of them come to school when they are menstruating and at times they do ask for permission to either absent or leave early under the excuse of headache and or abdominal pains (KII, male teacher, Kumbungu).

Yes, menstruation affect their class participation in the sense that, they always become timid and at times their mood in the class changes; they tend not to be active and appear moody and do not participate or get involved in class activities which directly affect their end of term results (KII, female teacher, Kumbungu).

Some of them tell you they are sick because they experience headache, abdominal pains, dizziness, nausea which affect their class participation, their confidence in class and even

Table 3: Association of sociodemographic factors and menstrual hygiene management of adolescent schoolgirls.

Characteristics	Good (%) MHM	Poor (%) MHM	Crude odds ratio (95% CI)	p value[1]	Adjusted odds ratio (95% CI)	p value[1]
Age group (years)						
10-13	10 (62.50)	6 (37.50)	0.97 (0.33, 2.90)		0.72 (0.21, 2.44)	
14-16	57 (41.61)	80 (58.39)	2.28 (1.34, 3.88)	0.006	2.61 (1.49, 4.55)	$p < 0.001$
17-19	60 (61.86)	37 (38.14)	1		1	
Age at menarche						
10-13	63 (48.09)	68 (51.91)	1.26 (0.76, 2.07)	0.369		
14-17	64 (53.78)	55 (46.22)	1			
Father's occupation						
Other[2]	19 (35.19)	35 (64.81)	1		1	
Farmer	84 (53.16)	74 (46.84)	0.48 (0.25, 0.91)	0.018	0.42 (0.21, 0.82)	0.005
Unemployed	24 (63.16)	14 (36.84)	0.32 (0.13, 0.75)		0.24 (0.10, 0.61)	
Mother's occupation						
Other[2]	20 (46.51)	23 (53.49)	1			
Farmer	34 (48.57)	36 (51.43)	0.92 (0.43, 1.97)	0.151		
Trader	37 (63.79)	21 (36.21)	0.49 (0.22, 1.10)			
Unemployed	36 (45.57)	43 (54.43)	1.04 (0.49, 2.19)			
Have television/radio						
Yes	70 (53.03)	62 (46.97)	1			
No	57 (48.31)	61 (51.69)	1.21 (0.73, 1.99)	0.456		
Earn money for yourself						
Yes	37 (56.06)	29 (43.94)	1			
No	90 (48.91)	94 (51.09)	1.33 (0.76, 2.35)	0.319		
Receive regular money for menstrual care products						
Yes	61 (58.65)	43 (41.35)	1		1	
No	66 (45.52)	79 (54.48)	1.70 (1.02, 2.83)	0.041	1.81 (1.06, 3.09)	0.028

MHM = menstrual hygiene management; CI = confidence interval. [2]Others include tailor, formal sector employee, daily labourer, butcher, imam, and mason. [1]p values are from the likelihood ratio test.

their movement in the class since they don't want to get soiled by the blood (KII, female teacher, Kumbungu).

4. Discussion

We found that approximately half of the girls were engaged in good menstrual hygiene management and about forty percent of them reported menstrual-related school absenteeism. After controlling for the effect of other factors, there remained evidence that the age of the schoolgirls, their father's occupation, and receipt of allowance for menstrual care products were associated with their menstrual hygiene management. Evidence shows that menstrual hygiene practices vary between girls of different ages [20] and this may explain why girls between the ages of 14 and 16 had almost 3-fold increased odds of poor menstrual hygiene management compared to those in the older age group. This is perhaps due to older girls' better knowledge about menstrual products, its use, and storage as they would have had more opportunity to learn from their peers and family compared to younger girls. A study in India found that older girls use more appropriate menstrual care products, change absorbent materials more frequently, and bath frequently during menstruation [20].

Our findings showed that most of the girls who were engaged in good hygiene practices received allowance from parents for menstrual care products, and girls who did not receive regular allowance for sanitary products were nearly 2 times more likely to engage in poor menstrual hygiene management compared to those who received allowance for sanitary products, which is consistent with similar studies in Ethiopia [19] and India [20]. In low- and middle-income settings, the cost of sanitary products is one of the major barriers to good hygiene practices during menstruation. It has been observed that family socioeconomic status influence girls' choice of menstrual care products, and this may further explain the association between fathers' occupation and the menstrual hygiene management of the girls. A study in India reported that girls from low socioeconomic families use unsanitary or substandard menstrual absorbents and lack access to hygiene facilities to manage menstruation [20].

A greater number of the girls in this study used commercial sanitary pads as compared to other menstrual absorbent materials during their last period before this study, which is contrary to the findings of studies in Ethiopia [10] and Mali [9] where adolescent girls used clothes, old cotton fabric, and rags as absorbent materials. The use of proper menstrual absorbent material will probably reduce the feeling of

Table 4: Adolescent schoolgirls' reasons for missing school during menstruation ($n = 101$).

Reasons[a]	Number	Percent (%)
Afraid of staining clothing	71	70.30
Afraid of being teased	71	70.30
Pain	83	82.18
Lack of private space to manage period at school	61	60.40
Lack of disposal facilities for used pad/cloth	50	49.50
I do not have a sanitary pad	64	63.37
Cultural restrictions	30	29.70
Religious restrictions	17	16.83
My parents asked me not to go to school	26	25.74
My teacher told me not to come to school	19	18.81

[a] Multiple responses were allowed and the percentage is greater than 100.

discomfort, prevent leakages and stains, and reduce their risk of infection during menstruation. However, only 45.2% of the girls changed their menstrual pads three or more times in a day, which is inconsistent with a study in Senegal where more than half (54.7%) of the study participants changed their menstrual absorbent materials at least three times in a day [21]. Not changing pads frequently enough, especially if they are inserted into the vagina, can introduce or support the growth of unwanted bacteria [3]. In India, Torondel et al., found that frequent changing of absorbent material was protective against bacterial vaginosis [22].

Sommer and Connolly encourage girls and women to wash the area around the vagina at least twice a day with mild soap and plain water when menstruating [2]. This practice was reported in nearly two-thirds of the schoolgirls in this study. Frequent washing of the genitals during menstruation reduces the incidence of reproductive tract infections. A study in India reported bacterial vaginosis and candida infection in women who practiced lower frequency of personal washing during their periods [22].

Consistent with the findings of a study in Zambia [23], many of the girls in this study were not engaged in good disposal practices as the majority of them disposed of their used absorbent materials in toilets (pit toilets). This method of disposal may be preferred because girls do not want others to see their used pads and probably because of the lack of dustbins in school toilets. In Zambia, Chinyama et al. found that girls disposed of their used pads in latrines because they were afraid their used pads could be used for witchcraft against them [23]. Nonetheless, improper disposal of blood-stained menstrual absorbent materials can contaminate the environment and spread diseases [4].

Menstrual-related school absenteeism was reported in less than half of the girls in this study, which is in contrast with similar studies in Ethiopia [10] and Uganda [24] but consistent with studies in Indonesia [15], South Africa [25], and Bangladesh [26]. Schoolteachers revealed that girls who attend school when menstruating feel shy to participate in school activities and exhibit poor concentration in class and loss of self-confidence. Several studies in low- and middle-income countries reported similar findings on the participation of girls in school activities during their periods [14–16]. In Nepal, Morrison et al. found that during their period of menstruation most girls are uncomfortable sitting near the front of the classroom and would never raise their hand to answer questions or write on the board [16]. The most frequently reported reasons for menstrual-related absenteeism in this study were menstrual pain, fear of staining clothing, and fear of being teased by colleagues, which are similar to findings reported in earlier studies [14–16]. These concerns together with the occasional school absenteeism may cause some girls to lag in their curricular activities particularly in complex and abstract subjects and may eventually lead to dropout [27]. The decreased attention span and poor concentration among adolescent schoolgirls during menstruation may be linked to the discomfort associated with menstruation, particularly dysmenorrhoea and excessive bleeding, as well as the mental stress during menstruation, mainly due to constant worry that others may know about their menstruation [28]. Education, undoubtedly, is a means of empowering women and girls, and for this reason, the barriers preventing women and girls from realising their right to education must be acknowledged and fully eliminated [12].

5. Limitations

The study has several limitations that should be considered when interpreting the findings. Firstly, data on school facilities, household income, parental education, and other potential risk factors for poor menstrual hygiene management were not collected. Data on these factors could have provided a deeper understanding of how girls manage menstruation in school, whether there was a supportive school environment and how household income influences the hygiene practices of girls. Secondly, this was a cross-sectional study and recall bias might have been introduced by the nature of the design. Thirdly, information about the class activities and school performance of the girls during menstruation were collected from classroom teachers and this could have been overstated. Finally, menstrual hygiene practices were self-reported by the adolescents, and reporting bias cannot be ruled out even though efforts were made to minimise it.

6. Conclusion

Approximately half of the girls were engaged in good menstrual hygiene practices, and about forty percent of them reported menstrual-related school absenteeism. We found evidence that the age of the schoolgirls, their father's occupation, and receipt of allowance for menstrual care products were associated with their menstrual hygiene management. Further research on the impact of menstruation and its management on the academic performance of adolescent schoolgirls is recommended. The study further recommends large-scale studies on the reproductive health effects of poor menstrual hygiene practices to fully understand the effects of menstrual hygiene management beyond school attendance and academic performance.

Abbreviations

KII: Key Informant Interviews
MHM: Menstrual Hygiene Management.

Acknowledgments

The authors would like to thank the Kumbungu District Director of Education and the headteachers of all the five Junior High Schools in Kumbungu. In addition, I would like to thank the teachers and students for their cooperation.

References

[1] S. House, T. Mahon, and S. Cavill, "Menstrual hygiene matters: a resource for improving menstrual hygiene around the world. First Edit," WaterAid, London, UK, 2012.

[2] M. Sommer and S. Connolly, "Growth and changes," Grow and Know, Inc., Cambodia, 2012, https://www.unicef.org/cambodia/Growth_and_Changes_lowres.pdf%0A%0A.

[3] H. Alberda, "Menstrual Health: Training Manual," The Netherlands, 2018https://simavi.org/wp-content/uploads/2018/10/MH-Manual-Digitaal-DEF.pdf%0A%0A.

[4] Water Supply & Sanitation Collaborative Council and Government of India, "WASH and Health for Menstrual Hygiene Management: Training of Trainers Manual v1.0," Water Supply & Sanitation Collaborative Council, London, UK, 2013, https://www.wsscc.org/wp-content/uploads/.../ToT-manual-Jul15-update-EN-web.pdf%0A%0A.

[5] UNICEF, *Sharing Simple Facts: Useful Information about Menstrual Health and Hygiene*, UNICEF India, New Delhi, India, 2008.

[6] T. Rheinländer and M. Wachira, *Emerging Issue Brief: Menstrual Hygiene An Ancient - but Ignored Global Health Problem of All Women*, Global Health Minders, 2015, http://ghm-menstrualhygiene-brief.pdf.

[7] UNESCO, *Puberty Education & Menstrual Hygiene Management. Booklet 9*, United Nations Educational, Scientific and Cultural Organization, Paris, France, 2014, https://www.susana.org/en/knowledge-hub/resources-and-publications/library/details/2213.

[8] R. Kaur, K. Kaur, and R. Kaur, "Menstrual hygiene, management, and waste disposal: practices and challenges faced by girls/women of developing countries," *Journal of Environmental and Public Health*, vol. 2018, Article ID 1730964, 9 pages, 2018.

[9] V. Trinies, B. Caruso, A. Sogoré, J. Toubkiss, and M. Freeman, "Uncovering the challenges to menstrual hygiene management in schools in Mali," *Waterlines*, vol. 34, no. 1, pp. 31–40, 2015.

[10] T. K. Tegegne and M. M. Sisay, "Menstrual hygiene management and school absenteeism among female adolescent students in Northeast Ethiopia," *BMC Public Health*, vol. 14, no. 1, article 1118, 2014.

[11] Swedish International Development Cooperation Agency [Sida], "Menstrual hygiene management," in *Health: Both a prerequisite and an outcome of sustainable development*, pp. 1–3, Swedish International Development Cooperation Agency, Stockholm, Sweden, 2016.

[12] C. Mathiaud, "Menstrual hygiene matters: menstrual hygiene insecurity (MHI) and the need for a global recognition of adequate menstrual hygiene management (MHM) as a fundamental right for all women and girls," France, 2014, https://www.graduatewomen.org/wp-content/.../30.04.18_MH-Day_Advocacy-Report.pdf%0A%0A.

[13] UNICEF, "Supporting the rights of girls and women through menstrual hygiene management (MHM) in the East Asia and Pacific Region good practice guidance note," UNICEF East Asia and Pacific Regional Office (EAPRO), Bangkok, Thailand, 2016, https://www.unicef.org/eapro.

[14] J. Hennegan, C. Dolan, M. Wu, L. Scott, and P. Montgomery, "Measuring the prevalence and impact of poor menstrual hygiene management : a quantitative survey of schoolgirls in rural Uganda," *BMJ Open*, vol. 6, no. 12, article e012596, 2016.

[15] E. Kennedy, W. Suriastini, A. Macintyre et al., "Menstrual hygiene management in Indonesia: understanding practices, determinants, and impacts among adolescent school girls," Indonesia, 2015, https://www.burnet.edu.au/system/asset/file/2034/2015_Menstrual_hygiene_management_Indonesia_FINAL_REPORT_February_2015_low_res.pdf.

[16] J. Morrison, M. Basnet, A. Bhatta, S. Khimbanjar, and S. Baral, "Analysis of menstrual hygiene practices in Nepal: the role of WASH in schools programme for girls education 2016," Nepal, 2018, https://www.unicef.org/nepal/reports/analysis-menstrual-hygiene-practices-nepal.

[17] Ghana Statistical Service (GSS), "2010 population & housing census. District analytical report: Kumbungu district," Accra, Ghana, 2014, https://www.statsghana.gov.gh/docfiles/2010_District_Report/Northern/Kumbungu.pdf%0A%0A.

[18] V. Kasiulevičius, V. Šapoka, and R. Filipavičiūtė, "Sample size calculation in epidemiological studies," *Geron*, vol. 7, no. 4, pp. 225–231, 2006.

[19] S. P. Upashe, T. Tekelab, and J. Mekonnen, "Assessment of knowledge and practice of menstrual hygiene among high school girls in Western Ethiopia," *BMC Women's Health*, vol. 15, no. 1, p. 84, 2015.

[20] S. Omidvar and K. Begum, "Factors influencing hygienic practices during menses among girls from South India-a cross sectional study," *International Journal of Collaborative Research on Internal Medicine & Public Health*, vol. 2, no. 12, pp. 411–423, 2010.

[21] WSSCC and UN Women, *Menstrual hygiene management: behaviour and practices in the Louga Region, Senegal*, Water Supply and Sanitation Collaborative Council and UN Women West Africa Sub Regional Office, Geneva, Switzerland, 2014.

[22] B. Torondel, S. Sinha, J. R. Mohanty et al., "Association between unhygienic menstrual management practices and prevalence of lower reproductive tract infections: a hospital-based cross-sectional study in Odisha, India," *BMC Infectious Diseases*, vol. 18, no. 1, p. 473, 2018.

[23] J. Chinyama, J. Chipungu, C. Rudd et al., "Menstrual hygiene management in rural schools of Zambia: a descriptive study of knowledge, experiences and challenges faced by schoolgirls," *BMC Public Health*, vol. 19, no. 1, p. 16, 2019.

[24] R. Boosey, G. Prestwich, and T. Deave, "Menstrual hygiene management amongst schoolgirls in the Rukungiri district of Uganda and the impact on their education: a cross-sectional study," *Pan African Medical Journal*, vol. 19, p. 253, 2014.

[25] M. Kgware, *Menstruation and Menstrual Hygiene Management in Selected Kwazulu-Natal Schools*, C. Martin, Ed., South Africa, Oxfam, 2016.

[26] M. U. Alam, S. P. Luby, A. K. Halder et al., "Menstrual hygiene management among Bangladeshi adolescent schoolgirls and risk factors affecting school absence: results from a cross-sectional survey," *BMJ Open*, vol. 7, no. 7, article e015508, 2017.

[27] Ten VTA and et al.V. T. A. Ten, Europe External Policy Advisors, Brussels, Belgium, 2007, https://www.ircwash.org/resources/menstrual-hygiene-neglected-condition-achievement-several-millennium-development-goals.

[28] WaterAid, "Is menstrual hygiene and management an issue for adolescent school girls? WaterAid/Anita Pradhan A comparative study of four schools in different settings of Nepal," Kupondole, Lalitpur, Nepal, 2009, https://www.wateraid.org/nepal.

6

Intended Pregnancy as a Predictor of Good Knowledge on Birth Preparedness and Complication Readiness: the Case of Northern Ethiopia Pregnant Mothers

Haile Zewdu Tsegaw,[1] Endeshaw Admassu Cherkos,[2] Marta Berta Badi,[2] and Muhabaw Shumye Mihret[2]

[1]*Maternity Ward, Gondar University Comprehensive and Specialized Referal Hospital, Ethiopia*
[2]*Department of Midwifery, College of Medicine and Health Sciences, University of Gondar, Ethiopia*

Correspondence should be addressed to Muhabaw Shumye Mihret; muhabawshumye@gmail.com

Academic Editor: Hind A. Beydoun

Background. Maternal mortality remains unacceptably high in developing countries. One key strategy to reduce such mortality is utilization of birth preparedness and complication readiness (BP/CR) and creating awareness of BP/CR is an important step for pregnant women, their families, and the community. However, there was limited to no evidence regarding the community's awareness on BP/CR in the study area. Therefore, this study aimed to assess knowledge on BP/CR and associated factors among pregnant women in Debremarkos town, Northwest Ethiopia, 2017. *Methods.* A Community based cross-sectional study was conducted from July 1 to 30/2017. A total of 441 pregnant women were included in the study. Structured and pretested questionnaire was administered through face to face interview to collect the data. Simple random sampling technique was used to select the study participants. The data were entered in to Epinfo version 7.0 and then exported to SPSS version 20.0 for analysis. Both bivariate and multivariable logistic regression model were fitted. Crude and adjusted odds ratio with 95 % confidence interval have been computed and variables with p-value < 0.05 were considered statistically significance. *Results.* The proportion of pregnant women having good knowledge on birth preparedness and complication readiness was found to be 45.2 with 95%CI (40.4, 50.0). In the multivariable analysis, having history of childbirth (AOR=2.17;95%CI:1.18,4.00), having intended pregnancy (AOR=2.13;95%CI: 1.16, 3.90), being governmental employee (AOR=6.50; 95%CI: 2.50, 16.87), and having Antenatal care visits (AOR=5.50; 95%CI:2.2,13.70) were factors which were independently and significantly associated with good knowledge on birth preparedness and complication readiness. *Conclusion.* Proportion of pregnant women having good knowledge on birth preparedness and complication readiness was low. Putting emphasis on intended pregnancy and antenatal care visit was recommended.

1. Introduction

Reduction of maternal mortality has been continued to be a global top public health identified problem [1]. About 830 women daily and 303,000 women annually die from pregnancy and/or childbirth-related complications globally by the year 2015. Almost all of these deaths occurred in low-resource settings, and most could have been prevented [2, 3]. It remains unacceptably high in least developed regions especially in West & Central Africa (WCA) and Sub-Saharan Africa (SSA). According to the United Nations Children's Fund (UNICEF) 2017 report, maternal mortality ratio (MMR) was 216 in globe, 679 in WCA, and 546 in SSA per 100, 000 live births [4]. As a SSA country, Ethiopia has also been suffered from similar problem [5–7]. According to Ethiopian Demographic Health Survey (EDHS) 2016 report, MMR in Ethiopia was 412/100,000 live births [8].

To reduce high maternal mortality, World Health Organization (WHO) in cooperation with its partners has been designing various strategies and standards [9, 10]. From the strategies, birth preparedness and complication readiness (BP/CR) is among the key strategies which have been intended to promote the timely use of skilled maternal and neonatal care [11, 12]. BP/CR is the process of planning for normal birth and anticipating the actions needed in case of an emergency [13]. Moreover, it encourages the pregnant women, the families, and the community at large to have an active preparation to prevent delay in receiving basic emergency obstetric and neonatal care (BEmONC) [14]. Every pregnant woman may face the risk of unpredictable and sudden complications that could end in death or injury [15]. Hence, pregnant women, their family, and the community need to plan for the care needed during the antepartum, intrapartum, and postpartum period and prepare themselves to take action in emergencies [16].

The main components of the BP/CR include recognizing danger signs, identifying skilled birth attendant, saving money, identifying mode of transport, identifying where to go in case of complications, and identifying a blood donor [17]. However, lack of advanced planning for use of skilled birth attendant for normal birth [18] and particularly inadequate preparation for rapid action in the event of obstetric complication are well documented factors contributing to delay in receiving skilled obstetric care [19–21]. Despite its significance, large number of pregnant women and their families may not be aware of the components of BP/CR which in turn may bring about low practice of BP/CR.

Despite the great potential of BP/CR in reducing the maternal and newborn deaths, there is a dearth of evidence on what proportions of women are aware of BP/CR in the study area. Moreover, it is crucial to identify the factors contributing for the woman's knowledge on BP/CR within the community context to design effective BP/CR awareness strategies. In doing so, this study was aimed to assess knowledge on BP/CR and its associated factors among pregnant women living in Debremarkos town.

2. Methods

A community based cross-sectional study was conducted from July 1 to 30/2017 in Debremarkos town, Northwest Ethiopia. The town which is located at 300 kilometers away from Addis Ababa-the capital city of Ethiopia is found at the Northwest direction and 265 kilometers away from Bahir Dar—the capital city of Amahara National regional state in the Southeast direction. It is also the administrative town of the East Gojam Zone which is among 11 Zones of Amhara national regional state. According to the Ethiopian population projection report for all regions at Woreda level conducted from 2014 to 2017, the total population of the town was estimated to be 92,470. Among these, about 45,732 were males and 46,738 were females [22]. From these, women in the reproductive age group were 14,618 and the numbers of households in the town were estimated to be 14,528.

In Ethiopia particularly in Debremarkos town, antenatal care (ANC) services are not active. In connection to this, health care providers have not gone to women's homes to provide formal ANC service even if the women do not attend the clinic. However, the health extension workers (HEWs) are anticipated to go home to home for awareness creation and community mobilization. Accordingly, HEWs are responsible to educate pregnant women, the family and even the community at large about birth preparedness and complication readiness; danger signs during pregnancy; childbirth and postpartum period; the importance of having ANC visit; when and how to get the skilled health care providers by moving home to home and/or arranging a discussion forum in the community in collaboration with the local governmental leaders and/or religious leaders. As far as duties for provision of ANC services are concerned, midwives are primarily responsible at the health centers and/or hospitals, whereas, health extension workers provide ANC services at health post (i.e., the smallest unit of health facility). Moreover, there is a consultancy and/or referral system across different health professionals and levels of health facilities. Accordingly, upon indications, HEWs at health posts refer cases to health centers and/or hospitals where midwives welcome and manage them. Depending on the type and severity of the problems, midwives may consult professionals who specialized in either Clinical Midwifery (Msc), Integrated Emergency Obstetrics and Surgery (Msc), or obstetrics and gynecology (doctors). In addition, midwives may refer eligible cases to higher level of health facilities as necessary.

All residents of Debrmarkos town's pregnant women (i.e., those pregnant women who have been living for at least six months in the town at the time of interview) were included in the study.

Single population proportion formula was used to calculate the sample size by assuming 50%, proportion of pregnant women having good knowledge on BP/CR; 95%, confidence interval; 5 %, margin of error; and 10%, nonresponse rate. Based on these assumptions, the total sample size was calculated using the following formula:

$$N = \frac{Z_{\alpha/2}{}^{2} . p\,(1\text{-}p)}{D^2} = \frac{(1.96)^2 * (0.5)\,(0.5)}{(0.05)^2} = 384 \quad (1)$$

where N= required sample size, Z= confidence level at 95% (at standard value of 1.96), p= estimated proportion (50%), and d = margin of error at 5 % (standard value of 0.05). Upon substitution of the given values in the above formula, the calculated minimum sample size was found to be 384. By adding 15% nonresponse rate, the total sample size turned to be 441.

First, the list of total number of pregnant women was obtained from HEWs in Debremarkos town. Then, study participants were selected using simple random sampling technique using computer generating method. Afterward, the data collectors have employed a map that the town health extension workers have been using, to get the selected mothers. Moreover, the data collectors and supervisors have been guided by HEWs whenever they faced difficulties of getting the selected pregnant woman.

Sociodemographic and obstetric related variables such as age, marital status, religion, ethnicity, husband's educational status, husband's occupation, family monthly income, parity, gravidity, age at 1st marriage, age at first pregnancy, desired number of children, antenatal care (ANC) visit in the current

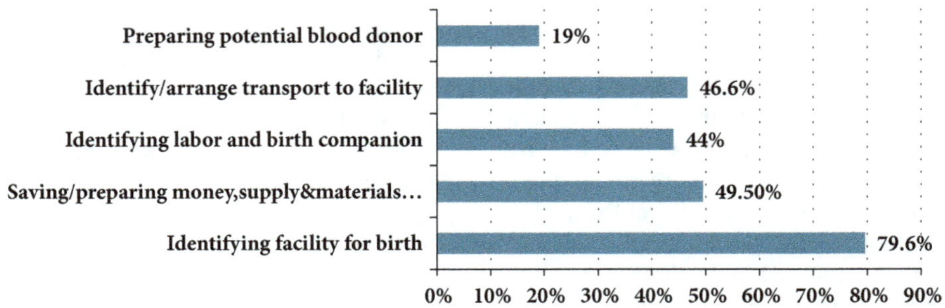

FIGURE 1: BP/CR elements mentioned by pregnant women in Debre Markos town, 2017.

pregnancy, and place of ANC visit in the current pregnancy and intended pregnancy were included. In addition, knowledge on BP/CR ('Good' or 'Poor') was assessed based on some criteria.

A selected pregnant woman was labeled as having good knowledge on BP/CR if she mentioned at least three out of the following five components of BP/CR: identified health facility for childbirth, saved money for birth, arranged transportation, arranged accompany, and arrange potential blood donor.

The data were collected using structured questionnaire through face to face interview. Six midwifery professionals were involved in data collection process. These included six unemployed midwives having diploma in midwifery as the data collectors and one midwife having Bsc in clinical midwifery as a supervisor. The questionnaire was adapted from previous similar research articles [19, 23]. It was first developed in English and then translated to local language (i.e., Amharic) and then back to English to facilitate the understanding of the respondents. A one-day training was provided for the data collectors and a supervisor regarding the objectives of the study, way of approach to the community, sampling techniques, sampling procedures, client privacy issue, client confidentiality issue, client informed and voluntary participation, data collection method, and significance of the study. Then after that, a pretest was conducted on 5% of sample size at Finoteselam, which is a nearby town for the study area, before the actual data collection started. The purpose and objectives of the study were clearly stated in the first page of the questionnaire which the interviewers have explained for participants. During data collection, there was a close communication among the data collectors, a supervisor, and a principal investigator. The collected questionnaires were checked for completeness and on spot corrective measures were taken both by data collectors and supervisors. Daily meeting has been conducted among the data collectors, a supervisor, and a principal investigator for discussion regarding presenting difficulties and to assess the progress of data collection.

Data were checked, coded, and entered into Epi-info7 then exported to SPSS version 20 software package for further analysis. Frequencies and cross tabulations were used to summarize descriptive statistics. The data were presented by texts, tables, and graphs. Furthermore, binary logistic regression was used to identify factors associated with knowledge on BP/CR. Thereafter, variables were fitted to multivariable logistic regression using backward likelyhood ratio method. Both crude odds ratio (COR) and adjusted odds ratio (AOR) with the corresponding 95%CI were computed to show the strength of the association. In addition, model fitness was checked using Hosmer and Lemeshow goodness of a fit test and the model test P-value was found to be 0.13. Finally, statistically significant association of variables was claimed based on AOR with its 95% CI and p-value <0.05.

3. Results

3.1. Sociodemographic Related Characteristics. A total of 436 pregnant women were participated in the study area. The participants' response rate was 98.9%. The mean age of respondents were 28.5 (SD ±6.8) and 67.7% of the women were within the age range of 18 -24 years. Majority (92.7%) of participants were Orthodox Tewahido Christian by religion. Moreover, three-fourth (77.5%) of respondents reported that they had an average family monthly income of more than 90 US Dollar. More than half (60%) of the male partners had attended education of college whereas 229 (52%) of male partners had been employed in governmental organizations [Table 1].

3.2. Obstetric Characteristics of the Respondents. About 200 (45.9%) and 198 (45.4%) of respondents were primiparous and nulliparous, respectively. Considerable number (6.9%) of respondents reported that they had gotten their first marriage at the age of <18 years. More than half (51.5%) of the participants' first pregnancies were within the age range of 18-24. Substantial (84.2%) of the current pregnancies were intended [Table 2].

3.3. Knowledge on Birth Preparedness and Complication Readiness. The proportion of pregnant mothers having good knowledge on BP/CR was found to be 45.2% with 95%CI (40.4, 50.00). More than nine-tenth (92.2%) of mothers mentioned at least one element of BP/CR. Majority (79.6%) of pregnant women had identified the health facility where they planned to give birth at time of interview [Figure 1].

In addition, about 405 (92.9%) of the pregnant women previously had heard about BP/CR; of them 73.8% heard from health professionals, 15.8% from mass media, and 10.4% from relatives and/or friends.

TABLE 1: Socio demographic related characteristics of pregnant women in Debre Markos town, 2017 (N=436).

Characteristics	Frequency	Percent
Mother's age		
18-24	325	74.54
>24	111	25.46
Mother Ethnicity		
Amhara	427	97.7
Tigre	4	0.9
Oromo	5	1.1
Mother education		
Unable to read & write	49	11.2
Can read &write via informal education	38	8.7
Primary	81	18.6
Secondary	99	22.7
College & above	169	38.8
Mother occupation		
Civil servant	170	39
Private employee	74	17
Daily labored	34	7.8
House wife	158	36.2
Husband education		
Un able to read & write	19	4.4
Can read to &write	21	4.8
Primary school	47	10.8
Secondary	87	20
College & above	262	60
Husbands occupation		
Civil servant	229	52
Private	141	32.3
Daily labored	66	15
Family Monthly income (in US dollar)		
< 36	45	10.3
36-90	53	12.2
>90	338	77.5

3.4. Knowledge on Danger Signs of Antepartum, Intrapartum, Postpartum, and Newborn. Most (93.1%) of the respondents mentioned at least one key danger sign during pregnancy and 352 (80.7%) mentioned at least two danger signs of pregnancy. Three hundred ninety-nine (91.5%) of the respondents mentioned at least one and 326 (74.8%) of participants mentioned at least two danger signs during labor and childbirth. Three hundred seventy-one (85%) and 332 (76.2%) of pregnant women mentioned at least one and at least two danger signs during postpartum period, respectively, whereas about 347 (79.6%) and 239 (54.8%) of pregnant women mentioned at least one and at least two newborn danger signs, respectively [Table 3].

3.5. Factors Associated with Birth Preparedness and Complication Readiness. Based on the findings from bivariate logistic regression analysis, mother's educational status, mother's occupation, family monthly income, intended pregnancy, parity, and ANC visit have been associated with knowledge on BP/CR. However, in the multivariable logistic regression analysis, mother's occupation, intended pregnancy, parity, and ANC visit for the current pregnancy have remained statistically significantly associated with good knowledge on BP/CR.

Accordingly, the odds of having good knowledge on BP/CR were 6.50 times higher among governmental employed mothers than others (AOR=6.50; 95% CI: 2.50, 16.87). Likewise, mothers having current intended pregnancy were 2.1 times more likely to have good knowledge on BP/CR as compared with their congruent(AOR =2.10; 95% CI: 1.16, 3.90). Moreover, mothers having ANC visit in the current pregnancy were 5.50 times more likely to have good knowledge on BP/CR than those mothers who had no ANC visit (AOR =5.50, 95%CI; 2.20,13.70). Similarly, pregnant women with history of childbirth were 2.6 times (AOR =2.60, 95% CI; 1.18, 4.00) more likely to have good knowledge on BP/CR than a nulliparous pregnant women (Table 4).

Table 2: Obstetric characteristics of pregnant women in Debremarkos town, 2017.

Characteristics	Number	Percent
Age at 1st marriage		
<18	30	6.9
18-24	295	67.7
>24	111	25.5
Age at 1st pregnancy		
<18	9	2.1
18-24	226	51.5
>24	201	46.1
Gravidity		
1	200	45.9
2-4	223	51.1
≥5	13	3
Parity		
0	198	45.4
1	136	31.2
2-4	77	17.7
≥5	25	5.7
Desired Number of children in life		
1-2	39	8.9
3-4	347	79.6
5-6	50	11.5
ANC visit		
Yes	253	58
No	183	42
Place of ANC visit (n=253)		
Hospital	59	23.3
Health center	194	76.7

4. Discussion

This community based cross-sectional study was conducted to assess knowledge towards BP/CR and associated factors among pregnant women living in Debremarkos town. The odds of good knowledge on BP/CR were higher among mothers who were governmentally employed, got the current pregnancy intentionally, had ANC follow-up during the current pregnancy and had history of previous childbirth.

In the current study, the proportion of mothers having good knowledge on BP/CR was 45.2%. This finding is comparable with the study conducted in Mpwapwa District Tanzania (43.1%) [24], Indore city India (47.8%) [25],Tewale teaching Hospital Ghana (43.7%) [26] and Morang district Nepal (45.2%) [27]. This result is also in line with the local studies taken place in various part of Ethiopia such as Dere Teyara district Eastern Ethiopia (42.8%) [28], Tehulederie district Northeast Ethiopia (44.6%) [29], Kofale District Southeast Ethiopia (41.3%) [30] and Kucha District Southern Ethiopia (44%) [31].

However, the result of this study found to be higher than studies carried out in Ruhengeri hospital Rwanda (22.3%) [32], Urban Lagos state Nigeria (31.6%) [33], East Pokot District Midwest Kenya (28%) [34], Ife central local Government Nigeria (34.9%) [35], Tharaka Nithi county Kenya (20.3%) [36], Jamnagar district India (32.2%) [37], Uttar Dinjpur District West Bengal (34.5%) [38], five hard-to-reach districts in Bangladish (24.5%) [39] and Mbarara District Uganda (35%) [40]. This figure is also higher than as compared with researches have done at different parts of Ethiopia such as Duguna Fango District South Ethiopia (18.3%) [41], Jimma Zone Southeast Ethiopia (23.3% [42], Arbaminch Zuria District Southern Ethiopia (30%) [43] and Aleta Wondo district South Ethiopia (17%) [44].

This disparity in magnitude might be secondary to variation in study settings. From these perspective, those participants who were selected from rural settings less likely have accessed for information, media and even healthcare services than those who were from urban areas. Moreover, this discrepancy might be resulted due to variation in respondent's sociodemographic characteristics. The current study finding revealed that more than 38% of respondents have attended college or university education. In contrary, other studies pointed out that only smaller number (13.4% or below), of participants could attend at college or university level of education [34, 41, 43]. Similarly, about nine-tenth of respondents in the current study were able to read and write. On the contrary, more than half number of study

TABLE 3: Danger signs of antepartum, intrapartum, postpartum, and new born mentioned by pregnant mothers in Debrmarkos town, Northwest Ethiopia, 2017.

Variables	Number	Percent
Elements of danger sign during pregnancy		
Vaginal bleeding	382	87.6
Severe headache	305	70
Blurred vision	197	45.2
Reduced /absent fetal movement	59	13.5
Knowledge on danger sign during labor and childbirth		
Excessive vaginal bleeding	362	83
Severe headache	249	57.1
Convulsion	205	47
Unconsciousness	85	19.5
Prolonged labor	75	17.2
Retained placenta	27	6.2
Knowledge on danger sign during postpartum period		
Severe headache	292	67
High fever	154	35.3
Foul smelling vaginal discharge	36	8.3
Knowledge on newborn danger sign		
Very low birth weight	210	48.2
Convulsion	196	45
Lethargy /unconsciousness	177	40.6
Breathing difficulty	175	40.1

participants in the previous studies had never attended any formal education [34, 39, 44]. This is also true for male partners' educational status [43]. Empirical evidences pointed out that educational status has direct proportional relationship with the general health care seeking behavior and decision making power of the individuals. Furthermore, this dissimilitude might be attributed to the variation in occupation of study participants. In the current study, considerable proportion,(39%), of respondents are governmental employees whereas more than 85% of respondents in the previous studies were non-governmental employer and/or with no paid work [40, 41]. Thus, employees pose great opportunity to meet multidisciplinary professionals thereby share a number of experiences and they are likely having comprehensive awareness on health related information. In connection to this, the disparity could be explained by variation in proportion of study participants who have attended ANC visit for the indexed pregnancy. In the current study, nearly three-fifth,(58%), of the pregnant women had ANC visit unlike that of only 44% in other study [44]. Finally, this disagreement might be resulted to the variation in measurement of the outcome variables; the current study has counted those participants who mentioned, practiced or intended to practice the BP/CR components while other respondents were aiming exclusively on the practice aspect [39, 43].

On the other hand, the findings of the current study are lower as compared with a study conducted in Debre birhan town Ethiopia (65.9%) [45], Mizan-Tepi Ethiopia (66%) [19], Northern Ghana (74.3%) [46], Federal Police Referral Hospital Ethiopia (53.3%)[23], Chamwino district Central Tanzania (58.2%) [47], Edo state Nigeria (87%) [48], Nepal (65%) [49], Imo state Nigeria (77%) [50], Migori county Kenya(56%) [51], Kericho county Kenya(70.5%) [52], Chiro zonal Hospital East Ethiopia (56.7%) [53], Urban Anambra state Nigeria (54.5%) [54], Kamineni Hyderabad (71.5%) [55], and Cross River State Southeastern Nigeria (70.6%) [32].

This difference might be explained by variation in the study design since some of the previous studies were institutional based [32, 51–55]. Furthermore, the difference in magnitude could be accredited to dissimilarity in number of ANC attendants. This is true even among community based studies since more than 95% study participants in the previous studies have had ANC follow-up [47, 49, 50] while the number of respondents were only 58% in the current study at the time of interview. Hence, ANC attendees are more likely to have better awareness as well as access for knowledge and advice on BP/CR from health care providers.

In the current study, intended pregnancy had significant association with good knowledge on BP/CR. This finding was also supported by local studies conducted at Debre birhan [45] and Jimma Zone [42]. From the above results, we can deduce that intended pregnancies have enormous advantages on accessing the information, care, and follow-up services for the pregnancy. This could be due to the fact that mothers having intended pregnancy more likely seek health related information by either reading different magazines, asking friends/relatives, attending health programs from media,

TABLE 4: Bivariate and Multivariable logistic regression analysis for factors associated with knowledge on BP/CR among pregnant women at Debre Markos town, Northwest Ethiopia, 2017(n=436).

Variables	Knowledge on BP/CR		COR(95%CI)	AOR(95%CI)
	Good	Poor		
Mother's age				
18-24	202	**123**	1.21(0.42,3.76)	1.13(0.21,4.26)
>24	64	**47**	1	1
Mothers educational status				
Able to read &write	181	206	1.81(3.05,9.31)	1.32(0.52,2.21)
Unable to read &write	16	33	1	1
Mothers occupation				
Government	95	75	2.50(1.60, 3.93)	**6.50(2.5,16.87)****
Private employee	35	39	1.78(1.01,3.12)	1.5(0.79,2.87)
Daily labor	14	20	1.39(0.65,2.96)	1.4(0.60,3.2)
House wife	53	105	1	1
Husband education				
Can read to &write	217	200	1.21(0.42,12.71)	1.15(0.32,9.46)
Un able to read & write	9	10	1	1
Husbands occupation				
Civil servant	128	101	1.12(0.53,1.82)	1.05(0.36,1.49)
Private	74	67	0.98(0.28,3.74)	0.74(0.17,3.64)
Daily labored	35	31	1	1
Monthly income (US Dollar)				
<39	14	31	1	1
39.00-90.00	18	35	1.14(0.49, 2.66)	1.18(0.48,0.93)
>90.00	165	173	2.11(1.08,4.11)	1.54(0.75,3.20)
Intended Pregnancy				
Yes	177	190	2.28(1.30,3.99)	**2.13(1.16,3.90)***
No	20	49	1	1
Parity				
One or more	118	120	1.48(2.61,9.63)	**2.17(1.18,4.0)***
Nulipara	79	119	1	1
ANC follow up for current pregnancy				
Yes	190	205	4.5(1.95,10.4)	**5.50(2.20,13.70)****
No	7	34	1	1
Gravidity				
Primigravida	102	98	1.10(0.83,6.48)	1.04(0.72,2.47)
Multigravida	115	121	1	1
Place of ANC visit(n=253)				
Hospital	36	23	1.41(0.73,1.38)	1.37(0.69,1.25)
Health center	102	92	1	1
Desired number of children				
1-4	202	184	1.19(0.63,3.71)	1.13(0.57,2.18)
5 or above	24	26	1	1

*=P-value <0.05, **=P-value <0.01, and 1= reference category.

or attending the recommended ANC follow-up at health facilities where they could get enough information about BP/CR than their counterparts.

Women's occupation was a significant and independent factor of knowledge on BP/CR. In this study, those government employees had higher probability of having good knowledge on BP/CR than housewives. This finding was also in agreement with studies conducted in Pune City India [56], Goba district Ethiopia [57], Migori county Kenya [51], and Tharaka Nithi county Kenya [36]. This could be due to the fact that government employees are more educated and have access for different media and information sources than the general population.

ANC visit for the current pregnancy was significantly associated with knowledge on BP/CR. Those pregnant women who had ANC follow-up for their current pregnancy had better knowledge on BP/CR than a woman who did not start ANC follow-up for the current pregnancy. This finding was in accordance with the study done in Debre Birhan Ethiopia [45], Bahir Dar Ethiopia [58], Duguna Fango district South Ethiopia [41], Chamwino District Central Tanzania [47], Indore City India [25], Aleta Wondo District South Ethiopia [44], and Lekhnath Municipality Nepal [59]. This could be due to the fact that women who had ANC follow-up had greater chance of getting health professional's advice and education on BP/CR as part of the ANC service than a woman who did not attend ANC.

Being parous was found to be independent predictor of good knowledge on BP/CR that those women with history of childbirth had higher chance of having good knowledge on BP/CR than nulliparous women. This finding was also consistent with studies conducted in sub-Saharan Africa Austere [60] and Goba district Ethiopia [57]. This might be due to the fact that woman who had history of previous child birth may have better anticipations of the pregnancy related complications than a woman with no child birth experience.

5. Limitations

The magnitude of good knowledge on BP/CR might be underestimated since mothers' knowledge status on BP/CR could be increased throughout the pregnancy period. Hence, those mothers who had poor knowledge at time of interview might have good knowledge at the end of the pregnancy.

6. Conclusion

In this study, proportion of pregnant women having good knowledge on BP/CR was found to be low. Having intended pregnancy, having history of previous childbirth, being governmental employee and having ANC visit for the current pregnancy were factors which associated independently with good knowledge on BP/CR among pregnant women. Hence, stakeholders would better design strategies that encourage women to have planned pregnancy, to attend ANC visit during pregnancy, and to engage in governmental work which in turn may enhance women's knowledge on BP/CR.

Abbreviations

ANC: Antenatal care
AOR: Adjusted odds ratio
BP/CR: Birth preparedness and complication readiness
COR: Crude odds ratio
MMR: Maternal mortality ratio
SDG: Sustainable development goal
SSA: Sub-Saharan Africa
WCA: West & Central Africa
WHO: World Health Organization
HEWs: Health Extension Workers.

Consent

Participants were informed about the purpose of the study, the importance of their participation, and their right to withdraw at any time. Informed consent was obtained prior to data collection. Study participants were interviewed at their homes individually to maintain their privacy. The information obtained from the study subjects was also kept anonymised to maintain confidentiality.

Authors' Contributions

Haile Zewdu Tsegaw and **Muhabaw Shumye Mihret** handled conception and design, acquisition of data, analysis and interpretation of data, drafting the article, critical revision of the article, and final approval of the version to be published. **Endeshaw Admassu Cherkos** and **Marta Berta Badi** also handled conception and design, acquisition of data, analysis and interpretation of data, revised the subsequent of drafts of manuscript, and final approval of the version to be published. All authors contributed equally to this research.

Acknowledgments

The authors would like to thank University of Gondar for ethical letter and financial support. Their gratitude also goes to all data collectors and study participants. They would also like to express their gratitude to Debremarkos town health office for writing permission letter. The research was supported by a grant from University of Gondar, College of Medicine and Health Science. The granting agency did not have a role in the design; collection, analysis, and interpretation of data; or in writing the manuscript.

References

[1] UNDP, "Sustainable Development Goals," 2015.

[2] WHO, *Trends in Maternal Mortality: 1990 to 2015 Estimates by WHO, UNICEF, UNFPA, World Bank Group and the United Nations Population Division*, 2015.

[3] L. Alkema, D. Chou, D. Hogan et al., "Global, regional, and national levels and trends in maternal mortality between 1990 and 2015, with scenario-based projections to 2030: a systematic analysis by the Un Maternal Mortality Estimation Inter-Agency Group," *The Lancet*, vol. 387, no. 10017, pp. 462–474, 2016.

[4] UNICEF, "SOWC-Statistical Table," 2017.

[5] G. A. Tessema, C. O. Laurence, Y. A. Melaku et al., "Trends and causes of maternal mortality in Ethiopia during 1990-2013: Findings from the Global Burden of Diseases study 2013," *BMC Public Health*, vol. 17, no. 1, 2017.

[6] Ethiopian Federal Ministry of Health, *The Health Sector Transformation Plan (HSTP)*, 2016.

[7] Ethiopian Federal Ministry of Health, *Health Sector Development Program IV 2010/11 – 2014/15*, 2010.

[8] Program D, *Ethiopia Demographic and Health Survey 2016 Key Indicators Report*, Central Statistical Agency, 2016.

[9] WHO, UNICEF, and AMDD, *Monitoring Emergency Obstetric Care: A Handbook*, 2009.

[10] WHO, UNFPA, UNICEF, ICM, ICN, FIGO et al., "Definition of Skilled Health Personnel Providing Care during Childbirth: the 2018 Joint Statement by WHO, UNFPA, UNICEF,ICM, ICN, FIGO and IPA:Making Pregnancy Safe: The Critical Role of The Skilled Attendant," *International Journal of Gynecology & Obstetrics*, 2018.

[11] WHO, *Standards For Improving Quality of Maternal and Newborn Care In Health Facilities*, 2016.

[12] WHO, *WHO Recommendations on Health Promotion Interventions for Maternal And Newborn Health*, 2015.

[13] EFMOH, *Basic Emergency Obstetric & Newborn Care (BEmONC)*, 2018.

[14] E. Otolorin, P. Gomez, S. Currie, K. Thapa, and B. Dao, "Essential basic and emergency obstetric and newborn care: From education and training to service delivery and quality of care," *International Journal of Gynecology and Obstetrics*, vol. 130, no. 2, pp. S46–S53, 2015.

[15] Ministry of Health, *Emergency Obstetric & Nweborn Care (EmONC) Improvement Plan 2016 - 2020*, Kingdom of Cambodia Nation-Religion-King, 2016.

[16] A. Banke-Thomas, K. Wright, O. Sonoiki et al., "Assessing emergency obstetric care provision in low- and middle-income countries: a systematic review of the application of global guidelines," *Global Health Action*, vol. 9, no. 1, p. 31880, 2016.

[17] WHO, *Working with Individuals, Families,and Communities to Improve Maternal and Child Health*, 2010.

[18] UNHCR, *Reproductive Health - Emergency Obstetric Care (EmOC) Standard*, The UN Refiguee Agency Public Health section, 2018, https://emergency.unhcr.org.

[19] A. Henok, "Knowledge towards Birth Preparedness and Complication Readiness among Mothers Who Attend Antenatal Care at Mizan-Aman General Hospital, South West Ethiopia," *Journal of Health, Medicine and Nursing*, vol. 15, 2015.

[20] M. Kyei-Onanjiri, M. Carolan-Olah, J. K. Awoonor-Williams, and T. V. McCann, "Review of emergency obstetric care interventions in health facilities in the Upper East Region of Ghana: A questionnaire survey," *BMC Health Services Research*, vol. 18, no. 1, 2018.

[21] T. Bhandari and G. Dangal, "Emergency Obstetric Care: Strategy for Reducing Maternal Mortality in Developing Countries," *Nepal Journal of Obstetrics & Gynaecology*, vol. 9, no. 1, pp. 8–16, 2014.

[22] A. Austin, H. Gulema, M. Belizan et al., "Barriers to providing quality emergency obstetric care in addis ababa, ethiopia: healthcare providers' perspectives on training, referrals and supervision, a mixed methods study," *BMC Pregnancy and Childbirth*, vol. 15, no. 1, article no. 74, Article ID 15034835, 2015.

[23] S. Tiku, "Awareness on Birth Preparedness and Complication Readiness Among Antenatal Care Clients in Federal Police Referral Hospital Addis Ababa, Ethiopia," *American Journal of Health Research*, vol. 3, no. 6, p. 362, 2015.

[24] F. August, A. B. Pembe, E. Kayombo, C. Mbekenga, P. Axemo, and E. Darj, "Birth preparedness and complication readiness- a qualitative study among community members in rural Tanzania," *Global Health Action*, vol. 8, no. 1, Article ID 26922, 2015.

[25] S. Agarwal, V. Sethi, K. Srivastava, P. K. Jha, and A. H. Baqui, "Birth preparedness and complication readiness among slum women in Indore city, India," *Journal of Health, Population and Nutrition*, vol. 28, no. 4, pp. 383–391, 2010.

[26] S. Suglo, *Birth Preparedness Among Pregnant Women Attending Antenatal Clinic At Tamale Teaching Hospital*, UCC, Library, 2016.

[27] D. Prativa and S. Mangala, "Knowledge on birth preparedness and complication readiness in Eastern Region of Nepal," *International Journal of Nursing and Midwifery*, vol. 8, no. 10, pp. 75–80, 2016.

[28] B. D. Isaac, B. D. Dego, and Z. R. Baruch, "Birth preparation practices and recognition of danger signs among pregnant women in Ethiopia," *African Journal of Nursing and Midwifery*, vol. 4, no. 2, pp. 603–612, 2016.

[29] D. B. Endeshaw, L. D. Gezie, and H. Y. Yeshita, "Birth preparedness and complication readiness among pregnant women in Tehulederie district, Northeast Ethiopia: A community-based cross-sectional study," *BMC Nursing*, vol. 17, no. 1, 2018.

[30] A. Tafa, D. Hailu, J. Ebrahim, M. Gebrie, and N. Wakgari, "Birth Preparedness and Complication Readiness Plan among Antenatal Care Attendants in Kofale District, South East Ethiopia: A Cross Sectional Survey," *Diversity & Equality in Health and Care*, vol. 15, no. 1, pp. 23–29, 2018.

[31] Z. G. Abate, M. Kote, M. G. Abate, and M. Tilahun, "Birth Preparedness Among Antenatal Clients in Rurar Health Centers in Kucha Woreda, Gamo-Gofa Zone, Southern Ethiopia," *Journal of Health, Medicine and Nursing*, vol. 35, 2017.

[32] J. E. Ekabua, K. J. Ekabua, P. Odusolu et al., "Awareness of Birth Preparedness and Complication Readiness in Southeastern Nigeria," *International Scholarly Research Network*, vol. 2011, Article ID 560641, 6 pages, 2011.

[33] B. Oni, O. Odukoya, A. Okunowo, O. Ojo, and Y. Abatan, "A comparative assessment of the awareness of danger signs and practice of birth preparedness and complication readiness among pregnant women attending rural and urban general hospitals in Lagos State," *Sahel Medical Journal*, vol. 19, no. 4, p. 206, 2016.

[34] K. E. Kasmai, O. M. Akpa, and O. Olayemi, "Birth Preparedness and Complication Readiness Among Pokot Nomadic Pastoralists' Pregnant Women in East Pokot District, Midwest- Kenya," *American Journal of Biomedical and Life Sciences*, vol. 6, no. 1, pp. 17–23, 2018.

[35] E. A. Abioye Kuteyi, J. O. Kuku ICL, J. A. Ogundipe, T. Mogbeyteren, and M. A. Banjo, "Birth Preparedness and Complication Readiness of Pregnant Women Attending the Three Levels of Health Facilities in Ife Central Local Government, Nigeria," *Journal of Community Medicine and Primary Health Care*, vol. 23, 2011.

[36] E. G. Makunyi, *Birth Preparedness Among Women In Tharaka Nithi County, Kenya*, 2014.

[37] K. A. Nimavat, A. D. Mangal, S. V. Unadkat, and S. Yadav, "A study of birth preparedness of women in Jamnagar district, Gujarat, India," *International Journal of Community Medicine and Public Health*, vol. 3, no. 9, pp. 2403–2408, 2016.

[38] D. K. Mukhopadhyay, S. Mukhopadhyay, S. Bhattacharjee, S. Nayak, A. K. Biswas, and A. B. Biswas, *Status of Birth Preparedness and Complication Readiness in Uttar Dinajpur District, West Bengal*, 2018.

[39] M. Moinuddin, A. Christou, D. M. E. Hoque et al., "Birth preparedness and complication readiness (BPCR) among pregnant women in hard-to-reach areas in Bangladesh," *PLoS ONE*, vol. 12, no. 12, 2017.

[40] J. K. Kabakyenga, P.-O. Östergren, E. Turyakira, and K. O. Pettersson, "Knowledge of obstetric danger signs and birth preparedness practices among women in rural Uganda," *Reproductive Health*, vol. 8, article 33, 2011.

[41] M. Gebre, A. Gebremariam, and T. A. Abebe, "Birth preparedness and complication readiness among pregnant women in Duguna Fango District, Wolayta Zone, Ethiopia," *PLoS ONE*, vol. 10, no. 9, 2015.

[42] G. T. Debelew, M. F. Afework, and A. W. Yalew, "Factors affecting birth preparedness and complication readiness in Jimma Zone, Southwest Ethiopia: a multilevel analysis," *The Pan African Medical Journal*, vol. 19, article 272, 2014.

[43] E. Andarge, A. Nigussie, and M. Wondafrash, "Factors associated with birth preparedness and complication readiness in Southern Ethiopia: a community based cross-sectional study," *BMC Pregnancy and Childbirth*, vol. 17, no. 1, p. 412, 2017.

[44] M. Hailu, A. Gebremariam, F. Alemseged, and K. Deribe, "Birth preparedness and complication readiness among pregnant women in Southern Ethiopia," *PLoS ONE*, vol. 6, no. 6, Article ID e21432, 2011.

[45] A. Hailemariam, *Assessment of Magnitude and Factors Associated with BirthPreparedness and Complication Readiness among Pregnant WomenAttending Antenatal Care Services at Public Health Facilities in Debrebirhan Town. (USA)*, vol. 16, 2015.

[46] P. K. Affipunguh and A. S. Laar, "Assessment of knowledge and practice towards birth preparedness and complication readiness among women in Northern Ghana: a cross-sectional study," *International Journal of Scientific Reports*, vol. 2, no. 6, p. 121, 2016.

[47] D. Bintabara, M. A. Mohamed, J. Mghamba, P. Wasswa, and R. N. Mpembeni, "Birth preparedness and complication readiness among recently delivered women in chamwino district, central Tanzania: a cross sectional study," *Reproductive Health*, vol. 12, no. 1, 2015.

[48] E. A. Tobin, A. N. Ofili, N. Enebeli, and O. Enueze, "Assessment of birth preparedness and complication readiness among pregnant women attending Primary Health Care Centres in Edo State, Nigeria," *Annals of Nigerian Medicine*, vol. 8, no. 2, 2018.

[49] R. Karkee, A. H. Lee, and C. W. Binns, "Birth preparedness and skilled attendance at birth in nepal: Implications for achieving millennium development goal 5," *Midwifery*, vol. 29, no. 10, pp. 1206–1210, 2013.

[50] M. Ohamaeme, J. Egwurugwu, E. Dike, G. Eberendu, and B. Chinko, "Assessment of Birth Preparedness and Complication Readiness (BP/CR) among Pregnant Women in Orlu Local Government Area of Imo State, Nigeria," *Journal of Advances in Medicine and Medical Research*, vol. 24, no. 3, pp. 1–12, 2017.

[51] C. Joyce, O. Grace, and M. Waithira, "Factors Affecting Birth Preparedness among Pregnant Women Attending Public Antenatal Clinics in Migori County, Kenya," *Biomedical Journal of Scientific & Technical Research*, vol. 3, no. 4, 2018.

[52] K. O. Phanice, A. F. Yaw, and O. Peter, "Birth Preparedness and Complication Readiness among Women Attending Antenatal Care Clinic in Health Facilities within Bureti Sub County of Kericho County, Kenya," *American Journal of Medicine and Medical Sciences*, vol. 6, no. 4, pp. 123–128, 2016.

[53] S. Bekele and T. Alemayehu, "Knowledge, Attitude and Practice on Birth Preparedness and Complication Readiness Among Pregnant Women Attending Antenatal Care at Chiro Zonal Hospital Eastern Ethiopia," *Ethiopian Journal of Reproductive Health (EJRH)*, vol. 10, 2018.

[54] U. Umeh, C. Onwasigwe, E. Adinma, and C. Nnebue, "Knowledge of Birth Preparedness and Complications Readiness: An Urban- Rural Comparison of Maternal and Child Health Clinic Attendees in Anambra State, Nigeria," *Asian Journal of Medicine and Health*, vol. 11, no. 2, pp. 1–10, 2018.

[55] V. Kamineni, A. Murki, and V. Kota, "Birth preparedness and complication readiness in pregnant women attending urban tertiary care hospital," *Journal of Family Medicine and Primary Care*, vol. 6, no. 2, pp. 297–300, 2017.

[56] M. R. Chavan and M. S. Upendra, "To Assess the Knowledge and Attitude of the AntenatalMothers Towards Self-Preparedness During Pregnancy and Delivery in Selected Areas of Pune City with a Viewto Develop Self Instructional Module," *Scintific Research*, vol. 5, no. 1, pp. 2277–8179, 2016.

[57] D. Markos and D. Bogale, "Birth preparedness and complication readiness among women of child bearing age group in Goba woreda, Oromia region, Ethiopia," *BMC Pregnancy and Childbirth*, vol. 14, no. 1, p. 282, 2014.

[58] Y. Bitew, W. Awoke, and S. Chekol, "Birth Preparedness and Complication Readiness Practice and Associated Factors among Pregnant Women, Northwest Ethiopia," *International Scholarly Research Notices*, vol. 2016, Article ID 8727365, 8 pages, 2016.

[59] P. K. Hari, L. B. K. NirmalaNeupane, and A. Ajaya, "Birth preparedness and complications readiness among women in LekhnathMuniciaplity, Nepal," *Global Journal of Medicine and Public Health*, vol. 4, no. 3, 2015.

[60] J. C. Joshua Sumankuuro and W. Shaoyu, "Factors influencing knowledge and practice of birth preparedness andcomplication readiness in sub-saharan Africa: a narrativereview of cross-sectional studies," *International Journal Of Community Medicine And Public Health*, vol. 3, no. 12, pp. 3297–3307, 2016.

7

The Prevalence of Traditional Malpractice during Pregnancy, Child Birth and Postnatal Period among Women of Childbearing Age in Meshenti Town, 2016

Haileyesus Gedamu, Adane Tsegaw, and Etsubdink Debebe

School of Nursing, Bahir Dar University, Bahir Dar, Ethiopia

Correspondence should be addressed to Etsubdink Debebe; nonina7@yahoo.com

Academic Editor: Hind A. Beydoun

Background. Cultural practices, beliefs, and taboos are often implicated in determining the care received by mothers during pregnancy and child birth which is an important determinant of maternal mortality. *Objective.* To assess prevalence of cultural malpractice during pregnancy, child birth, and postnatal period among women of childbearing age in Meshenti town, Amhara region, northwest Ethiopia, in 2016. *Methods.* Community based cross-sectional study was conducted among women of reproductive age group interviewed during the study period from May 10 to June 17, 2016. Total sample size was 318 women of reproductive age group. Systematic sampling technique was conducted. *Result.* Overall, 50.9% of the respondents had cultural malpractices during their pregnancy. Out of 318 women, 62 (19.5%) practiced nutrition taboo, 78 (24.5%) practiced abdominal massage, 87 (29.7%) delivered their babies at home, 96 (32.8%) avoided colostrums, 132 (45.2%) washed their baby before 24 hr after delivery, and 6 (6.9%) cut the cord by unclean blade. *Conclusion and Recommendation.* The findings of this study show that different traditional malpractice during perinatal period is still persisting in spite of modern developments in the world. Health education and promoting formal female education are important to decrease or avoid these cultural malpractices.

1. Introduction

Tradition represents the sum total of all behaviors that are learned, shared by a group of people, and transmitted from generation to generation. It includes language, religion, types of food eaten and methods of their preparation, childrearing practices, and all other values that hold people together and give them a sense of identity and distinguish them from other groups [1, 2].

Women all over the world are confronted with many difficult choices during pregnancy and child birth. Cultural practices, beliefs, and taboos are often implicated in determining the care received by mothers during pregnancy and child birth which is an important determinant of maternal mortality. Every day, at least 800 women die worldwide from the complications of pregnancy and child birth. These deaths are mainly due to obstetric problem which easily could be prevented if the mothers get the appropriate care they deserve during their pregnancy, delivery, and postnatal period [3, 4].

It has been recognized that violence and trauma, malpractice during pregnancy and childbirth, low social status, gender discrimination, and lack of awareness in ANC follow-up at nearby health facilities are direct and indirect medical causes of maternal mortality [5–7]. Harmful traditional practices that affect children and women are female genital mutilation, milk teeth extraction, food taboo, uvula cutting, forbidding food and fluids during diarrhea, keeping babies from exposure to sun, and feeding newborn babies with fresh butter [8, 9]. In Ethiopia, the great majorities of women deliver at home (90%) and follow the cultural birth customs. These create problems for several years associated with harmful cultural practices at each individual community and home during delivery [10, 11].

United Nations (UN) agencies and human right bodies started addressing harmful traditional practice in the early 1990s but there was little progress. There are now a number of important international instruments endorsed by most of the governments and could serve as a basis for a struggle against harmful traditional practice [12, 13]. In addition to deep-rooted beliefs, customs, and rational attitudes, lack of knowledge and being unaware of the effects of the practices help to maintain these problems. Sometimes a harmful practice is so deeply rooted that it seems impossible to change [14, 15].

In the world, there are many traditional malpractices during pregnancy, labor, and postnatal period. In Turkey and Iran, women use traditional practices to reduce engorgement of the breast and to increase the amount of breast milk [16–18].

In Guatemala, Guatemalan women believe speedy delivery can be induced by drinking a liquid created by boiling a purple onion in beer and in Niger, Muslim tradition allows only a woman's husband to touch her genitals, so midwives in this African nation facilitate labor by offering the mom-to-be herbal drinks and sprinkling herbs over her abdomen. Foods that are good sources of energy and protein are not allowed to be consumed by pregnant women for reasons such as difficult and prolonged labor due to fears of a large baby. Similarly, sources of vitamins and minerals are restricted during pregnancy mainly due to the fear of offensive discharges during delivery and skin diseases on the body. Studies conducted in central, eastern, and southern parts of Ethiopia have reported that food items that are white in color such as milk, fatty meat, porridge, potato, banana, clean vegetables, colostrums, and fruits are prohibited to be consumed by pregnant/lactating women and children [10, 19–21].

Another research done in Bangladesh on usage of colostrum and duration to initiate breastfeeding revealed that 90% of the mothers reported feeding their newborn colostrum. 59% of mothers initiated breastfeeding within 4 hours and 88% within 12 hours of parturition [22].

2. Methods and Materials

2.1. Study Area. The study was conducted in Meshenti town, west Gojjam zone, Amhara region, northwest Ethiopia. Meshenti was one of the towns found around Bahir Dar which has a total population of 6006, among those 2697 were males and 3309 were females. In addition, it has 1397 households and a total of reproductive age women (15–49 years) of 1418. The town has one health center and it has 1 Kebele; it is 555 km away from Addis Ababa and 12 km away from Bahir Dar.

Many harmful traditional practices have been performed in the study area. Therefore, this investigation revealed the evidence based occurrence of traditional malpractice during pregnancy, child birth, and postnatal period among women of child bearing age.

2.2. Study Design and Period. The community based cross-sectional study design was conducted from June 10 to June 17, 2016.

2.3. Source Population. The source population was all women of reproductive age group (15–49 years).

2.4. Study Population. The study population was all women in reproductive age (15–49 years) who experienced at least one pregnancy.

2.5. Inclusion and Exclusion Criteria

2.5.1. Inclusion. All reproductive age women who experience at least one pregnancy were included.

2.5.2. Exclusion. Women who had severe medical and mental illness and could not communicate verbally during data collection were excluded.

2.6. Sample Size Determination and Sampling Technique

2.6.1. Sample Size Determination. The sample size was calculated by using the following single population proportion formula:

$$n = (z)^2 \times \frac{p(1-p)}{w^2}, \quad (1)$$

where z^2 is the confidence limit of the study (95%), p is the proportion of study population (38.3%), w is margin of error or desired precision (5% or 0.05), and n is total sample size.

Let us take $p = 38.3\%$ which is prevalence rate for home delivery which is most common traditional malpractice during delivery at Limmu Genet town, Oromia region, southwest Ethiopia [23].

The required sample size for this study "n" at confidence interval of 95% and marginal error of 5% will be determined by using population proportion formula: $n = (1.96)^2 0.383(1-0.383)/(0.05)^2 = 364$. With correction formula $n/1 + n/N$ (where n is the sample size we calculate as 364 and N is total population), our sample size becomes 289 and then, with 10% nonresponse rate, a total of 318 study participants were recruited.

2.6.2. Sampling Technique and Procedure. The sampling technique was systematic random sampling which was conducted by considering list of households. The sampling interval was calculated using $k = N/n$ (1397/318) = 4th, where k is sampling interval, N is number of households in Meshenti town, and n is sampling size.

The first sample was selected by using lottery method among the first four households and then assessed every 4th house. In households with no eligible person, we went to the next house. But for households with more than one eligible individual, one of the individuals was selected randomly.

2.7. Data Collection. Data was collected by using structured questionnaire by face-to-face interview. The questionnaire includes sociodemographic characteristics, reproductive health part, and traditional malpractice. Questionnaire that addressed the objective of the study was gathered and adapted. The questionnaire was prepared in English and translated to Amharic version to facilitate the understanding. Data collection was carried out by five data collectors from preparatory students trained on the study and data collection.

2.8. Data Quality Assurance. Pretest of questionnaires was done one week before the actual survey and it was carried out with similar study population in Merawi town for 1 day on 5% of sample size and the necessary modification was made before being applied on study subjects. The data was collected carefully by the trained data collector and principal investigators to get the reliable and necessary information according to the aim of the study. The principal investigator made an ongoing checkup each day during the data collection to ensure the quality of data by checking filled questionnaires for their completeness and internal consistency. The quality of data collection process was monitored by giving a clear attention to the data. All the collected data was checked and rechecked and we made the necessary correction each day; when there were difficulties occurring during the data collection, explanation and discussion with the respondents were done and unclear questions were explained briefly by using respondent native language.

2.9. Data Processing and Analysis. The collected data was entered and analyzed by using SPSS version 20. Calculation was calculated by using a calculator and Microsoft Excel and statistical analysis was done by principal investigator. Finally description, tables, graphs, and charts were used to present the finding.

3. Ethical Consideration

Ethical clearance was obtained from Bahir Dar University CMHS Ethical Review Board before data collection. Written and oral consent were obtained from the study population during data collection. The right was given for the study population to refuse or stop or withdraw at any time of data collection. The confidentiality of the respondents was ensured, where any person name did not appear on research documents and respondents were informed about the aim of the study.

4. Result

4.1. Sociodemographic Characteristics. A total of 318 participants were included in the study and response rate was 100%. Regarding the sociodemographic characteristics of the respondents, 100 (31.4%) were in the age group of 25–29. The majority of them were orthodox (252) (79.2%) and Amhara (314) (98.7%) by religion and ethnicity, respectively. Out of 318, 260 (81.8%) were married and 137 (41.1) were illiterate and 70 (22%) completed grades 1–8. Concerning occupation, 211 (66.4%) were housewives (Table 1).

4.2. Traditional Malpractices during Pregnancy. Generally in Meshenti town, 50.9% of pregnant women are involved in traditional malpractice during their pregnancy. Out of these, 62 (19.5%) had nutritional taboo, 139 (43.7%) used the mother's drink "telba" during their pregnancy, and 48 (15.1%) and 43 (13.5%) practiced abdominal massage and drank "kosso," respectively (Table 2).

4.3. Traditional Malpractices during Child Birth. Generally in Meshenti town, 37.9% of mothers are involved in traditional malpractice during their child birth. From these, 6.3% of the mothers have traditional malpractice like abdominal massage and uterine massage and the other 29.7% have home delivery.

Table 1: Sociodemographic characteristics of respondents among women of childbearing age in Meshenti town, Bahir Dar Zuria woreda, Amhara region, June 2016.

Characteristics	Category	Frequency	Percent (%)
Age	15–19	15	4.7
	20–24	89	28.0
	25–29	100	31.4
	30–34	50	15.7
	35–39	34	10.7
	40–44	14	4.4
	45–49	16	5.0
	Total	*318*	*100.0*
Religion	Orthodox	252	79.2
	Muslim	64	20.1
	Protestant	2	.6
	Total	*318*	*100.0*
Ethnicity	Amhara	314	98.7
	Oromo	2	.6
	Tigre	2	.6
	Total	*318*	*100.0*
Educational status	Have no formal education	172	44.1
	G 1–8	70	22.0
	G 9–12	53	16.7
	12+	23	7.2
	Total	*318*	*100.0*
Marital status	Married	260	81.8
	Single	18	5.7
	Divorced	24	7.5
	Widowed	16	5.0
	Total	*318*	*100.0*
Occupational status	Housewife	211	66.4
	Employee	25	7.9
	Merchant	45	14.2
	Student	6	1.9
	Other	31	9.7
	Total	*318*	*100.0*

Out of 87 (29.7%) mothers who delivered their last child at home, most of them were assisted by their family (37) (42.5%), untrained traditional birth attendant (UTTBA) (29) (33.3%), neighbors (12) (13.8%), and trained traditional birth attendant (TTBA) (9) (10.3). Among 87 (29.7%) home deliveries, the cord was cut by using unboiled new blade (66) (75.9%), boiled new blade (14) (16.1%), unboiled blade used before (6) (6.9%), and boiled blade used before (1) (1.1%). From the 87 home deliveries, 84 of them had their umbilical cord tied using boiled thread (71) (84.5%), unboiled thread (10) (11.9%), and other material (3) (3.6%) (Table 3).

For home-delivery mothers, the majority (43%) of them were assisted by their family whereas 10% of them were assisted by traditional trained birth attendants (Figure 1).

TABLE 2: Traditional malpractice during pregnancy in Meshenti town, 2016.

Variables	Frequency	Percent (%)
Nutritional taboos	62	19.5
Abdominal massage	48	15.1
Drinking telba	139	43.7
Drinking kosso	43	13.5
Abdominal massage and drinking telba	20	6.3
Abdominal massage and drinking kosso	10	3.1
Drinking telba and drinking kosso	1	.3
Other	6	1.9
I don't know	51	16

TABLE 3: Traditional malpractice during delivery in Meshenti town, 2016.

Variables	Frequency	Percent (%)
Traditional malpractice		
Abdominal massage		
Yes	8	2.73
No	0	0
Uterine massage		
Yes	7	2.39
No	0	0
Abdominal and uterine massage		
Yes	5	1.7
No	0	0
Total	*20*	*6.82*
Place of delivery		
Home	87	29.7
Health facility	206	70.3
Total	*293*	*100*
Method used to expel placenta		
Spontaneously	76	87.4
Uterine massage	11	12.6
Total	*87*	*100*
Instrument used to cut cord		
Boiled new blade	14	16.1
Unboiled new blade	66	75.9
Unclean blade used before	6	6.9
Boiled blade used before	1	1.1
Total	*87*	*100*
Umbilical cord tied		
Yes	84	96.6
No	3	3.4
Total	*87*	*100*
Material used to tie umbilical cord		
Boiled thread	71	84.5
Unboiled thread	10	11.9
Other	3	3.6
Total	*84*	*100*

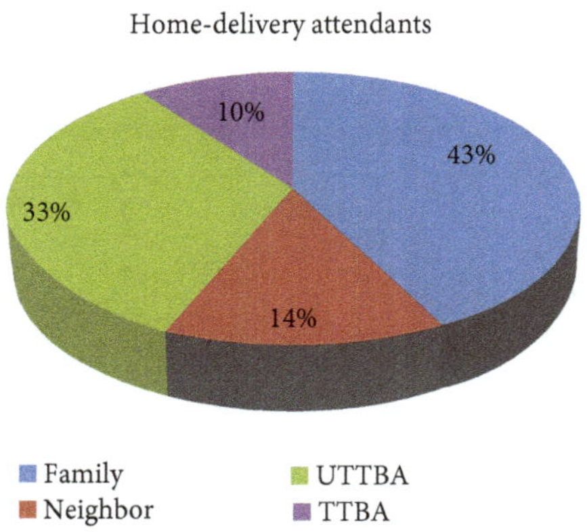

Figure 1: Distribution of birth attendants for women who deliver at home in Meshenti town, northwest Ethiopia, Amhara region, June 2016.

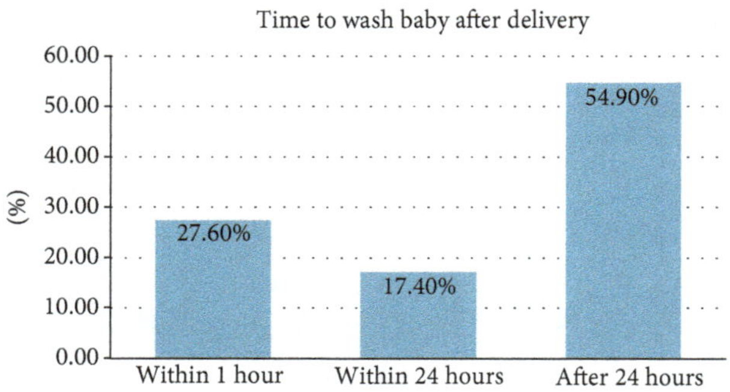

Figure 2: Time period of washing babies after delivery among reproductive aged women in Meshenti town, west Gojjam, northwest Ethiopia, June 2016.

Table 4: Traditional malpractice during postnatal period in Meshenti town, 2016.

Variables	Frequency	Percent (%)
What was applied on the stump of umbilicus		
Nothing	174	54.4
Cow dung	4	1.4
Butter	98	30.4
Other	17	5.8
Total	*293*	*100*
What was given to the child immediately after delivery		
Butter	60	20.5
Cow milk	5	1.7
Water	7	2.4
Nothing	210	71.7
Other	11	3.8
Total	*293*	*100*
Time to start breastfeeding		
Within 1 hour	219	74.7
Within 24 hours	51	17.4
After 24 hours	23	7.8
Total	*293*	*100*
Avoiding colostrum		
Yes	197	67.2
No	96	32.8
Total	*293*	*100*

4.4. Traditional Malpractices during Postnatal Period. Generally in Meshenti town, 76.1% of the mothers are involved in traditional malpractice during their postnatal period. From these 293 mothers, 96 (32.8%) mothers avoided colostrum and 98 (30.4%) of the mothers applied butter on their child umbilicus after delivery. some of the respondents started breastfeeding within 24 hr and 23 (7.8%) after 24 hr. On the other hand, 81 (27.6%) mothers washed their babies immediately after delivery (Table 4).

The majority of babies delivered at Meshenti town had their bodies washed after 24 hrs (Figure 2).

5. Discussion

This community based study has attempted to assess the prevalence of traditional malpractices during pregnancy, delivery, and postnatal period in Meshenti town, west Gojjam zone, Amhara region, northwest Ethiopia. The result of the study revealed that, from the total of 318 respondents, 100 (31.4%) of the women were of the age range of 25–29 years and majority were married and illiterate: 260 (81.8%) and 137 (43.1%), respectively. This result was in line with a research done at north Arbaminch, south Ethiopia, where 36% of the women were aged 25–29 and 90.8% and 53.6% were married and illiterate, respectively [23].

Our study reveals that the prevalence of nutritional taboo was 19.5%. This result was slightly similar to a study conducted in Lemmu genet town with prevalence of 19.1% [24]. The result was also lower than that of a study conducted in Shashemene with the prevalence of 49.8% [21]. The possible reason for the variation of the results was different characteristics in study population. The food items that are avoided during pregnancy, based on our research, are vegetables (6 times), meat (2 times), paper (34 times), "genfo" (9 times), sugar cane (16 times), and "ergo" (7 times); a research done in Shashemene shows vegetables (17 times) and meat (63 times) which is very high [21]. The major reasons for avoiding these food items during pregnancy were that the food may plaster the fetal head or make the baby fat and difficult to deliver.

As Guatemala women believe that drinking liquid (which is prepared by boiling purple onion in beer) is very helpful to induce labor, our research also shows that Meshenti women drink telba to facilitate their labor [19].

Our study revealed that the prevalence of home delivery was 29.7% which was lower than that of the study conducted in Lemmu genet town, Oromia region, Jimma zone, 38.3% [24]; however, our study was comparable with a study conducted in south Gondar zone, Debretabor town, where the prevalence was 29.6% [25]. Out of 29.7% of the home delivered babies, most of them were attended by family (42.5%) and untrained traditional birth attendants (33.3%) which is higher and lower than the study conducted in Debretabor town, south Gondar zone, 13%, and south Arbaminch, north Ethiopia, 79.4%, respectively [23, 25].

This investigation also revealed that prevalence of avoiding colostrum was 32.8% which was lower than study conducted in Bangladesh with the prevalence of 41% [22]; and the result was lower than the study conducted in Raya Kobo district, northeastern Ethiopia, with the prevalence of 13.5% [26]. In this study, 132 (45%) of the mothers washed their babies before 24 hours after delivery that is higher than the research done at Lemmu genet town, Oromia region, Jimma zone, which was 28.4% [24]. This may cause negative impact on the newborn baby like hypothermia.

About 6.9% of respondents used unsterile material to cut the umbilical cord during home delivery which was higher than the study conducted in South Gondar zone, Debretabor town, which was 0.6% [25].

A study conducted at Debretabor governmental health institution shows that 213 (60%) have started breastfeeding within one hour, 109 (30.7%) within 24 hr, and 33 (9.3%) after 24 hours (d). But our study revealed that 219 (74.7%) have started breastfeeding within one hour, 51 (17.4%) within 24 hr, and 23 (7.8%) after 24 hours [25].

Based on our study, 24.5% (78) of the mothers had abdominal massage during pregnancy which was relatively similar to a research done at Lemmu genet town, Oromia region, Jimma zone, with prevalence of 22% [24] and higher when compared to a research done at Debretabor governmental health institution, south Gondar zone, Debretabor town, 12.1% [25]. The possible reason to do such a practice is to avoid striae and to relieve back pain that occurred during pregnancy.

6. Conclusion

The prevalence of cultural malpractice in the study area was found to be high. Therefore, health education focusing on problems of cultural malpractice is recommended to reduce or avoid the consequences of the malpractice.

Authors' Contributions

All authors participated in proposal conception and designing the proposal, data collection, and analysis and wrote the manuscript. Finally, the paper was approved by all authors.

Acknowledgments

The authors would like to express their deepest and heartfelt appreciation to Bahir Dar University for providing the chance of carrying out this project. They also thank the Meshenti town administration officer and community for their cooperativeness and their valuable information to this work. Last but not least, they would like to express their heartfelt thanks to all data collectors and supervisor for their valuable contribution.

References

[1] D. Asefa, E. Wassie, M. Getahun, M. Berehaneselassie, and A. Melaku, *Harm Full Traditional Practices for the Ethiopian Health Center Team*, Ethiopian public health training initiative (EPHTI) manual, Awasa College, 2005, Harm full traditional practices for the Ethiopian health center team. Ethiopian public health training initiative (EPHTI) manual. Awasa College.

[2] CSA, *Ethiopia Demographic and Health Survey*, Central statistical authority (CSA), Addis Ababa, Ethiopia, 2005.

[3] UNCHR, *Harmful Traditional Practices Affecting the Health of Women and Children*, Fact Sheet No. 23, UN Office of the High Commissioner for Human Rights (UNCHR), Geneva, Switzerland, 2006.

[4] WHO, *Maternal Mortality*, World health organization (WHO) Fact sheet, Geneva, Switzerland, 2014.

[5] J. Raelori, "Cultural child birth practice's, believes & tradition in Libya, 2009".

[6] Adolescent pregnancy cultural complex issue, 2008.

[7] P. Otoo, H. Habib, and A. Ankomah, "Food prohibitions and other traditional practices in pregnancy: a qualitative study in western region of ghana," *Advances in Reproductive Sciences*, vol. 3, no. 3, pp. 41–49, 2015.

[8] MHRC, *Cultural Practices and their impact on the enjoyment of human rights, Particularly the Rights of Women and Children in Malawi*, Malawi Human Rights Commission (MHRC), 2005.

[9] A. Dawit, W. Eshetu, G. Masresha, B. Misganaw, and M. Atsinaf, *Harmful Traditional Practices: Module for Ethiopian Health Center Team*, Ethiopian Public Health Training Institute, Awassa College, 2004, Harmful Traditional Practices: Module for Ethiopian Health Center Team , Ethiopian Public Health Training Institute, Awassa College.

[10] M. Neguse, D. Hailemariam, and G. Metike, "Assessment of safe delivery services utilization among WCBA North Gondar zone, North West Ethiopia," *Ethio journal health*, vol. 18, no. 3, pp. 145–152, 2004.

[11] EGLDAM, *Follow up National Survey on Harmful Traditional Practices in Ethiopia*, 2008.

[12] M. Zuberi, ssessment of violence against children in the eastern and southern Africa region: Results of initial desk review for the UN secretary general's study on violence against children, 2006.

[13] G. D. Alene and M. Edris, "Knowledge, attitudes and practices involved in harmful health behavior in Dembia district, Northwest Ethiopia," *Ethiopian Journal of Health Development*, vol. 16, no. 2, pp. 199–207, 2002.

[14] F. Worku and S. Gebresilassie, *Reproductive Health for Health Science Students*, Ethiopian Public Health Training Institute, University of Gondar, 2008, Reproductive Health for Health Science Students , Ethiopian Public Health Training Institute, University of Gondar.

[15] WHO, *WHO Regional Health Forum South-East Asia Region*, vol. 6, World health organization (WHO), 2008.

[16] https://www.ncbi.nlm.nih.gov/pubmed/8693724.

[17] A. Suheyla and V. Katabi, "Comparison of Cultural Practices Used in Pregnancy Postpartum Periods among Women in Turkey & Iran," 2008.

[18] A. McKinley, "Traditions from around the world; from conception to birth and beyond, ancient traditions and cultural beliefs have always shaped the art of motherhood," 2010, https://www.pnmag.com.

[19] Ethiopian public health training initiative (EPHTI), *Pediatrics & Child Health Lecture Note for Health Science Students*, Jimma University, 2003.

[20] N. Zepro, "Food taboos and misconceptions among pregnant women of shashemene district, ethiopia," *Science Journal of Public Health*, vol. 3, no. 3, pp. 410–416, 2015.

[21] D. J. Holman and M. A. Grimes, "Colostrum feeding behaviour and initiation of breast-feeding in rural Bangladesh," *Journal of Biosocial Science*, vol. 33, no. 1, pp. 139–154, 2001.

[22] G. Ayele, "Prevalence and associated factors of home delivery in arbaminch zuria district, southern ethiopia: community based cross sectional study," *Science Journal of Public Health*, vol. 3, no. 1, p. 6, 2015.

[23] T. Tola and A. Tadesse, "Cultural malpractices during pregnancy, child birth and postnatal period among women of child bearing age in limmu genet town, southwest Ethiopia," *Science Journal of Public Health*, vol. 3, no. 5, 2015.

[24] K. Zenebe, H. Alem, A. Merga, G. Abate, and H. Taha, "prevalence of cultural malpractice and associated factors among women attending mch clinic at debretabor governmental health institution south gondar, amhara region, north west Ethiopia," *Gyneco and Obstet*, vol. 6, no. 10, 2015.

[25] M. Legesse, M. Demena, F. Mesfin, and D. Haile, "Factors associated with colostrum avoidance among mothers of children aged less than 24 Months in Raya Kobo district, North-eastern Ethiopia: Community-based cross-sectional study," *Journal of Tropical Pediatrics*, vol. 61, no. 5, Article ID fmv039, pp. 357–363, 2015.

[26] T. Rowen, N. Prata, and P. Passano, "Evaluation of a traditional birth attendant training programme in Bangladesh," *Midwifery*, vol. 27, no. 2, pp. 229–236, 2011.

8

Factors Associated with Modern Contraceptive Use among Married Women Attending Comprehensive Health Centers (CHCs) in Kandahar, Afghanistan

Mirwais Saheem,[1] Muhammad Haroon Stanikzai,[2] Najeeb Rahimy,[3] Najibullah Fazli,[4] Ghulam Mohydin Mudasir,[3] and Hadia Sayam[5]

[1]*Master of Public Health Program, Faculty of Medicine, Kandahar University, Kandahar, Afghanistan*
[2]*Public Health Department, Faculty of Medicine, Kandahar University, Kandahar, Afghanistan*
[3]*Para Clinic Department, Faculty of Medicine, Kandahar University, Kandahar, Afghanistan*
[4]*Internal Medicine Department, Faculty of Medicine, Kandahar University, Kandahar, Afghanistan*
[5]*Para-clinic Department, Malalay Institute of Higher Education, Kandahar, Afghanistan*

Correspondence should be addressed to Muhammad Haroon Stanikzai; haroonstanikzai1@gmail.com

Academic Editor: Vikas Roy

Background. Modern contraceptives are highly effective and reliable methods of preventing unintended pregnancies and reducing maternal deaths. Only 22 percent of currently married women use modern methods of contraceptives in Afghanistan. This study assessed the factors associated with modern contraceptive use among married women attending comprehensive health centers (CHCs) in Kandahar Province. *Methods.* This was an institution-based cross-sectional study that included 325 married women who attended randomly selected comprehensive health clinics in Kandahar between September and October 2019. The total sample size was allocated proportionally to selected health clinics based on the recent 3-month average patients load. We used a consecutive sampling method to select study participants. Data were collected in a structured questionnaire, which included information on respondents' demographic, socioeconomic, reproductive, and contraceptive experiences. Data was analyzed using SPSS 21.00 statistical software. We used descriptive statistics such as tables and proportions to present data. Binary and multiple logistic regression analyses were carried out to determine factors associated with modern contraceptive use. *Results.* Out of 325 married women, 127 used modern contraceptives with a prevalence of 39.1% (95%CI = 33.7%–44.6%). The results indicated that the area of residence (AOR = 2.61, 95% CI 1.43-4.78) and ever use of contraceptives (AOR = 14.92, 95% CI 6.88-32.34) are associated with modern contraceptive use among married women attending comprehensive health centers in Kandahar. *Conclusion.* This study found that modern contraceptive use was higher than reported on the national level. The most persistent factors associated with modern contraceptive use in this study were urban residence and ever use of contraceptives. As a policy measure, family planning programs should be prompted to the rural residency in Kandahar Province.

1. Background

The Maternal Mortality Ratio (MMR) in Afghan women continues to be a major public health concern and remains the highest in the region. It is estimated to be 638 deaths per 100000 live births in 2017. Afghanistan also has one of the world's highest fertility rates (4.5), and related to this is the high infant mortality rate. In Afghanistan, only 22 percent of currently married women used any contraceptive method in 2017 [1]. Contraceptive use encompasses potential benefits in terms of maternal health, economic developments, educational advances, and women empowerment. Therefore, it is considered one of the most successful interventions of the last 50 years.

The World Health Organization (WHO) defines contraceptives as a principal strategy that promote maternal and child health through adequate birth spacing and avoiding unintended pregnancies [2, 3]. Globally, it is estimated that 62 percent of married women or in union women of reproductive age (15-49) were using some form of contraceptive and 58 percent a modern method of contraceptive in 2017. The proportion of contraceptive use varies significantly by region ranging from a low 36 percent in Africa to a high 75 percent in North America [4].

Family planning is a vital component of comprehensive health care. Unintended pregnancies and inadequate birth spacing have significant adverse health effects. It can deteriorate women's health and raise neonates' risk of adverse health outcomes [5, 6]. WHO and other international organizations recommend 2-3 years of birth spacing to reduce child mortality and also improve maternal health [2]. However, recent studies have suggested that 3-5 years of birth spacing might be more advantageous [4–6].

Contraceptive use is affected by many factors such as socioeconomic factors including women' age, education, residency, and occupation [7–10]; reproductive factors including marital age, gestational age, gravidity, parity, and birth spacing [8–10]; and other factors including awareness regarding contraceptives, poor access to healthcare, access to media, and various disease-related issues [7–9, 11–15]. Understanding the factors influencing contraceptive use among those married women who are at risk for unintended pregnancies is essential for the development of effective family planning programs. Given Afghanistan's high fertility and MMR background, this study was aimed at determining the proportion of modern contraceptive use and elucidating factors that are associated with modern contraceptive use among married women who visit comprehensive health centers (CHCs) in Kandahar Province.

2. Methods

2.1. Study Setting and Period. This institution-based study was conducted in four out of thirteen randomly selected CHCs in Kandahar Province between September and October 2019. The data was collected from the outpatient departments of two rural (Sarkari Bagh and Mandisar) and two urban (Balakarz and Dr. Amirjan) CHCs. These comprehensive health clinics provide a wide range of primary healthcare services including general medical consultation, vaccination, and family planning services.

2.2. Study Design and Population. This was an institutional-based cross-sectional study recruiting consecutive married women attending CHCs for routine healthcare.

For inclusion and exclusion criteria, we included consenting married women attending selected CHCs for healthcare services. Pregnant women, women aged 15-49 who were not married, and those who were unable to respond due to serious illness or unwillingness to participate in the study were excluded.

2.3. Sample Size and Sampling Procedures. A total of 325 married women were included in the study and estimated by a single population proportion formula ($n = Z^2 P(1 - P)/(d)^2$) with the assumptions of the proportion of modern contraceptive use in Kandahar ($P = 28.6\%$) [1], 95% confidence interval, the margin of error 5%, design effect of 1.0, and 10% nonresponse rate.

With regard to the sampling methods, four (2 rural and 2 urban) out of thirteen health clinics were randomly included in the study. The possible number of study participants between health clinics was allocated proportionally based on the recent 3-month average patient load. We consecutively included consenting married women who visited outpatient departments of selected CHCs for healthcare services on all working days during the study period.

2.4. Data Collection Methods. We used a structured and pretested questionnaire to collect the required information. The questionnaire was first prepared in English; later, it was translated into the local language (Pashtu) by experts and back to English to ensure that meanings of translation were not lost during translation. Three female clinical nurses collected data after being trained by the principal investigators. During training, the questionnaire was pretested on 20 participants in a different setting (Kandahar medical faculty teaching hospital) with the aim of estimating the time required to complete the questionnaire and revising the poorly structured questions. It was estimated that each interview would take up to 10-15 minutes. The data collection process was closely monitored to ensure that questionnaires were correctly filled.

2.5. Variables

2.5.1. Independent Variables. The variables were grouped into three categories: sociodemographic, socioeconomic, and reproductive variables.

2.5.2. Dependent Variables. The outcome variable in this study was the current use of a modern contraceptive method by married woman or her partner.

2.6. Operational Definitions

2.6.1. Contraceptive Use. "The percentage of women married aged 15 to 49 who are currently using, or whose husband is using, at least one modern method of contraception, regardless of the method used" [2, 3].

2.6.2. Modern Methods of Contraception. They included "female and male sterilization, oral hormonal pills, the intra-uterine device (IUD), the male condom, injectables, the implant (including Norplant), vaginal barrier methods, the female condom and emergency contraception" [2, 3].

2.7. Data Analysis. The collected data were entered and coded using Microsoft Excel (2019) and analyzed using IBM SPSS version 21 [16]. We carried out descriptive statistics for frequencies. Both bivariate and multivariate analyses were carried out to find an association between dependent and independent variables. All variables with a P value < 0.25 in bivariate analysis were included in the multivariate analysis to control the confounding effects. The P value of <0.05 was considered statistically significant.

TABLE 1: Sociodemographic characteristics of married women attending comprehensive health centers in Kandahar, Afghanistan, 2019 ($n = 325$).

Variable	Frequency	Percentage (%)
Age (completed years)		
1. <20	24	7.4
2. 20-25	118	36.3
3. 26-34	117	36.0
4. ≥35	66	20.3
Residence		
1. Urban	162	49.8
2. Rural	163	50.2
Women educational status		
1. No formal education	298	91.7
2. Basic	15	4.6
3. Secondary	7	2.2
4. High school graduate	5	1.5
Husband level of education		
1. No formal education	261	80.5
2. Basic	25	7.5
3. Secondary	13	4.0
4. High school graduate	26	8.0
Women occupation		
1. Formally employed	16	4.9
2. Unemployed/housewife	309	95.1
Husband occupation		
1. Formally employed	190	58.5
2. Unemployed	135	41.5
Number of household members		
1. 1 to 4	54	16.6
2. 5 or more	271	83.4
Household monthly income in Afghanis		
1. 5000-10000	70	21.5
2. >10000	215	66.2
3. Do not disclose	40	12.3

2.8. *Ethical Consideration.* The study was approved by the Ethical and Research committee, Faculty of Medicine, Kandahar University. Administrative approval was obtained from the Kandahar public health directorate. In addition, after explaining the purpose of the study, informed written consent was obtained from all study participants.

3. Results

3.1. *Sociodemographic Characteristics of the Study Participants.* A total of 325 married women were included in the analysis making a response rate of 93.3%. The mean age of the respondent was 28 (±7.1) with minimum and maximum values of 15 and 49, respectively. Of the total, 118 (36.3%) respondents were of the age range 20 to 25 years. With regard to educational status, 298 (91.7%) respondents and 261 (80.5%) of respondents' husbands had no formal education. Most of the respondents (309, 95.1%) did not have a formal occupation and were housewives. More than half (215, 66.2%) of households had more than 10000 (Afghani) monthly income. Table 1 shows the sociodemographic information of study participants.

TABLE 2: Reproductive variables of married women attending comprehensive health centers in Kandahar, Afghanistan, 2019 ($n = 325$).

Variable	Frequency	Percentage (%)
Age at marriage		
1. <18	165	50.8
2. ≥18	160	49.2
Years in marriage		
1. <5	74	22.8
2. ≥5	251	77.2
Number of living children		
1. No child	15	4.6
2. 1 to 4	166	51.1
3. 5 or more	144	44.3
Age at the 1st child		
1. <18	117	37.5
2. ≥18	193	62.5
Child mortality experience		
1. Yes	53	16.3
2. No	272	83.7
Antenatal care visits		
1. Yes	250	76.9
2. No	75	23.1
Postnatal care visits		
1. Yes	271	83.4
2. No	54	16.6

3.2. *Reproductive Characteristics of the Study Participants.* The mean age of respondents at marriage was 17.3 (±3.2). Overall, 165 (50.8%) participants out of 325 were married before the age of eighteen. Of the 310 respondents with children, 161 (51.1%) had one to four children. Of all the study participants, 250 (76.9%) and 271 (83.4%) had ANC and PNC visits, respectively. The detailed characteristics of the respondent's reproductive variables are shown in Table 2.

3.3. *Knowledge and Practice Pattern of Contraceptives.* The results regarding knowledge and practice patterns of the participants on contraceptives are presented in Table 3. Of the total, 307 (94.5%) stated that they had knowledge about contraceptives. About half (49.2%) of the study participants had known more than one method. Other common methods known were pills (76, 24.8%), injectables (55, 17.9%), condoms (13, 4.2%), and intrauterine devices (IUD) (12, 3.9%). The main sources of information on contraceptives were health facilities (188, 61.2%) and peers (68, 22.1%).

Table 3: Knowledge and practice patterns of contraceptives by respondents.

Variable	Frequency	Percentage (%)
Knowledge of contraceptives		
1. Yes	307	94.5
2. No	18	5.5
Source of information ($n = 307$)		
1. Health facility	188	61.2
2. Media	6	2.0
3. Parents (mother-in-law)	45	14.7
4. Peers	68	22.1
Contraceptive methods known ($n = 307$)		
1. Pills	76	24.8
2. Condoms	13	4.2
3. Injectable	55	17.9
4. IUD	12	3.9
5. More than one	151	49.2
Currently using contraceptives		
1. Yes	127	39.1
2. No	198	60.9
Type of method used ($n = 127$)		
1. Pills	45	34.9
2. Condoms	26	20.6
3. Injectable	36	28.6
4. IUD	19	15.1
5. More than one	1	0.8
Where do respondents acquire their contraceptives ($n = 127$)		
1. Public hospital	92	72.6
2. Pharmacy	35	27.4
Ever use of contraceptives		
1. Yes	176	54.2
2. No	149	45.8
Reasons for using contraceptives ($n = 176$)		
1. Prevents unintended pregnancies	34	19.2
2. Prevents STIs	2	1.1
3. Helps to space children	138	78.5
4. Prevention of anemia	2	1.1
Experienced any side effects ($n = 176$)		
1. Yes	114	64.5
2. No	62	35.5
Side effects experienced ($n = 114$)		
1. Vaginal bleeding	28	24.6
2. Abdominal pain	10	8.9
3. Headache	34	29.9
4. Weight gain	18	16.1
5. Hypertension	18	16.1
6. More than one	5	4.4
Reasons for not using contraceptives ($n = 149$)		
1. Against religion	51	34.2
2. Opposition from husbands	24	16.2
3. Fear of side effects	25	16.8
4. Want to have more children	37	20.8
5. No knowledge	18	12.0

Other sources of information were parents (45, 14.7) and media (6, 2%).

Of all the study participants, 127 (39.1%, 95%CI = 33.7% –44.6%) had currently used at least one of the modern contraceptive methods, varying from 50.6% to 27.6% in urban and rural settings, respectively (Figure 1).

Concerning the type of method used, 45 (34.9%) were on pills, 36 (28.6%) were on injectables, 26 (20.6%) were on condoms, and 19 (15.1%) were using IUD. The majority (72.6%) of the participants acquired their contraceptives from public health facilities. With regard to the ever use of contraceptives, 176 (54.2%) participants reported that they had at least used one of the contraceptive methods. Major reasons for using contraceptives were child spacing (78.5%) and prevention of unintended pregnancies (19.2%). Of the 176 ever contraceptive users, 114 (64.5%) participants have experienced side effects. Among 149 nonusers, common reasons for not using contraceptives stated were religious prohibition (51, 34.2%), wanting to have more children (37, 20.8), and fear of side effects (25, 16.8%).

3.4. Factors Associated with Modern Contraceptive Use. We conducted the bivariate analysis for all independent variables. Multiple logistic regression analysis was done for those variables with a P value of <0.25 in bivariate analysis. The results of multiple logistic regression showed that married women from the urban residence had 2.61 times higher odds of currently using contraceptives than the odds of married women with rural residence (AOR = 2.61, 95% CI:1.43-4.78). This study also found that married women with previous contraceptive use had 14.92-fold higher odds of currently using contraceptives compared to those who had not used contraceptives in the past. Table 4 summarizes the results of bivariate and multivariable analyses.

4. Discussion

This cross-sectional study investigated the factors associated with modern contraceptive use among married women attending comprehensive health clinics in Kandahar Province. Understanding the factors influencing contraceptive use is of particular importance in countries like Afghanistan that have been affected by high MMR and infant mortality rate (IMR). This is a unique study providing a picture of both urban and rural populations.

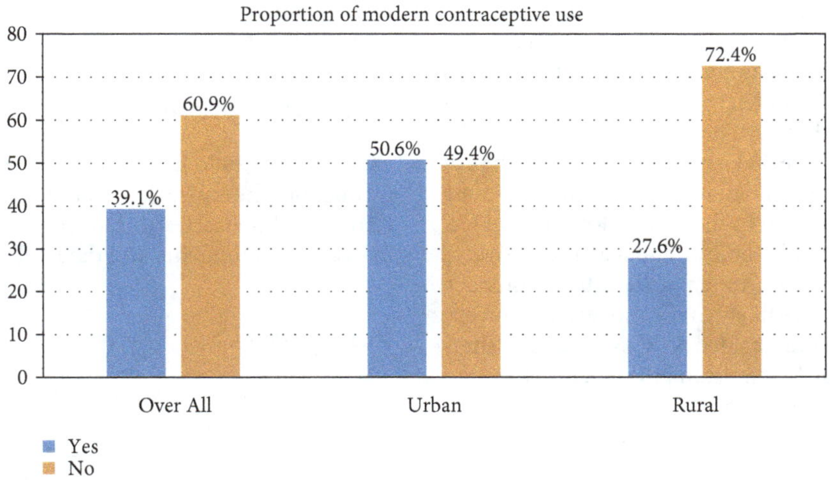

FIGURE 1: Proportion of contraceptive use among married women attending comprehensive health clinics in Kandahar Province, Afghanistan, 2019.

TABLE 4: Factors associated with modern contraceptive use among married women attending comprehensive health centers in Kandahar Province, 2019 (crude and adjusted odds ratio).

Independent variable	Categories	Contraceptive use Yes	Contraceptive use No	Crude odds ratio (95% CI)	Adjusted odds ratio (95% CI)
Residency	Urban	82	80	2.68 (1.69-4.26)	2.61 (1.43-4.78)
	Rural	45	118	1	1
Husband education	Educated	38	26	2.82 (1.61-4.94)	—
	Uneducated	89	172	1	—
Husband occupation	Employed	87	103	2.00 (1.25-3.19)	—
	Unemployed	40	95	1	—
Household income	5000-10000	21	49	1	—
	>10000	98	117	1.95 (1.09-3.48)	—
Years in marriage	1 to 4	17	57	1	—
	5 or more	110	141	2.61 (1.44-4.74)	—
ANC visit	Yes	108	142	2.24 (1.25-3.99)	—
	No	19	56	1	—
Previous contraceptive use	Yes	113	63	17.29 (9.20-32.49)	14.92 (6.88-32.34)
	No	14	135	1	1

The findings revealed that the prevalence of modern contraceptive use was 39.1%, varying from 50.6% to 27.6% in urban and rural settings, respectively. This finding was higher than reported on the national level [1] and other studies conducted in Afghanistan [15, 17, 18]. This overestimation can be explained by the fact that married women visiting health clinics for seeking healthcare are more likely to use contraceptives than their counterparts. This may be the case as these health facilities are rendering family planning services. In this study, modern contraceptive use was lower than that of other studies conducted in India (52.2%) [9], Pakistan (49.7%) [10], Iran (72.9%) [11], and the United Arab Emirates (61.8%) [12]. This variation in contraceptive use reported in studies could be attributed to variation in cultural attitudes towards contraceptive use, access and availability of contraceptives in the study area, socioeconomic status, research design, and other nonexplored factors.

In this study, the main methods of modern contraception are oral contraceptive pills (34.9%) and injectables (28.6%), which is inconsistent with a prior study conducted in Afghanistan [15]. Major reasons cited for using modern contraceptives were child spacing and women's desire to prevent unintended pregnancies. These findings were consistent with the study conducted in Afghanistan [15] and similar studies conducted in Ethiopia [7] and Ghana [8]. On the other hand, religious prohibitions and wanting to have more children were the common reasons for not using modern contraceptives. This finding is in line with studies from Bangladesh [13] and Ethiopia [14].

In our study, the common source of information and acquiring contraceptives by married women were health facilities. This finding is consistent with the national report [1] and with a recent research report conducted in Afghanistan [15]. Since educational level was not associated with contraceptive use, all women of reproductive age including educated ones should receive health education on family planning. It is also imperative that a massive public health program aimed at improving awareness on the family planning methods should be undertaken in the light of low health literacy among the general population in Kandahar Province.

This study revealed that women with urban residency were nearly three times more likely to use modern contraceptives than women from rural residency. This finding is similar to that of a study from Afghanistan [15] and other studies from Pakistan [4] and Bangladesh [13]. The possible reasons for high use in urban dwellings include better socioeconomic status of women and cultural disparity. Furthermore, limited access and availability of family planning services in the rural area might further limit the use of modern contraceptives. In the current study, women who ever used contraceptives were more likely to use contraceptives, which is also supported by studies conducted in Uganda [19], Pakistan [20], and Bangladesh [21].

Factors shown to be associated with modern contraceptive use in previous studies such as age, income, education, parity, and occupation of married women were not associated in this study [8, 9, 11–15]. This may indicate possible differences in age, income, education, parity, and occupation of study participants.

5. Limitations of the Study

This study found crucial factors for modern contraceptive use in married women. The findings of this study, however, should be considered in light of its limitations. Since this study was an institutional-based one, the proportion of modern contraceptive use might have been overestimated and may not reflect what is going on at the community level. The cross-sectional nature of the study limits the causality effects between variables.

6. Conclusion

In this study, the proportion of modern contraceptive use among married women was 39.1 percent, which suggests an increase from the past studies. Urban residency and ever use of contraceptives were the factors associated with modern contraceptive use. As a policy measure, family planning programs should be prompted to the rural residence in Kandahar Province. Improving availability and access in rural areas are highly recommended to enhance modern contraceptive use. The results also suggest the need for qualitative research to divulge more information on religious and cultural beliefs influencing modern contraceptive use.

Authors' Contributions

HS, MS, and HS designed the study. HS, NR, and MS analyzed the data and prepared the initial manuscript. NF and GM advised the whole research. All authors discussed the results and critically commented on the manuscript at all stages. All authors read and approved the final manuscript.

Acknowledgments

The authors would like to acknowledge the support provided throughout the entire data collection period by the Baran and Kandahar Public Health Directorate. We also would like to thank the respondents and data collectors of the study.

References

[1] Central Statistics Organization/Afghanistan, Ministry of Public Health/Afghanistan, and ICF, *Afghanistan Demographic and Health Survey 2015*, Central Statistics Organization, Kabul, Afghanistan, 2017, http://dhsprogram.com/pubs/pdf/FR323/FR323.pdf.x.

[2] World Health Organization, *Reproductive Health. Family Planning: A Global Handbook for Providers: Evidence-Based Guidance Developed through Worldwide Collaboration*, Johns Hopkins Ccp-Info, Geneva, Switzerland, 2007.

[3] D. Hubacher and J. Trussell, "A definition of modern contraceptive methods," *Contraception*, vol. 92, no. 5, pp. 420-421, 2015.

[4] United Nations, Department of Economic and Social Affairs, Population Division, *Family Planning and the 2030 Agenda for Sustainable Development*, United Nations, New York, NY, USA, 2019, https://www.un.org/en/development/desa/population/publications/pdf/family/familyPlanning_DataBooklet_2019.pdf.x.

[5] S. Singh, G. Sedgh, and R. Hussain, "Unintended pregnancy: worldwide levels, trends, and outcomes," *Studies in Family Planning*, vol. 41, no. 4, pp. 241–250, 2010.

[6] R. Omani-Samani, M. Ranjbaran, M. Mohammadi et al., "Impact of unintended pregnancy on maternal and neonatal outcomes," *The Journal of Obstetrics and Gynecology of India*, vol. 69, no. 2, pp. 136–141, 2019.

[7] A. Mohammed, D. Woldeyohannes, A. Feleke, and B. Megabiaw, "Determinants of modern contraceptive utilization among married women of reproductive age group in North Shoa Zone, Amhara Region, Ethiopia," *Reproductive Health*, vol. 11, no. 1, 2014.

[8] P. A. Apanga and M. A. Adam, "Factors influencing the uptake of family planning services in the Talensi District, Ghana," *Pan African Medical Journal*, vol. 20, 2015.

[9] J. R. New, N. Cahill, J. Stover, Y. P. Gupta, and L. Alkema, "Levels and trends in contraceptive prevalence, unmet need, and demand for family planning for 29 states and union territories in India: a modelling study using the Family Planning Estimation Tool," *The Lancet Global Health*, vol. 5, no. 3, pp. e350–e358, 2017.

[10] M. Siddiqui, K. Fatima, S. N. Ali et al., "Prevalence and Predictors of Contraception Usage in Karachi, Pakistan," *Cureus*, vol. 12, no. 10, p. e11265, 2020.

[11] N. G. Gejo, A. A. Anshebo, and L. H. Dinsa, "Postpartum modern contraceptive use and associated factors in Hossana town," *PLoS One*, vol. 14, no. 5, article e0217167, 2019.

[12] N. Kanwal, J. Muttappallymyalil, S. Al-Sharbatti, and I. Ismail, "Contraceptive utilisation among mothers of reproductive age in Ajman, United Arab Emirates," *Sultan Qaboos University Medical Journal*, vol. 17, no. 1, pp. e50–e58, 2017.

[13] S. M. M. Kamal and M. A. Islam, "Contraceptive use: socioeconomic correlates and method choices in rural Bangladesh," *Asia Pacific Journal of Public Health*, vol. 22, no. 4, pp. 436–450, 2010.

[14] A. T. Beekle and C. McCabe, "Awareness and determinants of family planning practice in Jimma, Ethiopia," *International Nursing Review*, vol. 53, no. 4, pp. 269–276, 2006.

[15] S. Ajmal, A. Idris, and B. Ajmal, "Factors affecting contraceptive use and unmet need among currently married women in Afghanistan: further analysis of the 2015 Afghanistan Demographic and Health Survey," *Journal of Global Health Reports*, vol. 2, 2018.

[16] International Business Machines Corporation, *IBM SPSS Statistics for Windows, Version 21.0*, IBM Corporation, Armonk, NY, USA, 2012.

[17] A. K. Osmani, J. A. Reyer, A. R. Osmani, and N. Hamajima, "Factors influencing contraceptive use among women in Afghanistan: secondary analysis of Afghanistan Health Survey 2012," *Nagoya Journal of Medical Science*, vol. 77, no. 4, pp. 551–561, 2015.

[18] Z. Anwary, M. H. Stanikzai, W. M. Wyar, A. W. Wasiq, and K. Farooqi, "Anemia among women who visit Bost Hospital for delivery in Helmand Province, Afghanistan," *Anemia*, vol. 2021, Article ID 9358464, 6 pages, 2021.

[19] K. M. Sileo, R. K. Wanyenze, H. Lule, and S. M. Kiene, "Determinants of family planning service uptake and use of contraceptives among postpartum women in rural Uganda," *International Journal of Public Health*, vol. 60, no. 8, pp. 987–997, 2015.

[20] S. K. Azmat, W. Hameed, M. Ishaque, G. Mustafa, and A. Ahmed, "Post-abortion care family planning use in Pakistan," *Pakistan Journal of Public Health*, vol. 2, no. 2, pp. 6–8, 2011.

[21] S. Salway and S. Nurani, "Postpartum contraceptive use in Bangladesh: understanding users' perspectives," *Studies in Family Planning*, vol. 29, no. 1, pp. 41–57, 1998.

9

Adherence to Iron-Folate Supplementation and Associated Factors among Pastoralist's Pregnant Women in Burji Districts, Segen Area People's Zone, Southern Ethiopia: Community-Based Cross-Sectional Study

Negussie Boti,[1] Tezera Bekele,[1] Wanzahun Godana,[1] Eskeziyaw Getahun,[1] Feleke Gebremeskel,[1] Behailu Tsegaye,[2] and Bilcha Oumer[3]

[1]*Department of Public Health, College of Medicine and Health Sciences, Arba Minch University, Arba Minch, Ethiopia*
[2]*Department of Biomedical Sciences, College of Medicine and Health Sciences, Arba Minch University, Arba Minch, Ethiopia*
[3]*Department of Midwifery, College of Health Sciences, Arba Minch, Ethiopia*

Correspondence should be addressed to Negussie Boti; kahlidboti@gmail.com

Academic Editor: Stefania A. Nottola

Background. Iron deficiency anemia among pregnant women is one of the most common public health problems in developing country particularly in Ethiopia. Iron/folic acid supplementation with optimal adherence is the main cost-effective strategy for prevention and control of iron deficiency anemia in pregnant women. However, level of adherence to iron/folic acid supplementation and its associated factors were not well identified in study area. Therefore, the aim of this study was to determine the level of adherence to iron/folic acid supplementation and associated factors among pregnant women in Burji Districts, southern Ethiopia. *Methods.* A community-based cross-sectional study was conducted among 317 pregnant women in Burji Districts from March to April 2017 using interviewer administered questionnaires. Data were entered into Epi Info 3.5.1 and exported to SPSS version 20.0 for analysis. Binary and multivariable logistic regression was used to identify factors associated with iron/folic acid supplementation. Adjusted odds ratio (AOR) with 95% confidence interval (CI) and p-value <0.05 were used to declare statistical significance. *Results.* Among women participating in the study, 163(51.4%) were adherent to iron/folate acid supplementation. Factors significantly associated with adherence to iron and folic acid supplementation were maternal educational status (AOR: 2.47, 95% CI: 1.13-4.97), early registration for ANC (AOR: 2.49, 95% CI: 1.45 – 4.27), history of anemia during current pregnancy (AOR: 2.02, 95% CI: 1.09-3.72), and knowledge about iron and folic acid supplementation (AOR: 1.96, 95% CI: 1.02-3.76). Forgetfulness and fear of side effects were among the leading reasons of pregnant women for nonadherence to iron and folic acid supplementation. *Conclusions.* This study revealed that adherence to iron /folic acid supplementation was found to be 51.4%. Maternal educational status, early registration for ANC, history of anemia during current pregnancy, and knowledge about iron and folic acid supplementation were significant factors associated with adherence to iron/folic acid supplementation among pastoralist's pregnant women. Therefore, anemia prevention strategy should include strengthening giving awareness, counseling, strengthening community health education, and participation in health programs which are necessary to improve the uptake of iron/folic acid supplements.

1. Introduction

Anemia is a global public health problem affecting two billion people worldwide [1]. The primary cause of anemia is iron deficiency, a condition caused by inadequate intake or low absorption of iron, the increased demands during pregnancy, and loss of iron through menstruation [1–3].

Pregnant women are the most prone groups for IDA [4, 5]. During pregnancy, physiological iron requirements are the highest and the amount of iron absorbed from the diet is not sufficient to meet requirements during pregnancy [6, 7]. However, plasma expansion being increased in the second trimesters, the dietary intake of the two elements cannot meet the increased need during pregnancy which leads to IDA [6]. Anemia during pregnancy leads to low birth weight, lowered resistance to infection, poor cognitive development, and reduced work capacity [3, 8, 9].

Iron and folic acid supplementation have been the preferred intervention to prevent IDA among pregnant women that may help to improve maternal and fetal outcomes because it is essential to the normal development of the spine, brain, and skull of the fetus [1, 3]. Folate also supports the pregnant woman's expanding blood volume and growing maternal and fetal tissues [2, 7].

WHO recommends that in the first four weeks of pregnancy all pregnant women should be receive a standard dose of 30–60 mg iron and 400 μg folic acid beginning as soon as possible during the first trimester of pregnancy [1]. Accordingly, in Ethiopia, the national guideline for control and prevention of micronutrient deficiencies highlights the need of daily iron supplementation for at least 6 months during pregnancy and 3 months postpartum [3]. Iron-folic acid (IFA) adherence is the extent to which patients take medication or condition of sticking to dose and time for taking iron/folate supplements as prescribed by their healthcare providers or per recommendations [10, 11]. Women are said to adhere to an iron/folic acid supplement if they took 65% or more of the supplement, equivalent to taking the supplement at least 4 days a week [12]. However, oral iron-folate supplementation is hindered by different factors such as poor adherence to regimens, frequency of side effects, gastrointestinal side effects, inadequate supply of tablets, lack of counseling of pregnant women by health care providers concerning to the utilization of tablets and possible side-effects of the supplementation, poor utilization of ANC services, lack of knowledge on the IFA tablet, and lack of knowledge on anemia, but experts suggest that 1000 mg of iron is needed for mother and fetus during pregnancy [2, 13, 14].

Therefore, to control problem associated with IDA and its adverse health consequences affecting both pregnant mother and their neonate in Ethiopia especially in study area provision iron and folic acid supplementation is one of strategies to all pregnant during pregnancy. Therefore identifying the level of adherence and its determinants in high-risk groups, such as pregnant women, would be essential for evidence-based intervention. There is no updated data about the level of Adherence to IFAS among pregnant women in the study area. Therefore, the aim of this study is to determine the level of adherence and associated factors among pregnant women in Burji Districts, Southern Ethiopia.

2. Methods and Materials

2.1. Study Area and Design. This study was conducted in Burji District. Burji District is one of the five districts in Segen Area Peoples Zone of the Southern Nations, Nationalities, and Peoples Region (SNNPR) of Ethiopia. The administrative center of Burji is Soyama. Burji District has two urban and twenty-four rural kebeles. There are five health centers and twenty-four health posts, which provide routine antenatal care services to the community. Based on the 2007 Census conducted by the Central Statistical Agency of Ethiopia (CSA), this woreda has a total population of 55,681, of whom 27,207 are men and 28,474 women [15]. A community-based cross-sectional study design was conducted from March to April 2017.

2.2. Source and Study Populations. All pregnant women aged 15–49 years who were living in the district were the source population. The study population was pregnant women aged 15–49 years who were attending ANC and being supplied with the iron-folate supplement at least for a month during the data collection period. Pregnant women who were severely ill, those who had a mental illness, and who were living in the study area less than six months were excluded.

2.3. Sample Size Determination. The sample size was calculated using the single population approach and it was calculated using Epi Info version 7.02 statistical software package with the assumption of 95% confidence level ($Z\alpha/2=$ 1.96), 80% power ($Z\beta=$ 0.84), and P =74.9% on the proportion of adherence to iron-folic acid supplementation among the pregnant women, which was taken from a previous study conducted rural districts of Ethiopia [16]. Considering 10% nonresponse rate, the maximum sample size was 317 study participants.

2.4. Sampling Procedure. Simple random sampling technique was used to select study participants using average previous month's antenatal care users used as the sampling frame which is obtained from a community family folder. In Burji District, there were twenty-six kebeles; among those, eight kebeles were selected using a lottery method. A proportional to size allocation was employed to obtain the sample size for selected kebeles. Prior to the actual data collection being given, the list of study subjects was identified by using community health management information system (CHMIS) folder. Finally, the study participants were selected by using a simple random sampling method. If in case more than one eligible respondent is found in the household, only one respondent had been chosen by lottery method

2.5. Operational Definition

2.5.1. Adherence. Pregnant mothers took at least 65% of the expected dose of the iron-folate tablets in the previous week before the study, which is equivalent to consuming at least 1 tablet daily for 4 days in the week consecutively or consuming 20 tablets in a month daily without missing the prescribed doses [1, 17].

2.5.2. Knowledge of Iron-Folate Supplement. It was measured by summing up 8 multiple-choice items. A correct answer was given one mark, while a wrong answer was not given any mark. If the pregnant women scored median and above, then they have good knowledge and those pregnant women who scored below the median, they have poor knowledge [18].

2.6. Data Collection Procedure and Data Quality Control. Data were collected using structured questionnaire adapted from different peer-reviewed published works of literature [4, 17, 19]. A structured pretested interviewer administered questionnaire was developed in English and then translated into Amharic language for simplicity and then backtranslated to English language for its consistency by two different language expert individuals who speak both English and Amharic fluently. The questionnaire has four parts sociodemographics, obstetrics characteristics, health service-related characteristics, and client related characteristics which were used. Pretesting of the questionnaire was done on 5% of the sample at Arba Minch Zuriha district who was not included in the study; that was a week before commencement of the actual data collection. Based on the pretest, a questionnaire was corrected to ensure clarity, wording, and logic sequence and skip patterns. The data was collected by nine diploma health professionals and supervised by four trained health professionals who had BSc. Data collectors and supervisor were trained for one day on objectives of the study, how to keep confidentiality of information, the contents of the questionnaire, filling data collection format, and data quality management by the principal investigator. At the end of each day, questionnaires were reviewed and cross-checked for completeness, accuracy, and consistency by the supervisor and principal investigator and corrective measures were taken. The overall activity was supervised by the principal investigator of the study.

2.7. Data Processing and Analysis. The collected data were coded, cleaned, and entered by Epi-Info version 7.2 and exported to statistical package for social science (SPSS) version 20.0 for analysis. Descriptive statistics including tables and proportion were used to describe the data. Binary and a multivariable logistic regression analyses were performed to see the association between dependent and independent variables. Variables that showed association in binary logistic regression analysis and which have P-value less than 0.20 were entered into multivariable logistic regression analysis model. Finally multivariable logistic regression model is used for controlling confounding factors and to identify significant factors associated with dependent variable. An effort was made to assess whether the necessary assumptions for the application of multivariable logistic regression analysis were fulfilled. In this regard, the Hosmer and Lemeshow's goodness-of-fit test with large p-value ($p>0.05$) was checked to see good fitness. Multicollinearity and confounding effect was checked by using standard error. The variable without multicollinearity was entered into multivariable model. At the end AOR with 95% CI, P-value <0.05 was considered statistically significant.

2.8. Ethical Consideration. The study was conducted after getting ethical clearance from Arba Minch University, College of Medicine and Health Science Institutional Review Board (IRB). Support letter was obtained from Zonal Health Department as per the recommendation letter from the public health department. Verbal consent was secured from study participants after explaining the objective and purpose of the study to each study participant. The participants were also assured about the confidentiality.

3. Results

3.1. Socioeconomic and Demographic Characteristics of Pregnant Women. A total of 317 pregnant women whose age ranges from 18 to 49 years were interviewed. The mean age was found to be 25.6 with (±SD) 4.9 years and the majority of pregnant women, 270 (85.2%), were age group from 20 to 34 years. Two hundred thirty-eight (75.1%) of study participants have resided in the urban area. The majority, 248 (78.2%), was married. The majority, 188 (89.3%), of pregnant women had no formal education while 47 (14.8%) pregnant women had primary educational status, but the majority of husbands, 129 (40.7%), had primary educational status. About 292 (92.1%) mothers were housewives and 169 (53.3%) mothers had more than six children (Table 1).

3.2. Obstetric Related Characteristics of Pregnant Women. One hundred eighty (56.8%) and 178 (56.1%) were primigravidae and primiparous, while 137 (43.2%) and 95 (30%) were multigravida and multiparous. About 185 (58.4%) mothers visited the ANC clinic within the last 16 weeks of gestation. The majority of pregnant women, 217 (68.5%), visited ANC for follow-up more than four times in health institution. About 32 (10.1%) respondents had the history of abortion; also 12 (3.8%) respondents had the history of stillbirth. On current pregnancy, 141 (44.5%) pregnant women had the history of anemia (Table 2).

3.3. Knowledge of Pregnant Women about Anemia and IFAS. Accordingly, 170 (53.6%) respondents had good knowledge of anemia (scored median and above) and 147 (46.4%) respondents had poor knowledge of anemia (scored below the median). Out of all study participants, 148 (46.7%) respondents had good knowledge of IFAS (scored median and above) and 169 (53.3%) respondents had poor knowledge of IFAS (scored below the median).

3.4. Adherence to the Iron/Folate Supplementation Based on Pill Counting. Adherence to the iron/folate supplementation was measured based on pill counting [9]. The finding of this study reveals that one hundred sixty-three (51.4%) of pregnant women have adhered to IFAS (took ≥4 tablets per week or consuming 20 tablets in a month daily without missing the prescribed doses) and 154 (48.6%) did not adhere to IFAS (took <4 tablets per week or consuming table with missing the prescribed doses). The reasons for adherence were getting counseling from health extension worker (245, 86.5%), followed by fear of illness if not taking the supplement (106, 42.3%) and getting family support (43, 15.2%). The leading reason for not adhering was forgetfulness to take table, 135 (46.7%), then taking too many pills, 72(22.7%), followed by fear of side effects, 70 (45.4%). From those who express side effects, the commonest side effect was heartburn, 153 (48.3%), and vomiting, 137 (43.2 %) (Figure 1).

3.5. Factors Associated with Adherence to IFAS among Pregnant Women. The multivariable logistic regression showed that maternal educational status, time of ANC registration, knowledge of anemia, and knowledge of IFAS were

TABLE 1: Sociodemographic and economic characteristics of Pastoralist's pregnant mothers in Burji Districts, Segen Area Zone of Southern Nations, Nationalities and Peoples Region, Ethiopia, March-April 2017 (N=317).

Variables	Categories	Frequency(n)	Percent (%)
Age in years	15-19	22	6.9
	20-34	270	85.2
	≥35	25	7.9
Residence	Rural	79	24.9
	Urban	238	75.1
Marital status	Single	24	7.6
	Married	248	78.2
	Divorced	34	10.7
	Widowed	11	3.5
Maternal educational status	Have no formal education	188	89.3
	Primary	47	14.8
	Secondary and above	82	28.8
Husband educational status	Have no formal education	106	33.4
	Primary	129	40.7
	Secondary and above	82	25.9
Maternal Occupational status	Housewife/Farmer	292	92.1
	Merchants	12	3.8
	Employers	12	3.8
	Others	1	0.3
Number of lived children	1-3	45	14.2
	4-6	103	32.5
	>6	169	53.3

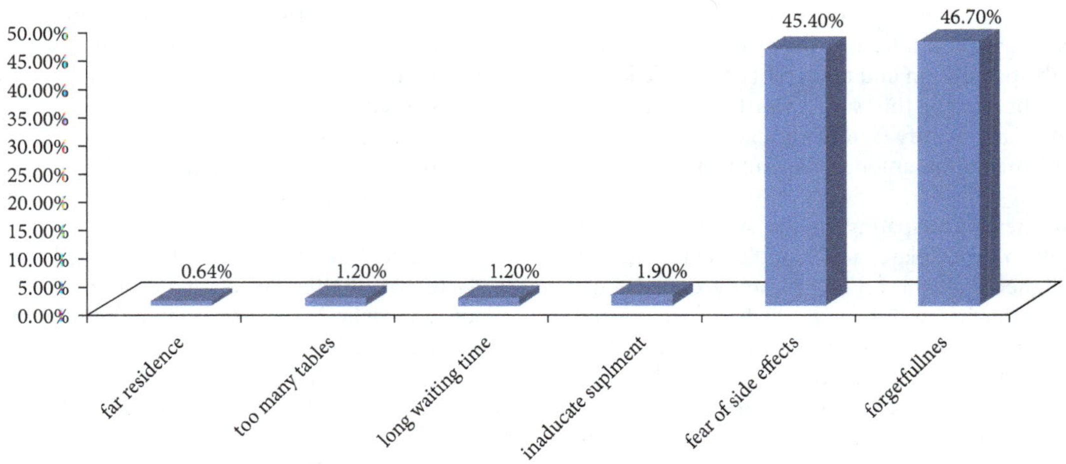

FIGURE 1: Reason for not adherence among Pastoralist's pregnant women in Burji Districts, Segen Area Zone of Southern Nations, Nationalities and Peoples Region, Ethiopia, March–April 2017.

statistically significant with adherence of IFAS. The pregnant women who had secondary and above education were nearly 2.5 times (AOR=2.47, 95% CI=1.13-4.97) more likely to have adhered to IFAS than those pregnant women who had primary education. The pregnant women who had early registration (≤16 weeks) for ANC were 2.49 times (AOR= 2.49, 95% CI=1.45 – 4.27 more likely to adhere to IFAS than those who had late registration (>16 weeks). The pregnant women who had the history of anemia during current pregnancy were 2 times (AOR= 2.02, 95% CI= 1.09-3.72) more likely to adhere to IFAS than those who did not have any symptom of illness. The pregnant women who had good knowledge of IFAS were nearly 2 times (AOR= 1.96, 95% CI= 1.02-3.76) more likely to have adhered to IFAS than those who had poor knowledge of IFAS (Table 3).

4. Discussion

Pregnant women are among the most vulnerable groups of iron deficiency anemia. The World Health Organization

TABLE 2: Obstetric related characteristics of Pastoralist's Pregnant mothers in Burji Districts, Segen Area Zone of Southern Nations, Nationalities and Peoples Region, Ethiopia, March-April 2017 (N=317).

Variables	Categories	Frequency(n)	Percent (%)
Number of pregnancy	Primigravida	180	56.8
	Multigravida	137	43.2
Number of deliveries	Nulliparous	44	13.9
	Primiparous	178	56.1
	Multiparous	95	30
Number of Visits	≤4	217	68.5
	>4	100	31.5
Gestational age at the start of ANC	First trimester	121	38.2
	Second trimester	177	55.8
	Third trimester	19	6
Time of registration	<16weeks (Early)	185	58.4
	≥16weeks (Late)	132	41.6
History of Abortion	Yes	32	10.1
	No	285	89.9
History of still birth	Yes	12	3.8
	No	305	96.2
History of Anemia on current pregnancy	Yes	141	44.5
	No	176	55.5

recommends giving all pregnant women a standard dose of 60mg iron and 400μg folic acid daily for 6-month duration. Iron and folic acid supplementation are among the feasible ways to prevent anemia during pregnancy. However, maternal adherence to iron and folic acid supplementation plays a major role in the prevention and treatment of iron deficiency anemia. Thus, the aim of this study was to determine the adherence status and identify factors associated with iron and folic acid supplementation among pregnant women who live in a study area.

Among women participating in the study, 163 (51.4%) were adherent to iron/folate acid supplementation. This finding was higher than the finding of study conducted in Mecha district, Northwest Ethiopia (20.4%) [19], the one conducted in North Western Zone of Tigray, Ethiopia (39.2%) [17], and the study conducted in Kenya (24.5%) [14]. This might be associated with increased knowledge of pregnant women about anemia and IFA supplementation (through medical advice and media).

In addition, the result of adherence found in this study was lower than result found in eight rural districts in SNNP, Ethiopia, 2014, which was 74.9% average level of adherence rate of pregnant women in the area [16] and the study was done in South India (64.7%) [20]. This inconsistency may be due to cultural, geographical location, and availability of drugs in the health center. Another might be that this study was done in rural-based area and the pregnant women may not get information from the health center and women in rural areas were probably less educated than those in urban areas which could have contributed to the lower level than the regional level. Also, there might be a misunderstanding of the need to take the tablets throughout pregnancy due to inadequate counseling and beliefs against consuming medications during pregnancy; that is, the medications may cause too much blood or a big baby, making delivery more difficult.

This study revealed that maternal education status had a significant association with adherence to iron and folic acid supplementation. Pregnant women who had secondary and above education were nearly 2.5 times more likely to adhere to IFAS than those pregnant women who had primary education. The finding is supported by other studies done in Mecha district, Northwest Ethiopia, Nepal, and Indonesia [18, 21, 22].

This might be associated with educated women who are likely to have better knowledge and access to information about iron deficiency anemia and therapy, the benefits of supplements, and pregnancy in general. Secondly, it might be due to the fact that education would increase the women's access to information through reading and understanding the benefit of the supplement. Third, it might be associated with the notion that education is more likely to enhance female awareness of micronutrient deficiency and ways to overcome these deficiencies. And it might be associated with the fact that educated women have greater ability to stick to health care inputs such as IFA which offer better care for both the infant and the mother.

The present study reveals that adherence was better observed among pregnant women who were early registered for antenatal care service as compared to late registered women. Accordingly, pregnant women who had early registration (≤16 weeks) for ANC were 2.49 times more likely to have adhered to IFAS than those who had late registration (>16 weeks). The result of this study is supported by other studies done in Tigray, Ethiopia, Indonesia, and India [17, 20, 21]. The reason might be that pregnant women who

TABLE 3: Factors associated with adherence to IFAS among Pastoralist's Pregnant women in Burji Districts, Segen Area Zone of Southern Nations, Nationalities and Peoples Region, Ethiopia, March-April 2017(N=317).

Variables	Categories	Adherence status		COR(95% CI)	AOR(95% CI)
		Adhered N (%)	Not Adhered N (%)		
Age	15-19	11(6.7)	11(7.1)	0.67(0.21,2.12)	0.83(0.27,2.53)
	20-34	142(87.1)	128(83.1)	0.60(0.26,1.39)*	1.24(0.29,5.23)
	≥35	10(6.1)	15(9.7)	1	**1**
Maternal educational status	Have No formal education	82(50.3)	106(68.8)	1	**1**
	Primary	31(19	16(10.4)	2.02 (1.19,3.43)*	0.77(0.34,1.71)
	Secondary and above	50(30.7)	32(20.8)	0.81 (0.38,1.71)	**2.47(1.13,4.97)****
Husband educational status	Have No formal education	44(27)	62(40.2)	1	1
	Primary	69(42.3)	60(39)	2.20 (1.22,3.97)*	1.46(0.72,2.94)
	Secondary and above	50(30.7)	32(20.8)	1.36(0.77,2.39)	2.10(0.92,4.39)
Maternal occupational status	Housewife	109(66.9)	113(73.4)	1	**1**
	Merchants	25(15.3)	25(16.2)	1.81(0.79,4.13)	1.98(0.82,4.79)
	Employers	29(17.8)	16(10.4)	1.88(0.97,3.65)*	2.13(0.94,4.37)
Family size	1-3	25(15.3)	20(13)	1	1
	4-6	54(33.1)	49(31.8)	1.13(0.56,2.29)	1.43(0.61,3.36)
	>6	84(51.5)	85(55.2)	1.27(0.65,2.45)	1.05(0.38,2.88)
Gravidity	Primigravida	98(60.1)	82(53.2)	1	1
	Multigravida	65(39.9)	72(46.8)	1.32(0.85, 2.07)*	1.17(0.52,2.61)
Trimester	First	58(35.6)	63(40.9)	1	1
	Second	98(60.1)	79(51.3)	0.74 (0.47,1.18)*	1.19(0.34,4.17)
	Third	7(4.3)	12(7.8)	1.58(0.58,4.28)	0.51(0.71,1.47)
Time of Registration	Early(≤16weeks)	100(61.3)	85(55.2)	1.29(0.82,2.02)*	**2.49(1.45,4.27)****
	Late(>16weeks)	63(38.7)	69(44.8)	1	**1**
History of Anemia	Yes	74(45.4)	67(43.5)	1.08(0.69,1.68)	**2.02(1.09,3.72)****
	No	89(54.6)	87(56.5)	1	1
Knowledge of Anemia	Good	84(51.5)	86(55.8)	1.19(0.76,1.85)	1.21(0.75,1.95)
	Poor	79(48.5)	68(44.2)	1	1
Knowledge of IFAS	Good	52(31.9)	27(17.5)	2.2(1.29,3.74)*	**1.96(1.02,3.76)****
	Poor	111(68.1)	127(82.5)	1	1

AOR = adjusted odd ratio; CI = confidence interval; COR = crude odd ratio; ** = statistically significant

had early registration for ANC services probably had better concern for their pregnancy and had more ANC visits which in turn leads to getting better medical advice and ultimately increased knowledge about anemia and iron and folic acid supplementation.

Similarly, a history of anemia during current pregnancy was associated with greater adherence to iron supplementation. Pregnant women who had a history of anemia during current pregnancy were 2.02 times more likely to have adhered to IFAS than those who did not have any symptom of illness. This finding was supported by study conducted in Tigray, Ethiopia, and study conducted in Mecha district, Western Amhara [17, 19]. This might be due to relief from symptoms and fear of further complications and the provider may give more emphasis to anemic clients on counseling compared to non-academic clients. Secondary it might be the fact that the number of iron/folic acid pills that should be taken according to the prescription will entirely depend on the frequency of illness that the mother had. If the mother did not have any symptom of illness, she would not take the amount of pills she should take.

Another factor that had a significant association with iron and folic acid supplementation adherence in this study was knowledge of iron and folic acid supplementation. Pregnant women who had good knowledge of IFAS were nearly 2 times more likely to adhere to IFAS than those who had poor knowledge of IFAS. This finding is supported by other studies done in eight rural districts of Ethiopia and India [16, 20]. The possible reason is that those pregnant women who had good knowledge of iron and folic acid supplementation were aware of the tablets importance, side effect, how it is taken, and complication if missed. Secondly, this might be associated with the fact that knowledge helps women to have a good perception of the benefits of taking iron tablets.

Forgetfulness and fear of side effect were the leading reason of pregnant women for nonadherence to iron and folic acid supplementation. The finding of this study is supported by other studies done in Ethiopia [4–6]. A possible explanation for forgetfulness was because most pregnant women in a rural part of Ethiopia were tired at night time because they spent the daytime with different activities. The majority of women have a misunderstanding about taking the tablets due to inadequate counseling because most of the community in rural part believes that consuming medications during pregnancy may make delivery more difficult. So better counseling might decrease the high occurrence of side effects by increasing the psychological tolerance of women to side effects of the tablet.

4.1. Strength and Limitations of the Study. The possible strength of this study was using a gold standard method of measuring the number of iron/folic acid uptake pills; counting method was used which is the best predictor of adherence rate. Limitation of this might be cross-sectional in nature or might be chicken egg dilemma and it does not test the hypothesis.

5. Conclusions

The finding of this study revealed that the adherence rate was 51.4%. Maternal educational status, early registration for antenatal care services, history of anemia during current pregnancy, and knowledge of pregnant women about iron and folic acid supplementation were significantly associated with pregnant women adherence to iron and folic acid supplementation. Forgetfulness and fear of side effects were among the leading reasons of pregnant women for nonadherence to iron and folic acid supplementation. Therefore, health professionals and responsible bodies should give attention to advising and counseling a pregnant woman on benefits and starting time of iron folate supplementation.

Abbreviations

ANC: Antenatal care
AOR: Adjusted odds ratio
CI: Confidence interval
COR: Crude odds ratio
IDA: Iodine deficiency anemia
IFA: Iron folic acid
IFAS: Iron folic acid supplementation
OR: Odds ratio
SNNPR: Southern Nations Nationalities Peoples Region
SPSS: Statistical Package for Social Science
WHO: World Health Organization.

Disclosure

Arba Minch University has no role in the design of the study, collection, analysis, and interpretation of the data and in writing the manuscript.

Authors' Contributions

Tazera Bekele has made substantial intellectual contributions to conception, design, and acquisition of data, analysis, and interpretation of data to this study. ***Negussie Boti*** has been involved in drafting the manuscript and revising it critically for important intellectual contents. ***Wanzahun Godana, Eskzyiaw Getahun, Feleke Gebremeskel, Behailu Tsegaye, and Bilcha Oumer*** have made substantial contributions to conception, design, analysis, and interpretation of data and participated in the critical review and editing of all the manuscript draft for scientific merit and depth. All authors read and approved the final manuscript and agreed to be accountable for all aspects of the work in ensuring that questions related to the accuracy or integrity of any part of the work are appropriately investigated and resolved.

Acknowledgments

The authors thank all the study participants and Arba Minch University for financial support.

References

[1] *WHO. Guideline: Daily iron and folic acid supplementation in pregnant women*, World Health Organization, Geneva, 2012.

[2] R. M. Burke, J. S. Leon, and P. S. Suchdev, "Identification, prevention and treatment of iron deficiency during the first 1000 days," *Nutrients*, vol. 6, no. 10, pp. 4093–4114, 2014.

[3] Fedreal Ministry of Health, *Implementation Guidelines for the Prevention and Control of Micronutrient Deficiencies*, FMOH, Ethiopia, 2014.

[4] S. Shewasinad and S. Negash, "Adherence and Associated Factors of Prenatal Iron Folic Acid Supplementation among Pregnant Women Who Attend Ante Natal Care in Health Facility at Mizan-Aman Town, Bench Maji Zone, Ethiopia, 2015," *Journal of Pregnancy and Child Health*, vol. 04, no. 03, 2017.

[5] T. W. Brhanie and H. Sisay, "Prevalence of Iron Deficiency Anemia and Determinants among Pregnant Women Attending Prevalence of Iron Deficiency Anemia and Determinants among Pregnant Women Attending Antenatal Care at Woldia Hospital, Ethiopia," *Journal of Nutritional Disorders & Therapy*, vol. 6, no. 4, 2016.

[6] J. Haidar, "Prevalence of anemia, deficiencies of iron and folic acid and their determinants in Ethiopian women," *International centre for diarrhoeal disease research, Bangladesh*, vol. 28, no. 4, pp. 359–368, 2010.

[7] H. Abdullahi, G. I. Gasim, A. Saeed, A. M. Imam, and I. Adam, "Antenatal iron and folic acid supplementation use by pregnant women in Khartoum, Sudan," *BMC Research Notes*, vol. 7, no. 1, article no. 498, 2014.

[8] M. Getachew, D. Yewhalaw, K. Tafess, Y. Getachew, and A. Zeynudin, "Anaemia and associated risk factors among pregnant women in Gilgel Gibe dam area, Southwest Ethiopia," *Parasites & Vectors*, vol. 5, no. 1, article no. 296, 2012.

[9] *Ethiopia. Mini Demographic and Health Survey*, Central Statistics Agency, Addis Ababa, Ethiopia, 2014.

[10] Y. B. Nisar and M. J. Dibley, "Earlier initiation and use of a greater number of iron-folic acid supplements during preg-

nancy prevents early neonatal deaths in Nepal and Pakistan," *PLoS ONE*, vol. 9, no. 11, 2014.

[11] S. Siabani et al., "Determinants of Adherence to Iron and Folate Supplementation among Pregnant Women in West Iran: A Population Based Cross-Sectional Study," *Quality in Primary Care*, vol. 25, no. 3, pp. 157–163, 2017.

[12] L. C. Almeida and M. A. Cardoso, "Recommendations for folate intake in women: Implications for public health strategies," *Cadernos de Saúde Pública*, vol. 26, no. 11, pp. 2011–2026, 2010.

[13] M. Juma, S. O. Oiye, and S. O. Konyole, "Predictors of optimum antenatal iron-folate supplementation in a low resource rural set-up in Eastern Kenya," *Journal of Public Health and Epidemiology*, vol. 7, no. 11, pp. 337–345, 2015.

[14] L. Dinga, A. Mwangi, and G. Abong, *Factors associated with adherence to iron/folate supplementation among pregnant women attending antenatal clinic at thika district hospital in kiambu county, Kenya*, 2013.

[15] Wikipedia contributors, *Burji special woreda. In Wikipedia, The Free Encyclopedia*, 2018.

[16] S. Gebremedhin, A. Samuel, G. Mamo, T. Moges, and T. Assefa, "Coverage, compliance and factors associated with utilization of iron supplementation during pregnancy in eight rural districts of Ethiopia: a cross-sectional study," *BMC Public Health*, vol. 14, article 607, 2014.

[17] A. Gebre, "Assessment of Factors Associated with Adherence to Iron-Folic Acid Supplementation Among Urban and Rural Pregnant Women in North Western Zone of Tigray, Ethiopia: Comparative Study," *International Journal of Nutrition and Food Sciences*, vol. 4, no. 2, p. 161, 2015.

[18] A. Arega Sadore, L. Abebe Gebretsadik, and M. Aman Hussen, "Compliance with iron-folate supplement and associated factors among antenatal care attendant mothers in Misha District, South Ethiopia: Community based cross-sectional study," *Journal of Environmental and Public Health*, vol. 2015, 2015.

[19] B. Taye, G. Abeje, and A. Mekonen, "Factors associated with compliance of prenatal iron folate supplementation among women in Mecha district, Western Amhara: a cross-sectional study," *Pan African Medical Journal*, vol. 20, article 43, 2015.

[20] P. Mithra, B. Unnikrishnan, T. Rekha et al., "Compliance with iron-folic acid (IFA) therapy among pregnant women in an urban area of South India," *African Health Sciences*, vol. 14, no. 1, 2014.

[21] C. R. Titaley and M. J. Dibley, "Factors associated with not using antenatal iron/folic acid supplements in Indonesia: The 2002/2003 and 2007 Indonesia Demographic and Health Survey," *Asia Pacific Journal of Clinical Nutrition*, vol. 24, no. 1, pp. 162–176, 2015.

[22] S. Begum, "Factors associated with adherence to Iron Folic acid supplementations during Pregnancy in Uttar Pradesh," *Indian Journal of Maternal and Child Health*, vol. 14, no. 2, 2012.

10

Comparison of Serum Inhibin B and Follicle-Stimulating Hormone (FSH) Level between Normal and Infertile Men in Yaoundé

Tchoula Mamiafo Corinne[1], **Pieme Constant Anatole**,[2] **and Ngogang Yonkeu Jeanne**[2]

[1]*Department of Biochemistry, Faculty of Sciences, University of Yaoundé I, PB 812 Yaoundé, Cameroon*
[2]*Department of Biochemistry, Faculty of Medicine and Biomedical Sciences, University of Yaoundé I, PB 1364 Yaoundé, Cameroon*

Correspondence should be addressed to Tchoula Mamiafo Corinne; tchoulacorinne@yahoo.fr

Academic Editor: Yuksel Agca

Objective. Hormones play a vital role in initiating and maintaining male reproductive function. The present study explores the influence and predictive ability of two reproductive hormones on semen quality among men who were partners in an infertile couple. *Design.* During our cross sectional study, men were recruited from private and public hospital and laboratories for clinical evaluation of fertility status. *Methods.* Fresh semen samples were assessed for quality (concentration, motility and morphology) according to the 2010 World Health Organization manual and the serum levels of hormones, including follicle-stimulating hormone (FSH), Inhibin B was measured (ELISA). *Results.* We found a significant difference in the two groups regarding sperm concentration ($p < 0.0001$), total sperm count ($p < 0.0001$), progressive motility ($p < 0.0001$), vitality ($p < 0.0001$) and the percentage of normal forms ($p = 0.043$). We found a strong and negative correlation between FSH and Inhibin B in the overall population, the normozoospermic reference group and the case group. Our study confirmed that Inhibin B was significantly and positively correlated with sperm concentration and leucocytes, and that FSH was negatively correlated to sperm concentration and vitality. *Conclusion.* Consistent with other studies, our results show strong association between semen quality and FSH and Inhibin B.

1. Introduction

Male infertility is found in 50% of infertile couples [1]. When reviewed, 55% of the reasons for infertility are found to be male-related and 35% to be female-related, while 10% constitutes infertility of unknown origin [2].

The etiology of declining male fertility can be related to falling androgen levels, decreased sexual activity, alterations in sperm motility and morphology, and deterioration in sperm quality and DNA integrity [3].

Previous studies have reported that circulating levels of specific reproductive hormones in men are associated with semen quality parameters [4]. In particular, Inhibin B and follicle-stimulating hormone (FSH) are thought to be markers of spermatogenesis and Sertoli cell function, and it has even been suggested that measuring the two hormones in serum could serve as a substitute for measuring semen quality or fecundability in epidemiologic studies [4].

Inhibin B is a heterodimeric glycoprotein composed of a common α-subunit and a specific βB-subunit [5]. In men, this protein is produced exclusively by the testis [5]. Inhibin B production is stimulated by the secretion of pituitary follicle-stimulating hormone (FSH). The resulting Inhibin B exerts a negative feedback on FSH secretion. Inhibin B also exerts a paracrine intratesticular effect [5]. The assessment of testicular function typically involves an initial endocrine assessment, in which serum FSH and total testosterone levels are routinely measured [6, 7]. When measured, Inhibin B levels correlate quite well with FSH concentrations in the vast majority of cases. However, the diagnostic accuracy of FSH is limited by the fact that some conditions do not lead to changes in FSH secretion [5]. FSH and Inhibin B are complementary tools in gonadal male conditions and andrological diagnostics [5, 8]. In particular, FSH and Inhibin B together are more sensitive than either alone in predicting the histological status of the testis and the presence of sperm in bioptic tissue [5].

This study is designed to study levels of follicle-stimulating hormone (FSH), and Inhibin B in blood serum, and their relation to seminal fluid functional parameters in a group of infertile patients.

2. Material and Methods

2.1. Subject Recruitment. The study population comprised healthy men referred for semen analysis to some private laboratories and health institutions. Our men subjects were members of infertile and fertile couples. For a given individual, the semen and blood samples were provided on the same day. All the participants gave their written informed consent.

2.2. Study Design. This cross-sectional study was carried out at six Public health institutions and Private laboratories of the Yaoundé Town. These centers are located in the political capital of Cameroon, and receive a large number of male patients living in Yaoundé and surrounding towns. A convenient sample of 240 infertile male patients, aged 18 years and above, were consecutively enrolled in the study during twelve months. But only 156 succeeded in providing both semen and blood samples. All the procedures used in this study were in accordance with the current revision of the Helsinki Declaration. A written and signed informed consent was provided by all the subjects. Consent forms and procedures, as well as survey protocol, were approved by the Cameroon National Ethics Committee (Reference number: 2015/04/572/CE/CNERSH/SP).

2.3. Interview Data. At enrollment standardized data collection forms were completed, including sociodemographic characteristics, the medical background, previous unions, chirurgical background, and sexuality.

2.4. Collection of Semen Samples. Semen was collected by masturbation into a sterile plastic specimen cup at the hospital or laboratory. Subjects were instructed to abstain from ejaculation for at least 72 hours prior to producing the semen sample. The actual abstinence period was recorded based on the information given by men at the time of the semen collection .The sample was liquefied for at least 30 minutes at 37°C, but no longer than 1 hour prior to performing a routine semen analysis, which included measurements of volume, pH, sperm concentration, sperm motility, progressive motility, and sperm morphology according to standard methodologies [9].

2.5. Evaluation of the Quality of Sperm. Before starting semen analysis, a period of time must be allowed for liquefaction. The normal liquefaction time is 30 minutes. If this is not done within this time, we will say that it is slow rather than normal. The semen volume, total sperm number, sperm concentration, motility, and vitality were interpreted according to the 2010 WHO guidelines.

Strict scoring criteria were used to classify men as having normal or subnormal morphology [9] as recommended by WHO guidelines. Kruger's classification identifies a single sperm anomaly. The anomaly is listed in order of importance as follows: acrosome, head, intermediate piece and flagella. As soon as an abnormality is identified, the spermatozoon is directly classified as "abnormal".

2.6. Determination of Biochemical Parameters. Venous blood samples were taken from the cubital vein. The samples were left for 30 min at room temperature, then centrifuged at 3000 rpm for 15 minutes at room temperature. The sera were transported to small Eppendorf tubes and stored at −20°C. The serum Inhibin B was determined in duplicate using the Inhibin B Gen II ELISA technic of Beckman Coulter (250 S. Kraemer Blvd. Brea, CA 92821 U.S.A.) which is an enzymatically amplified three-step "sandwich" assay. In the assay, calibrators, controls and samples are incubated in microtitration wells which have been coated with anti-activin B antibody [10]. Serum FSH levels were measured with a Microplate Immunoenzymometric assay of Monobind Inc. (IEMA/ELISA) (100 North pointe Drive, Lake Forest, CA 92630 U.S.A.).

2.7. Statistical Analysis. Data were coded and entered in Excel 2013, then analyzed using XLSTAT 2014. Semen parameters and hormone levels were expressed as the median (5th–95th percentiles). The Mann–Whitney U test was used to compare the reference and case groups.

Relationships between hormone levels and semen parameters were analyzed using Spearman's correlation test.

The evaluation of the parameters is based on the World Health Organization criteria.

Different aspects of semen analysis are discussed, such as enumeration of spermatozoa, viability, Kruger classification and interpretation of results.

Normozoospermia (reference group) corresponded to a total sperm count ≥20 million/ejaculate, progressive motility ≥32% (as defined in the 2010 WHO manual), and normal forms ≥15% (as defined in our laboratory).

A p value <0.05 was used to characterize significant results.

3. Results

3.1. Semen Characteristics and Hormone Level Distributions of the Study Population. We recruited a total of 240 men but only 156 of them actually provided blood and semen samples for analysis. Of these, 48 presented semen parameters within the reference limits and thus constituted the reference group (Normospermic). In contrast, 108 men presented at least one abnormal semen parameter (as defined above) and thus constituted the case group.

The mean age of our population was 37.101 ± 7.371 years and the majority classes were those aged 30–35 followed by those aged 40–45.

Our patients had on average one child and the type of infertility found was more secondary (53.846%).

Table 1 presents the semen characteristics and hormone level distributions of our population. We found a significant difference in the two groups regarding sperm concentration ($p < 0.0001$), total sperm count ($p < 0.0001$), progressive motility ($p < 0.0001$), vitality ($p < 0.0001$) and the percentage of normal forms ($p = 0.043$). No statistical difference has been

Table 1: Semen characteristics of the study population. Data are reported as the median (5th–95th percentiles). Comparison between the reference group and the case group was performed using a Mann–Whitney U test.

Characteristics of the population	Overall population	Reference group	Case group	Normal values	p
Age (years)	37 (26–50)	37.6 (27–49.6)	36.5 (23.8–48.8)	NA	0.385
Number of children	1 (0–4)	1 (0–4)	1 (0–5)	NA	0.471
Abstinence (days)	3 (2–6)	3 (2–6)	3 (3–7)	3–5 days	0.441
Semen volume (mL)	2.92 (0.96–5.5)	2.95 (0.72–5.6)	2.8 (1.2–4.46)	≥2 mL	0.923
pH	8.31 (7.5–9)	8.32 (7.6–9)	8.3 (7.5–9)	≥7,2	0.594
Viscosity	1 (0–3)	1 (0–3)	1 (0–3)	0	0.431
Sperm concentration (million/mL)	14.8 (0.2–70.2)	10.8 (0.03–54.6)	39.6 (2.1–78.8)	$\geq 20\times 10^6$/l	**<0.0001**
Total sperm count (million/ejaculate)	33 (0–194.08)	12.42 (0–109.1)	122.12 (14.83–300.28)	$\geq 40\times 10^6$	**<0.0001**
Progressive motility (%)	43.2 (2–76)	35.3 (0–72.6)	64 (45.6–80.6)	≥50%	**<0.0001**
Vitality (%)	53 (10.8–85.2)	45.8 (9.4–81.4)	72 (56.4–86.6)	≥50%	**<0.0001**
Normal forms (%)	85 (67–94)	84 (65.8–94)	87 (74.8–92.6)	≥85%	**0.043**

$p < 0.05$ was considered to be statistically significant. The significant values are $p < 0.0001$ and $p = 0.043$.

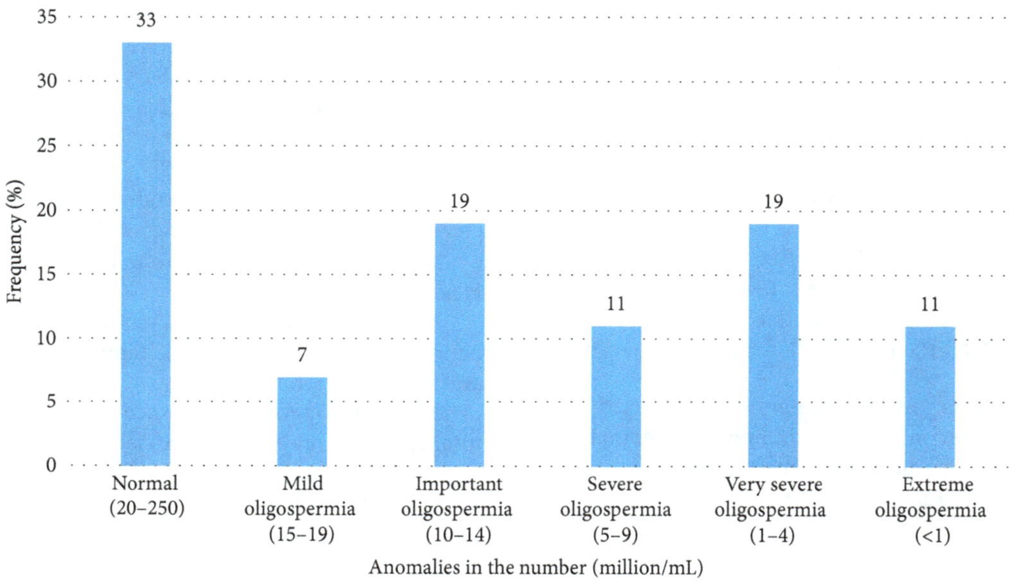

Figure 1: Distribution of the population according to anomalies in numbers.

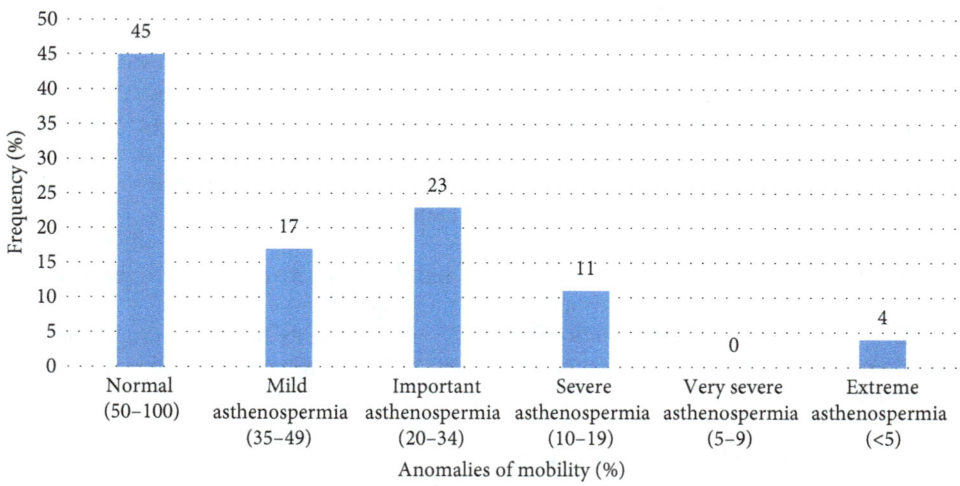

Figure 2: Distribution of the population according to mobility anomalies.

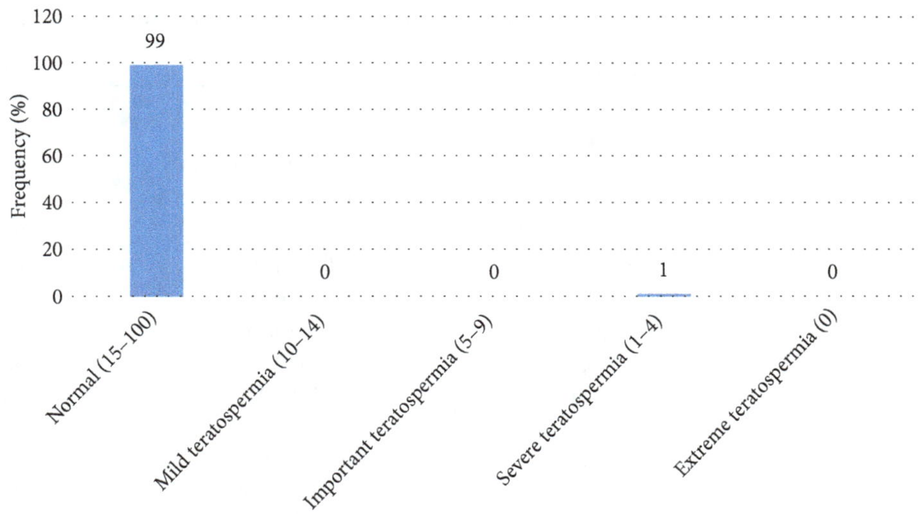

Figure 3: Distribution of the population based on morphology abnormalities.

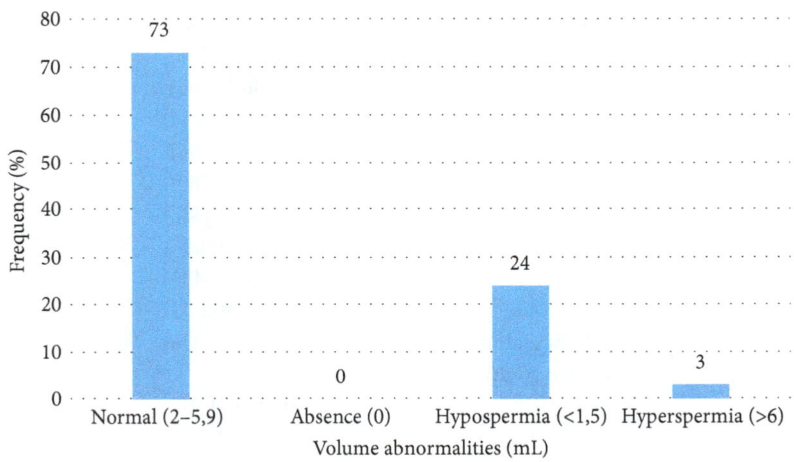

Figure 4: Distribution of the population according to volume anomalies.

Table 2: Distribution of the population according to the level of hormone FSH and Inhibin B.

Characteristics of the population	Overall population	Reference group	Case group	Normal values	p
Inhibin B (pg/mL)	139.1 (10.33–373.72)	153.2 (44.5–389.7)	125.94 (9.8–311.44)	>30 pg/mL	**0.013**
FSH (UI/L)	5.53 (0.2–29.4)	3.78 (0.1–34.93)	6.63 (0.24–28.62)	Young man: <5 UI/L Adult: 3–15 UI/L Andropause (>40 years): 37–100 UI/L	**0.020**

$p < 0.05$ was considered to be statistically significant. The significant values are $p = 0.013$ and $p = 0.020$ which is less than 0.05.

found regarding age, number of children, days of abstinence, semen volume, pH, and viscosity ($p > 0.05$).

Figure 1 presents the distribution of the population based on the anomalies in the number. It appears that in terms of frequency, patients with significant oligospermia were execo with those with very severe oligospermia (19%).

Concerning mobility abnormalities, (Figure 2) shows that 23% of patients had significant asthenospermia, 17% a mild asthenospermia and 11% a severe asthenospermia.

The abnormalities of morphologies are presented in Figure 3. We note that 99% of the patients had a normal sperm morphology.

The study of abnormalities in sperm volume (Figure 4) shows that 73% had a normal sperm volume, 24% were hypospermia, and 3% were hyperspermia.

Also, in a general point of view, about 46% of our infertile patients presented associations of the abnormalities cited above cited above (morphology, mobility, number and volume).

TABLE 3: Relationship between hormone levels and semen parameters. Correlation was done using spearman correlation test.

Semen parameters	Population	Inhibin B (r; p)	FSH (r; p)
	Overall population	0.139 (0.096)	−0.004 (0.966)
Semen volume (mL)	Reference group	**0.528*** **($p < 0.0001$)**	−0.284 (0.051)
	Case group	0.058 (0.553)	0.065 (0.504)
	Overall population	−0.049 (0.562)	0.024 (0.779)
Viscosity	Reference group	−0.045 (0.761)	0.102 (0.488)
	Case group	−0.083 (0.393)	−0.006 (0.949)
	Overall population	−0.117 (0.163)	0.159 (0.057)
pH	Reference group	−0.283 (0.052)	0.223 (0.127)
	Case group	−0.110 (0.258)	0.152 (0.116)
	Overall population	**0.183*** **(0.028)**	**−0.217*** **(0.009)**
Sperm concentration (million/mL)	Reference group	0.043 (0.771)	−0.001 (0.992)
	Case group	0.006 (0.948)	−0.113 (0.243)
	Overall population	**0.307*** **($p < 0.0001$)**	**−0.179*** **(0.032)**
Total sperm count (million/ejaculate)	Reference group	0.245 (0.093)	−0.045 (0.762)
	Case group	**0.261*** **(0.006)**	**−0.197*** **(0.041)**
	Overall population	0.103 (0.219)	**−0.197*** **(0.018)**
Vitality (%)	Reference group	−0.159 (0.280)	0.024 (0.869)
	Case group	−0.056 (0.565)	−0.112 (0.249)
	Overall population	0.072 (0.388)	−0.152 (0.069)
Progressive motility (%)	Reference group	0.046 (0.755)	−0.062 (0.674)
	Case group	−0.032 (0.744)	−0.036 (0.709)
	Overall population	0.088 (0.296)	0.005 (0.956)
Normal forms (%)	Reference group	0.041 (0.780)	0.064 (0.664)
	Case group	−0.084 (0.387)	−0.010 (0.922)
	Overall population	**0.227*** **(0.006)**	0.025 (0.764)
Leucocytes	Reference group	−0.103 (0.486)	−0.036 (0.805)
	Case group	**0.207*** **(0.032)**	0.006 (0.949)
	Overall population	−0.073 (0.386)	−0.004 (0.958)
Red blood cells	Reference group	/	/
	Case group	−0.030 (0.757)	0.075 (0.437)
	Overall population	−0.027 (0.747)	−0.040 (0.635)
Round cells	Reference group	**−0.301*** **(0.038)**	0.024 (0.872)
	Case group	0.070 (0.473)	0.067 (0.492)

$p < 0.05$, $p$was considered to be statistically significant. *Significant. The significant values in this table are $p < 0.0001$, $p = 0.028$, $p = 0.006$, $p = 0.032$, $p = 0.038$, $p = 0.09$, $p = 0.018$ and $p = 0.041$.

Table 2 shows the hormonal distributions of our population. We found that FSH was significantly higher in the case group ($p = 0.020$). In contrast, the level of Inhibin B was lower in the case group ($p = 0.013$).

The analysis of the hormone concentrations according to the age classes have shown a great increase of FSH with years ($p < 0.0001$) and a decrease of Inhibin B concentration ($p = 0.328$).

3.2. Correlations between Hormone Levels and Semen Parameters. Relationship between hormone levels and semen parameters have been studied in Table 3 and we have noticed in the **overall population**, a positive correlation between Inhibin B and sperm concentration ($p = 0.028$; $r = 0.183$), total sperm count ($p < 0.0001$; $r = 0.307$) and leucocytes ($p = 0.006$; $r = 0.227$); while a negative correlation between FSH and sperm concentration ($p = 0.009$; $r = -0.217$), total sperm count ($p = 0.032$; $r = -0.179$) and vitality ($p = 0.018$; $r = -0.197$). In the **reference group**, we noted a positive correlation between Inhibin B and the volume ($p < 0.0001$; $r = 0.528$) and a negative correlation between Inhibin B and the round cells ($p = 0.038$; $r = -0.301$). Finally, the **case group** showed positive correlation between Inhibin B and total sperm count ($p = 0.006$; $r = 0.261$) and leucocytes and a negative correlation between FSH and the total sperm count ($p = 0.041$; $r = -0.197$).

We found a strong and negative correlation between FSH and Inhibin B ($r = -0.477$; $p < 0.0001$) in the overall population, the normozoospermic group (reference group) ($r = -0.367$; $p = 0.011$), and the case group ($r = -0.511$; $p < 0.0001$).

We analyzed the relationship between semen parameters in our population. Table 4 shows that, in the overall population, **positive** correlation has been found between the volume and Total sperm count ($r = 0.235$) and leucocytes ($r = 0.187$); the sperm concentration and total sperm count ($r = 0.636$), vitality ($r = 0.540$), mobility ($r = 0.551$), red blood cells ($r = 0.232$), and

TABLE 4: Relationship between semen parameters in the overall population. Correlation was done using spearman correlation test.

Variables	Volume (mL)	Viscosity	pH	Sperm concentration (spz/ml)	Total sperm count (spz/ejaculate)	Vitality (1 h) %	Motility (1 h) %	Normal forms	Leucocytes	Red blood cells	Round cells
Volume (mL)	**1**	−0.087	**−0.215***	−0.122	**0.235***	0.138	0.160	0.097	**0.187***	−0.065	−0.005
Viscosity	−0.087	**1**	0.063	−0.025	−0.033	−0.027	−0.037	−0.122	**−0.192***	0.005	−0.087
pH	**−0.215***	0.063	**1**	−0.136	**−0.185***	−0.058	−0.069	0.121	−0.110	−0.043	−0.091
Sperm concentration (spz/ml)	−0.122	−0.025	−0.136	**1**	**0.636***	**0.540***	**0.551***	0.076	**−0.199***	**0.232***	**0.232***
Total sperm count (spz/ejaculate)	**0.235***	−0.033	**−0.185***	**0.636***	**1**	**0.525***	**0.520***	**0.249***	**0.238***	**−0.391***	−0.161
Vitality (1 h) %	0.138	−0.027	−0.058	**0.540***	**0.525***	**1**	**0.969***	**0.267***	0.044	−0.026	0.116
Motility (1 h) %	0.160	−0.037	−0.069	**0.551***	**0.520***	**0.969***	**1**	**0.269***	0.020	−0.018	0.148
Normal forms	0.097	−0.122	0.121	0.076	**0.249***	**0.267***	**0.269***	**1**	**0.231***	**−0.194***	−0.114
Leucocytes	**0.187***	**−0.192***	−0.110	**−0.199***	**0.238***	0.044	0.020	**0.231***	**1**	**−0.525***	**−0.226***
Red blood cells	−0.065	0.005	−0.043	**0.232***	**−0.391***	−0.026	−0.018	**−0.194***	**−0.525***	**1**	**0.614***
Round cells	−0.005	−0.087	−0.091	**0.232***	−0.161	0.116	0.148	−0.114	**−0.226***	**0.614***	**1**

$p < 0.05$ was considered to be statistically significant. *Significant. All the values marked with asterix (*) are significant ($p<0.05$).

TABLE 5: Relationship between semen parameters in the reference group. Correlation was done using spearman correlation test.

Variables	Volume (mL)	Viscosity	pH	Sperm concentration (spz/ml)	Total sperm count (spz/ejaculate)	Vitality (1 h) %	Motility (1 h) %	Normal forms	Leucocytes	Round cells
Volume (mL)	**1**	−0.078	−0.051	0.003	**0.286***	0.006	0.142	0.037	0.071	−0.151
Viscosity	−0.078	**1**	0.007	−0.118	−0.095	0.082	0.087	−0.145	−0.184	0.001
pH	−0.051	0.007	**1**	**−0.349***	**−0.296***	0.115	0.002	0.200	0.038	0.124
Sperm concentration (spz/ml)	0.003	−0.118	**−0.349***	**1**	**0.793***	−0.051	0.110	−0.129	0.115	−0.010
Total sperm count (spz/ejaculate)	**0.286***	−0.095	**−0.296***	**0.793***	**1**	−0.245	−0.031	−0.087	0.208	0.007
Vitality (1 h) %	0.006	0.082	0.115	−0.051	−0.245	**1**	**0.799***	−0.211	−0.027	0.211
Motility (1 h) %	0.142	0.087	0.002	0.110	−0.031	**0.799***	**1**	−0.072	0.104	0.267
Normal forms	0.037	−0.145	0.200	−0.129	−0.087	−0.211	−0.072	**1**	−0.045	−0.113
Leucocytes	0.071	−0.184	0.038	0.115	0.208	−0.027	0.104	−0.045	**1**	**0.654***
Round cells	−0.151	0.001	0.124	−0.010	0.007	0.211	0.267	−0.113	**0.654***	**1**

$p < 0.05$ was considered to be statistically significant. *Significant.All the values marked with asterix (*) are significant ($p<0.05$).

round cells ($r = 0.232$); the total sperm count and vitality ($r = 0.525$), motility ($r = 0.520$), normal forms ($r = 0.249$), and leucocytes ($r = 0.238$); the vitality and mobility ($r = 0.969$) and normal forms ($r = 0.267$); the motility and normal forms ($r = 0.269$); the normal forms and leucocytes ($r = 0.231$); the red blood cells and round cells ($r = 0.614$). On the other hand, we observed a **negative** correlation between the volume and pH ($r = -0.215$); the sperm concentration and leucocytes ($r = -0.199$); the total sperm count and pH ($r = -0.185$) and red blood cells ($r = -0.391$); the normal forms and red blood cells

TABLE 6: Relationship between semen parameters in the case group. Correlation was done using spearman correlation test.

Variables	Volume (mL)	Viscosity	pH	Sperm concentration (spz/ml)	Total sperm count (spz/ejaculate)	Vitality (1 h) %	Motility (1 h) %	Normal forms	Leucocytes	Red blood cells	Round cells
Volume (mL)	1	−0.072	**−0.235***	−0.109	**0.193***	0.101	0.121	0.084	**0.191***	−0.054	0.043
Viscosity	−0.072	1	0.061	0.059	−0.005	0.084	0.043	−0.131	**−0.214***	0.013	−0.112
pH	**−0.235***	0.061	1	−0.021	−0.179	−0.083	−0.072	**0.194***	**−0.206***	−0.051	−0.078
Sperm concentration (spz/ml)	−0.109	0.059	−0.021	1	**0.597***	**0.367***	**0.420***	0.070	**−0.258***	0.146	0.153
Total sperm count (spz/ejaculate)	**0.193***	−0.005	−0.179	**0.597***	1	**0.347***	**0.407***	0.141	0.145	**−0.313***	−0.125
Vitality (1 h) %	0.101	0.084	−0.083	**0.367***	**0.347***	1	**0.904***	0.089	−0.079	0.059	0.112
Motility (1 h) %	0.121	0.043	−0.072	**0.420***	**0.407***	**0.904***	1	0.163	−0.111	0.045	0.142
Normal forms	0.084	−0.131	**0.194***	0.070	0.141	0.089	0.163	1	0.146	−0.111	−0.109
Leucocytes	**0.191***	**−0.214***	**−0.206***	**−0.258***	0.145	−0.079	−0.111	0.146	1	**−0.392***	−0.158
Red blood cells	−0.054	0.013	−0.051	0.146	**−0.313***	0.059	0.045	−0.111	**−0.392***	1	**0.626***
Round cells	0.043	−0.112	−0.078	0.153	−0.125	0.112	0.142	−0.109	−0.158	**0.626***	1

$p < 0.05$ was considered to be statistically significant. * Significant. All the values marked with asterix (*) are significant ($p < 0.05$).

($r = -0.194$); the red blood cells and leucocytes ($r = -0.525$); the leucocytes and round cells ($r = -0.226$) and viscosity ($r = -0.192$).

As shown in Table 5, in the reference population the correlation between semen parameters showed a **positive** correlation between volume and total sperm count ($r = 0.286$); the total sperm count and sperm concentration ($r = 0.793$); the vitality and motility ($r = 0.799$); leucocytes and round cells ($r = 0.654$). We also noticed a **negative** correlation between pH and sperm concentration ($r = -0.349$) and total sperm count ($r = -0.296$).

Concerning the correlation between semen parameters in the case group (Table 6), it appears a **positive** correlation between volume and the total sperm count ($r = 0.193$) and the leucocytes ($r = 0.191$); the pH and normal forms ($r = 0.194$); the sperm concentration and total sperm count ($r = 0.597$), vitality ($r = 0.367$) and motility ($r = 0.420$); the total sperm count and vitality ($r = 0.347$) and motility ($r = 0.407$); the red blood cells and round cells ($r = 0.626$); vitality and motility ($r = 0.904$). We also found a **negative** correlation between the pH and volume ($r = -0.235$) and leucocytes ($r = -0.206$); Leucocytes and viscosity ($r = -0.214$); total sperm count and red blood cells ($r = -0.313$); sperm concentration and leucocytes ($r = -0.258$); Leucocytes and red blood cells ($r = -0.392$).

4. Discussion

Previous studies have reported that circulating levels of specific reproductive hormones in men are associated with sperm quality parameters [4]. In particular, Inhibin B and FSH are considered markers of Sertoli spermatogenesis and cell function. It has even been suggested that measurement of both hormones in serum may be a substitute for measuring sperm quality or fecundability in epidemiological studies [4].

The current study analyzes blood levels of Inhibin B and FSH and their relationship with semen parameters.

In line with previous studies [11, 12, 22–29] we found that the infertile men's group was older than the reference group (with majority age classes from 30 to 35 followed by 40 to 45). This is probably the age at which men feel the need to start a family. More than 58% of our population had an advanced age of paternity (>35 years). In addition, we observed a great increase of FSH with years and a decrease of Inhibin concentration. The literature describes a positive and significant correlation between age and number of children, duration of infertility and marital status. This could be explained by the fact that as men age, testicular function and metabolism deteriorate when the testes undergo age-related morphological changes such as decreased germ cell counts, Leydig cells, and Sertoli, as well as structural changes, including shrinkage of seminiferous tubules [30, 31].

In men inhibin is secreted from the testis as a product of Sertoli cells involved in the regulation of FSH secretion [33]. We found a strong and negative correlation between FSH and Inhibin B in the overall population, the case and the reference group. This corroborates very well the findings of Barbotin et al. [5], Jensen et al. [32], and Von Eckardstein et al. [33], stating that FSH and Inhibin B are complementary tools in gonadal male conditions and andrological diagnostics [5]. In particular, FSH and Inhibin B together are more sensitive than either alone in predicting the histological status of the testis and the presence of sperm in bioptic tissue [5]. FSH which is a gonadotropin that is produced and secreted by the anterior pituitary, acts on Sertoli cells in the seminiferous tubules to initiate spermatogenesis. Sertoli cells secrete Inhibin B, which is a protein hormone. Thus, as found in our study, an association between Inhibin B and sperm concentration was to be expected, since the regulation of both factors is dependent upon Sertoli cell function [4, 5, 14].

In the overall population and the case group, Inhibin B was significantly and positively correlated with sperm concentration while FSH was negatively correlated to sperm concentration. We could not observe this correlation in the normospermic group. These findings confirmed those of Jorgensen et al. in 2010 [15], Kumanov et al. in 2006 [16], Myers et al. in 2008 [17], Sikaris et al. in 2005 [18] and Grunewald et al. in 2013 [19]. Moreover, Barbotin et al. explained that associations between hormone levels and sperm count are stronger in studies of the general population [32, 34] or infertile men [4, 16, 17, 35] than in studies of fertile men [15, 17]. They were precise that it could be due to the marked interindividual differences in sperm count seen in populations of primarily normozoospermic and/or fertile men. In total, categories of men (fertile, infertile, and normozoospermic) represented overlap in semen qualities, suggesting that Inhibin B and FSH were not mainly markers of fertility but rather markers of semen quality and thereby fecundity. In addition, It has been suggested that Inhibin B may be a better predictor of spermatogenesis than FSH [33]. The clinical value of the Inhibin B assay is emphasized by the fact that in contrast to FSH, Inhibin B is produced inside the testis and might reflect close interactions between Sertoli and germ cells [33]. Thus, Inhibin B levels correlate directly with spermatogenesis and reflect testicular sperm production.

Although the known association between sperm motility and sperm concentration [17], we could not observe in our population a correlation between sperm motility and Inhibin B and FSH levels but we did observe the correlation between sperm concentration and vitality and mobility both in the overall population and the case group but not in the normospermic group. Considering their overall population, Tomlinson et al. [20] and Karabulut et al. [21] also found a strong correlation between the sperm concentration, the motility and the morphology. Our results are different from Barbotin et al. who observed in their population a relationship between sperm motility and Inhibin B and FSH levels. But just like us they found a strong relationship between sperm concentration and vitality and mobility both in the overall population and the case group but not in the normospermic group. This could be explained by the fact that they included a very large number of individuals compared to our sample size.

5. Conclusion

At the end of this study, our results showed lower values of semen parameters in the case group especially concerning the sperm concentration, the progressive motility, the vitality, and the percentage of normal forms.

The correlation of Inhibin B and FSH to the sperm parameters highlights their role as markers of spermatogenesis. The combination of FSH and Inhibin B is currently the best predictor of the presence of spermatozoa.

Authors' Contributions

Study concept and design: Ngogang Yonkeu Jeanne, Pieme Constant Anatole, and Tchoula Mamiafo Corinne. Data collection: Tchoula Mamiafo Corinne. Statistical analysis: Tchoula Mamiafo Corinne. Drafting: Tchoula Mamiafo Corinne. Manuscript revision: Ngogang Yonkeu Jeanne, Pieme Constant Anatole and Tchoula Mamiafo Corinne. Study supervision: Ngogang Yonkeu Jeanne.

Acknowledgments

This research did not receive any specific grant from any funding agency in the public, commercial or not-for-profit sector.

References

[1] T. G. Cooper, E. Noonan, S. von Eckardstein et al., "World Health Organization referencevalues for human semen characteristics," *Human Reproduction*, vol. 16, pp. 231–245, 2010.

[2] L. Speroff and M. A. Fritz, "Female infertility, Chapter 27," *Clinical Gynecologic Endocrinology and Infertility*, Lippincott Williams & Wilkins, 8th edition, 2010, syf: 1157.

[3] G. Sartorius and E. Nieschlag, "Paternal age and reproduction," *Human Reproduction*, vol. 16, pp. 65–79, 2010.

[4] J. D. Meeker, L. Godfrey-Bailey, and R. Hauser, "Relationships between serum hormone levels and semen quality among men from an infertility clinic," *Journal of Andrology*, vol. 28, no. 3, pp. 397–406, 2007.

[5] A.-L. Barbotin, C. Ballot, J. Sigala et al., "The serum Inhibin B concentration and reference ranges in normozoospermia," *European Journal of Endocrinology*, vol. 172, pp. 669–676, 2015.

[6] B. D. Anawalt, "Approach to male infertility and induction of spermatogenesis," *Journal of Clinical Endocrinology and Metabolism*, vol. 98, no. 9, pp. 3532–3542, 2013.

[7] Practice Committee of American Society for Reproductive Medicine, "Diagnostic evaluation of the infertile male: a committee opinion," *Fertility and Sterility*, vol. 98, no. 2, pp. 294–301, 2012.

[8] V. Mitchell, G. Robin, F. Boitrelle et al., "Correlation between testicular sperm extraction outcomes and clinical, endocrine and testicular histology parameters in 120 azoospermic men with normal serum FSH levels," *International Journal of Andrology*, vol. 34, pp. 299–305, 2011.

[9] Word Health Organization (WHO), *Laboratory Manual for the Examination of Human Semen and Sperm-Cervical Mucus Interaction*, University Press, Cambridge, 4th edition, 1999.

[10] H. Ludlow, S. Muttukrishna, M. Hyvönen, and N. P. Groome, "Development of a new antibody to the human inhibin/activing betaB subunit and its application to improvement Inhibin B ELISAs," *Journal of Immunological Methods*, vol. 329, no. 1–2, pp. 102–111, 2008.

[11] V. Subramanian, A. Ravichandran, N. Thiagarajan, M. Govindarajan, S. Dhandayuthapani, and S. Suresh, "Seminal

reactive oxygen species and total antioxidant capacity: Correlations with sperm parameters and impact on male infertility," *Clinical and Experimental Reproductive Medicine*, vol. 45, no. 2, pp. 88–93, 2018, pISSN 2233-8233, eISSN 2233-8241.

[12] Q. A. Makarim, S. A. Rana, and F. Muhammad-Baqir, "Relationship between lipid peroxidation and integrity of sperm plasma membrane in a sample of iraqi infertile men IOSR," *Journal of Pharmacy and Biological Sciences (IOSR-JPBS)*, vol. 12, no. 6 Ver. I, pp. 19–27, 2017.

[13] C. D. Okafor, S. C. Meludu, K. Nwaefulu, J. I. Ikechebelu, C. E. Dioka, and U. Obi, "Comparison of serum oxidative stress markers among male partners of fertile and infertile couple at Nnamdi Azikiwe University Teaching Hospital, Nnewi, Anambra State," *Nigeria Journal of Scientific and Innovative Research*, vol. 6, no. 4, pp. 126–128, 2017.

[14] F. H. Pierik, J. T. M. Vreeburg, T. Stijnen, F. H. De Jong, and R. F. A. Weber, "Serum Inhibin B as a marker of spermatogenesis," *Journal of Clinical Endocrinology and Metabolism*, 2006, jcem. endojournals.org at Medical Library Erasmus MC on December 11, 0021-972X/98/$03.00/0.

[15] N. Jorgensen, F. Liu, A. M. Andersson et al., "Serum inhibin-b in fertile men is strongly correlated with low but not high sperm counts: a coordinated study of 1,797 European and US men," *Fertility and Sterility*, vol. 94, no. 6, pp. 2128–2134, 2010.

[16] P. Kumanov, K. Nandipati, A. Tomova, and A. Agarwal, "Inhibin B is a better marker of spermatogenesis than other hormones in the evaluation of male factor infertility," *Fertility and Sterility*, vol. 86, no. 2, pp. 332–338, 2006.

[17] G. M. Myers, G. M. Lambert-Messerlian, and M. Sigman, "Inhibin B reference data for fertile and infertile men in Northeast America," *Fertility and Sterility*, vol. 92, pp. 1920–1923, 2009.

[18] K. Sikaris, R. I. McLachlan, R. Kazlauskas, D. de Kretser, C. A. Holden, and D. J. Handelsman, "Reproductive hormone reference intervals for healthy fertile young men: evaluation of automated platform assays," *Journal of Clinical Endocrinology and Metabolism*, vol. 90, pp. 5928–5936, 2005.

[19] S. Grunewald, H.-J. Glander, U. Paasch, and J. Kratzsch, "Age-dependent Inhibin B concentration in relation to FSH and semen sample qualities: a study in 2448 men," *Reproduction*, vol. 14, no. 5, pp. 237–244, 2013.

[20] M. J. Tomlinson, O. Moffatt, G. C. Manicardi, and D. Sakkas, "Interrelationships between seminal parameters and sperm nuclear DNA before and after density gradient centrifugation: implication for assisted conception. European society of human Reproduction and Embryology," *Human Reproduction*, vol. 16, no. 10, pp. 2160–2165, 2001.

[21] S. Karabulut, I. Keskin, and Y. Sagıroglu, "Relationship between semen parameters in samples obtained from sub-fertile," *Andrology (Los Angel)*, vol. 6, no. 1, 2017.

[22] F. Atig, A. Kerkeni, A. Saad, and M. Ajina, "Effects of reduced seminal enzymatic antioxidants on sperm DNA fragmentation and semen quality of Tunisian infertile men," *Journal of Assisted Reproduction and Genetics*, vol. 34, no. 3, pp. 373–381, 2017.

[23] A. Mehrotra, D. K. Katiyar, A. Agarwal, V. Das, and K. K. Pant, "Role of total antioxidant capacity and lipid peroxidation in fertile and infertile men," *Biomedical Research-India*, vol. 24, pp. 347–352, 2013.

[24] M. A. El-Taieb, M. A. Ali, and E. A. Nada, "Oxidative stress and acrosomal morphology: a cause of infertility in patients with normal semen parameters," *Middle East Fertility Society Journal*, vol. 20, no. 2, pp. 79–85, 2015.

[25] T. Kullisaar, S. Turk, K. Kilk, K. Ausmees, M. Punab, and R. Mandar, "Increased levels of hydrogen peroxide and nitric oxide in male partners of infertile couples," *Andrology*, vol. 1, no. 6, pp. 850–858, 2013.

[26] S. Benedetti, M. C. Tagliamonte, S. Catalani et al., "Differences in blood and semen oxidative status in fertile and infertile men, and their relationship with sperm quality," *Reproductive BioMedicine Online*, vol. 25, no. 3, pp. 300–306, 2012.

[27] Y. Gao, Y. Gao, L. Du, Z. Qin, and Z. Hu, "Zinc, lead, cadmium, malondialdehyde contents and superoxide dismutase activity in serum and seminal plasma in male infertility patients," *Journal of Reproductive Medicine*, vol. 21, pp. 43–46, 2012, Article in Chinese.

[28] M. B. Shamsi, R. Kumar, N. Malhotra et al., "Chromosomal aberrations, Yq microdeletion, and sperm DNA fragmentation in infertile men opting for assisted reproduction," *Molecular Reproduction and Development*, vol. 79, no. 9, pp. 637–650, 2012.

[29] O. Alejandro, A. Spira, and L. Multigner, "Contribution of environmental factors to the risk of male infertility," *Human Repoduction*, vol. 16, no. 8, pp. 1768–1776, 2001.

[30] S. Gunes, G. N. Hekim, M. A. Arslan, and R. Asci, " Effects of aging on the male reproductive system," *Journal of Assisted Reproduction and Genetics*, vol. 33, no. 4, pp. 441–454, 2016.

[31] D. Durairajanayagam, " Lifestyle causes of male infertility," *Arab Journal of Urology*, vol. 16, no. 1, pp. 10–20, 2018.

[32] T. K. Jensen, A. M. Andersson, N. H. Hjollund et al., "Inhibin B as a serum marker of spermatogenesis: correlation to differences in sperm concentration and follicle-stimulating hormone levels. A study of 349 Danish men," *Journal of Clinical Endocrinology and Metabolism*, vol. 82, no. 12, pp. 4059–4063, 1997.

[33] S. Von Eckardstein, M. Simoni, M. Bergmann et al., "Serum Inhibin B in combination with serum follicle-stimulating hormone (FSH) is a more sensitive marker than serum FSH alone for impaired spermatogenesis in men, but cannot predict the presence of sperm in testicular tissue samples," *Journal of Clinical Endocrinology and Metabolism*, vol. 84, pp. 2496–2501, 1999.

[34] M. L. Uhler, M. J. Zinaman, C. C. Brown, and E. D. Clegg, "Relationship between sperm characteristics and hormonal parameters in normal couples," *Fertility and Sterility*, vol. 79, pp. 1535–1542, 2003.

[35] F. H. Pierik, A. Burdorf, F. H. de Jong, and R. F. Weber, "Inhibin B: a novel marker of spermatogenesis," *Annals of Medicine*, pp. 3512–3520, 2003.

11

Involvement of Male Partners in Skilled Birth Care in the North Dayi District, Ghana

Farrukh Ishaque Saah[1] **Elvis Enowbeyang Tarkang,**[2] **Joyce Komesuor,**[2] **Eric Osei**[2] **Evelyn Acquah**[3] **and Hubert Amu**[2]

[1]*Department of Epidemiology and Biostatistics, School of Public Health, University of Health and Allied Sciences, Hohoe, Ghana*
[2]*Department of Population and Behavioural Sciences, School of Public Health, University of Health and Allied Sciences, Hohoe, Ghana*
[3]*Institute of Health Research, University of Health and Allied Sciences, Ho, Ghana*

Correspondence should be addressed to Farrukh Ishaque Saah; fsaahpnur14@uhas.edu.gh

Academic Editor: Hind A. Beydoun

Background. With more than half of the global maternal deaths occurring in sub-Saharan Africa, skilled attendance during childbirth is essential in achieving safer births and lower maternal mortalities. Given that societal ascriptions of gender roles strongly influence the utilisation of skilled care by women, male partner involvement in skilled birth is essential. We explored male partner involvement in skilled birth at the North Dayi District of Ghana. *Methods.* This qualitative study interviewed 14 mothers and their male partners, together with two health professionals. The participants were purposively recruited using in-depth interviews. Data collected were analysed manually, but thematically. *Result.* Male partners had inadequate knowledge of childbirth and the skilled birth process as well as possible complications arising during delivery. Even though the male partners demonstrated positive perception towards skilled birth and their involvement in the process, their actual involvement in skilled birth care was generally low. Factors which inhibited most of the male partners from getting involved in skilled birth care were health facility nonconduciveness and occupation. However, motivations to do so were marital commitment and sense of responsibility, past experience, nearness to health facility, and safety and survival of partner and baby. *Conclusion.* These findings imply that Ghana may not be able to meet the Sustainable Development Goal Three target of reducing its maternal mortality ratio from 216 to below 70 per 100,000 live births by 2030. Stakeholders in Ghana's health industry need to develop male accommodating skilled birth policies and approaches to promote male involvement in skilled birth care.

1. Introduction

The health of a woman during pregnancy and childbirth is essential in reducing maternal mortality and achieving the Sustainable Development Goals (SDGs) [1]. Inherent in goal three of the SDGs is a reduction in the global maternal mortality ratio from 216 per 100,000 live births in 2015 to below 70 per 100,000 live births by the year 2030. The goal is expected to be achieved by ensuring universal access to sexual and reproductive healthcare for all, especially women in their reproductive age. An important aspect of sexual and reproductive healthcare which the goal seeks to achieve is skilled birth [1].

Skilled birth is crucial in ensuring that women obtain quality care and deliver in a setting that is equipped for emergencies [2]. It is seen as a key strategy in the reduction of maternal complications and death [3]. During childbirth, the presence of a skilled birth attendant lessens the possibility of stillbirth or death resulting from complications such as sepsis, eclampsia, and obstructed labour by about 20% [3]. Globally, one in every four births (25%) occur without the assistance of a skilled birth attendant. This results in over 40 million unattended births, particularly in developing countries [3].

Societal ascriptions of gender roles for men and women strongly influence access to skilled birth care for pregnant women [4]. The gender division of roles in households usually makes male partners the heads of their households. Being the heads of their households, the male partners usually decide when and what means of accessing healthcare the family including the women should use [5]. Male partner involvement refers to "the various ways in which men relate to reproductive health problems and programmes, reproductive rights, and reproductive behaviour" ([6], p. 1). Male partner involvement in maternal healthcare also refers to the direct assistance provided by men to improve their partners' and children's health through the perinatal, antenatal, labour, and delivery period [7].

Notwithstanding the fact that male partner involvement plays a key role in the health outcomes of women, many societies and cultures treat pregnancy as solely a women's issue and this may have contributed to men not being invited to learn about and engage in matters related to women's and children's health [8]. Universal reproductive health programmes and services in developing countries have also over the years focused on education of women on maternal healthcare such as skilled birth [9]. Yet, in many of these societies, the decision-making authority regarding when and where to seek skilled birth care is vested in the male partner [9, 10]. Men are dominant in the decision-making process in the household [11]. Hence, women are left with little or no say in matters that affect their own lives, including their reproductive health such as delivery care [11].

Similarly, in Ghana, decisions regarding childbirth are the sole vesture of the male partner. Yet, programmes such as sexual and reproductive health education including care and support during pregnancy and childbirth have over the years mainly focused on women [9, 12]. Even efforts of the free-exemption policy for maternal care programme and Safe Motherhood Initiative geared towards involving men in maternal care and skilled birth are yet to be accepted by the populace [13]. This is because there are still deep-seated perceptions regarding male involving in maternal healthcare which posit that male partners have no active role to play in issues concerning delivery care [14].

In this study, the operational definition for the concept of male partner involvement in skilled delivery care was adapted from Kumar [6] and Ampt et al. [7] as responsibility of men with their partners in all aspects of the skilled delivery process and direct assistance provided by men to improve their partners' and children's health through the perinatal, antenatal, labour, and delivery period, respectively. The focus of male partner involvement in skilled delivery was, therefore, based on their readiness to provide emotional, financial, and physical support and accompany their female partners to facility as well as companying them during skilled delivery period.

The role of men in ensuring the safety of their partners during delivery cannot thus be overemphasised. Many studies have indicated positive impacts of male partner involvement in several reproductive health issues [15, 16]. It is important that the relationship between male partner involvement and skilled birth is also investigated to help increase skilled birth utilisation by pregnant women. There is, therefore, a need to ascertain the correlates of male partner involvement in skilled birth care in Ghana, hence this study.

2. Conceptual Framework

The study adapted two theories, Health Belief Model (HBM) and Healthcare Utilisation Model (HUM), as the conceptual framework. This was in recognition of the fact that both models have tenets which are very relevant to the study and compatible with the objectives of the study. Male partners' perceptions about skilled birth and their involvement in skilled birth process are, for instance, posited by the Health Belief Model. The perceived possibility of any complication arising during the delivery process influences the need to seek skilled birth care while comprehending the benefit of delivery by skilled attendant, as argued by Rosenstock [17] in relation to perceived threats (comprising perceived susceptibility and perceived seriousness) of a health condition. A male partner will therefore recognise the need to be involved in skilled birth if he realises that the threat posed by the delivery process to his partner and unborn child's life is severe (Figure 1).

Both the HBM and HUM recognise the role of knowledge in influencing male partner involvement in skilled birth care. Knowledge about the delivery process and skilled birth care as posited by the sociopsychological variables of the HBM, for instance, affects the kind of perceptions a male partner may have about skilled birth and his involvement in skilled birth care. It is also seen by the enabling factors of the HUM as having direct implications for male partners' involvement in the delivery process in that, as they gain knowledge about the process, their appreciation of the need to be involved also increases.

This study also sought to explore the factors influencing male partner involvement in skilled birth care, which the HUM groups into three categories: sociodemographic (predisposing) factors, health service-related (enabling) factors, and sociologic (reinforcing) factors. These factors shape the roles male partners play in the delivery process such as planning for transportation, blood donation if needed, birth preparedness, and supporting the spouse emotionally and psychologically.

The cues to action from the HBM are also relevant to the factors contributing to male involvement in skilled birth care. Mass media campaigns about skilled birth and its importance, advice from other members of the community, and death or some other form of complications from the delivery process of a family member or friend influence male partners' involvement. Also, health visitor's or a physician's explanation of the potential complications associated with delivery process to male partners as well as how skilled attendant at birth reduces chances of complications during delivery invariably affects their involvement in skilled birth.

The framework shows two possible outcomes of male partner involvement in skilled birth. First of all, it indicates that high male partner involvement stemming from knowledge of delivery process results in positive perception towards skilled birth care and involvement manifested through such actions as physical and emotional and financial support. This will lead to good maternal health outcomes while the opposite is true for low male partner involvement resulting from low knowledge, negative perceptions, and persistent factors which act as barriers (Figure 1).

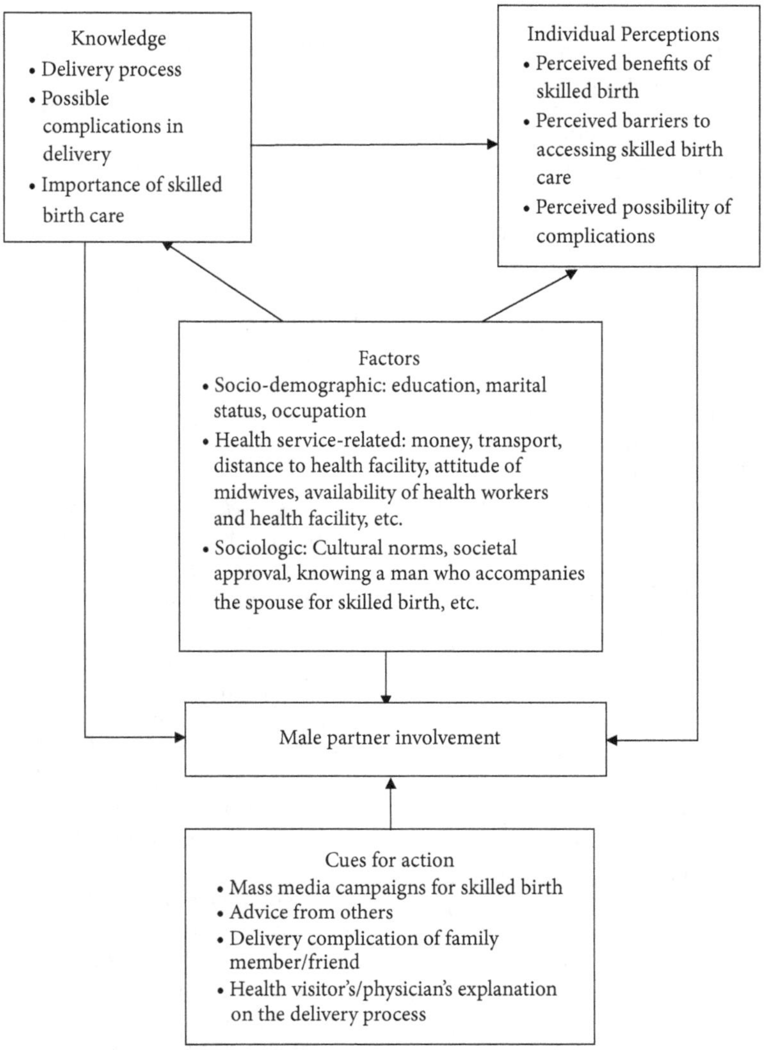

FIGURE 1: Conceptual framework. Source: adapted from Current Nursing (2012) and Andersen and Newman [18].

3. Materials and Methods

3.1. Setting. North Dayi is one of the 25 administrative districts in the Volta Region of Ghana [19]. It is bounded in the north by Kpando Municipality, in the south by South Dayi District, in the east by Afadzato South District, and in the west by the Volta Lake. The 2010 Population and Housing Census of Ghana reports that North Dayi has a population of 39,913, of which females constitute 53.3 % [19]. The Total Fertility Rate for the district is 3.3 births per woman. The General Fertility Rate of the district is 95.0 births per 1,000 women aged 15-49 years. North Dayi has one mission hospital (Anfoega Catholic Hospital), the only top-level facility, and four Community-Based Health Planning and Services (CHPS) zones made up of 23 CHPS compounds. It also has seven (7) health centres with 46 outreach points for rendering Reproductive and Child Health Services [19]. The district has many highlands, creating many hard to reach communities, with very poor road conditions. This makes accessibility to health facilities difficult especially for such communities.

3.2. Study Population and Design. This study was qualitative in nature, adopting an explanatory design. This design was adopted in order to identify the extent and nature of cause-and-effect relationship in relation to male involvement in skilled birth care [20]. The target population for this study comprises women attending CWC at Anfoega Catholic Hospital, their male partners, and midwives who assist the women during skilled birth.

3.3. Procedures. A purposive sampling procedure was used to identify women attending the Child Welfare Clinic (CWC) at the Anfoega Catholic Hospital. The male partners of the women were then traced to their homes. This was done by selecting the women based on the fact that they had undergone labour and delivery within the past five years. The purpose of using women attending CWC was to ensure that all participants have experienced the central phenomenon of this study, skilled birth. The midwife in charge of the maternity unit of the hospital and another midwife were also purposively included in the study. In all, 14 women attending

CWC and their male partners as well as two midwives were included, making a total sample size of 30 participants.

Data for the study were collected by the researcher with the support of two research assistants who were trained for two days to orient them on the purpose of the study and to acquaint them with the research instruments. Women attending Child Welfare Clinic were contacted after their individual sessions and the purpose of the study was explained to them. Those who agreed to participate were included in the study and then led the interviewers to their male partners to also be included. Appointment was booked with the health professional and the interview conducted at her place of convenience, the facility.

In-depth interviews via face-to-face interview procedure were used in collecting data from the participants using three in-depth interview guides. The interview guides were self-developed and used as the instruments for data collection from the three study population groups, women attending CWC, male partners, and the health professionals. Follow-up questions (probes) were asked when necessary in order to obtain detailed insight. The interviews were tape-recorded and notes taken to guarantee accuracy of data that will be collected. Each interview lasted for about 35 minutes.

3.4. Data Analysis. Data collected from the participants were analysed using manual thematic analysis. All the recorded interviews, including notes, were transcribed and those not in English were translated and transcribed into English. After this, the transcripts were read and edited by listening to the tapes again and resolving possible omissions and additions in the original transcripts. Codes were combined to form broader themes based on the research objectives as well as themes which emerged from the data itself. Quotes from the participants were used in presenting the data so as to substantiate issues discussed. A frequency table was, however, used to present the sociodemographic characteristics of the participants. Also, level of male partner involvement was determined by comparing roles of male partners played towards and during the skilled delivery period with the operational definition of male partner involvement in skilled delivery care as adopted for this study [6, 7].

3.5. Ethical Issues. Ethical approval for the study was granted by the Ghana Health Service Ethical Review Committee (Reference number: GHS-ERC: 63/05/17) before the study was conducted. Permission was taken from the District Health Management Team administration, community leaders (including chiefs and assembly members), and management of the hospital. Written consent was obtained from the participants before including them in the study. This study also ensured the highest level of confidentiality and anonymity in information disclosed to us.

4. Results

4.1. Sociodemographic Characteristics of Participants. Table 1 presents the sociodemographic characteristics of the 30 participants for this study. Of them, 46.7%, purposefully selected, were mothers, while 6.6% were health professionals and the rest were the male partners. The health professionals were a senior staff midwife and a medical doctor in charge of obstetrics. The participants were aged from 24 and 46 years. A comparative majority (43.3%) were in their late 20s while those who were 40 years and above constituted 6.7%. About 60% were cohabiting and 40% were married at the time of the study. About 73.3% of the participants were Christians and the rest were Muslims. Most of the participants were Ewes (70%) while Guans had the least representation with 10%. Level of education among the participants ranged from JHS to Degree.

4.2. Male Partners' Knowledge of Childbirth and the Skilled Birth Process

4.2.1. Knowledge of Childbirth and the Delivery Process. Responses from the female participants and their male partners as well as the health professionals point to the fact that male partners did not have adequate knowledge of childbirth and the delivery process. Concerning male partners not having or demonstrating having knowledge of childbirth and delivery process, a 22-year-old mother said, *"My partner did not do anything to show that he knows something about childbirth and the processes involved in it"*. A male partner, 33 years, also said, *"I don't have much knowledge on it (skilled birth), and I don't need to know because the doctors are there to help us"*.

4.2.2. Knowledge of Complications Occurring during the Delivery Process. Most of the male partners did not have adequate knowledge of the possible complications during delivery. A few of them were, however, aware of vaginal bleeding, prolonged labour, sepsis, swollen hands and feet, placenta retention, eclampsia, breached delivery, stillbirth, and the need for Caesarean section in some instances as some of the complication emanating from childbirth and the delivery process. Regarding male partners not having knowledge of possible complications that can arise during delivery, one of the health professionals, 29 years, for instance said, *"Not all of them are aware of the possible problems. Only a few of them do"*. A 32-year-old male partner also opined, *"No. I don't have any knowledge on this (complications occurring during delivery)"*. A mother, 24-year-old, also noted, *"He was able to identify when I lost appetite for food and got worried, but he doesn't know of any of the possible complications that can occur"*.

4.3. Perception of Male Partners Regarding Skilled Birth and Their Involvement in the Delivery Process

4.3.1. Perception of What Constitutes Male Partner Involvement. There were similarities in the way the women and their male partners perceived male partner involvement in skilled birth care. To both groups, it entails the man being present, providing support, and making provisions to ensure safe delivery, as well as making decisions as the head of the household, but in connection with ensuring a safe child birth, paying bills and providing money for feeding during the

TABLE 1: Sociodemographic characteristics of participants.

Sociodemographic variable	Frequency	Percentage (%)
Participant Type		
Mother	14	46.7
Male Partner	14	46.7
Health Professional	2	6.6
Age		
20-24	3	10.0
25-29	13	43.3
30-34	7	23.3
35-39	5	16.7
40+	2	6.7
Sex		
Male	15	50.0
Female	15	50.0
Marital status		
Co-habiting	18	60.0
Married	12	40.0
Religion		
Christian	22	73.3
Muslim	8	26.7
Ethnicity		
Ewe	21	70.0
Akan	6	20.0
Guan	3	10.0
Level of education		
JHS/Middle school	9	30.0
SHS/O' Level/A' Level	17	56.7
Tertiary	4	13.3

period. A 27-year-old mother, for instance, said, "*I think he is supposed to be beside me, to feel for me and to tell me 'sorry dear' in the period of labour pains*". Among the males, a 37-year-old partner stated,

> *I understand it (male partner involvement) to mean that the man should be present and take care of the woman during childbirth. It also implies accompanying your wife to the hospital and providing financial support to ensure the baby is born safely. Even making provisions for blood if she needs it during delivery process is my responsibility at that crucial time.*
>
> *- Male partner, 37 years*

The health professionals corroborated the perceptions of both the mothers and the partners regarding what male partner involvement in skilled birth care is. One of them noted,

> *It (male partner involvement) is about the woman's husband or spouse taking part in the labour and delivery process of their baby by involving himself in all the activities of the delivery process and providing the needed care and support to the woman.*
>
> *- Health professional, female, 29 years*

4.3.2. Perception of Skilled Birth. All the participants acknowledged that the male partners perceive skilled birth care as the best option for delivery. The majority linked their perceptions to the preparedness of the health facilities to attend adequately to complications that may arise during delivery. This view was expressed in the following quote:

> *Yes! it is good. Sometimes, in the house, they cannot take care of the woman because we, the house people don't know what is going on in the lady. But doctors or nurses at the hospital will know and do something else to make sure the woman and the baby are safe.*
>
> *- Male partner, 46 years*

A 24-year-old mother also said, "*He (her male partner) sees delivery at home as dangerous compared to delivery at the hospital. Home delivery does not have anything to detect complications like baby not turning right*". Even though the health professionals agreed that male partners perceive skilled birth as a better option compared to home delivery, they also added that some male partners have the view that a person who had previously given birth at home did not have to seek skilled birth care in subsequent deliveries. One of them opined,

> *They see it (skilled birth) to be the best option as compared to the home delivery especially because of the infections and complications that occur during delivery. For instance, today we had a case of a lady delivering at home before coming with bleeding. Some of them, however, think that when the lady has delivered at home before, it is not necessary for the lady to delivered at the hospital but sometimes it is not the best.*
>
> *– Health professional, female, 29 years*

4.3.3. Perception of Male Partner Involvement in Skilled Birth Process. Participants were asked questions which sought to elicit their perception of male partners' involvement in skilled birth care. To the participants, male partners being involved in the delivery process is a good thing and should be encouraged. One of the health professionals, for instance, had this to say:

> *I think it is an essential component of the delivery process and I think it really helps in the delivery. Most women who come with their partners you are able to see the difference between those who do not come with their partners. When it comes to finances, especially. When the partners are there, anything you ask they provide for. Otherwise they delay us in calling on the partner to get those items. Even though some of them their partners give them money, it almost always not enough. So, when the partner too come it shows that they are really prepared.*
>
> *– Health professional, female, 29 years*

A mother also said,

> *I see that his (male partner's) involvement is good and not time wasting as some people would want to make it look like. This is because when there is a problem during the delivery it is all his burden and so, if he is there with me, it makes things easier for me and he is also able to see what is going on.*
>
> *– Mother, 38 years*

A male partner had this to say:

> *It is a good thing that male partners get involve (in the skilled birth process). Sending someone else to lead her to the hospital or be with her, that person cannot get the needs of my wife that will be requested by the doctors and the nurses done the way I would want and do it. For instance, referrals will require my support to find a car or make the decision and the person may not be able to make that decision for me.*
>
> *– Male partner, 46 years*

4.4. Level of Male Partner Involvement in Skilled Birth. Generally, male partner involvement in skilled birth care was low. More than half of the women and their male partners, respectively, as well as the health professionals noted that the male partners were mostly not involved in the delivery process. They either delegated their roles of accompanying and staying with their partners to a female relative or limited those roles to providing financial support and decision-making regarding where the women should give birth. Regarding the fact that male partners were mostly not involved in the skilled birth process, a male partner had this to say:

> *I did not do much in the delivery process. Besides, the only thing I was supposed to do which I actually did was to give them money for everything needed for the delivery to take place successfully and the hospital bill.*
>
> *– Male partner, 32 years*

A mother also noted,

> *He was not involved at all. He only gave my sister money and asked her to take me to the hospital. In fact, he left for his work place. I did everything by myself and with my sister's support.*
>
> *–Mother, 28 years*

One of the health professionals remarked,

> *Their (male partners) involvement in the delivery process is very low in this area. Most of the men do not do anything else apart from providing money for the woman to buy things needed for the delivery process.*
>
> *– Health professional, female, 29 years*

Regarding male partners deciding the choice of place of delivery during the last birth, a 26-year-old mother said, "*It was my husband's decision for me to give birth at the hospital*". A male partner, 28 years, reported, "*As the man of the house, I was the one who took the decision for her (his female partner) to give birth at the hospital*". One of the health professionals also noted,

> *I think it is the husbands/partners who mainly take the decision regarding where the women should give birth when it is time (for the woman to give birth). We, the health professionals, also influence their decision. I think the health professionals help because they listen to us.*
>
> *–Health professional, female, 29 years*

4.5. Factors Influencing Male Partner Involvement in Skilled Birth Care. It emerged that factors which influenced male partner involvement in skilled birth care fall into two main categories. While some served as motivators for the involvement of a few of the male partners in the delivery process, others served as barriers inhibiting most of them from getting involved in the process.

4.5.1. Motivations for Male Partner Involvement in Skilled Birth Care. The major motivational factors for male partner involvement identified were marital or relationship commitment and male partner's sense of responsibility, past experience, partner's education and occupation, safety and survival of partner and baby, and nearness to health facility.

Concerning show of affection and relationship commitment, the male partners stated that it was because of the commitment they have towards their partners that they maintained the level of involvement during their partner's last delivery while the mothers interpreted that to mean show of love. A male partner noted,

> *I believe that once you're married, there are some things that you need to do to show affection towards your partner. If you love your wife, you have to do these things for her. From my elders, it is something a man should do and that is why I supported her.*
>
> *- Male partner, 46 years*

Regarding male partner's responsibility, the mothers whose male partners supported them said their partners considered it their responsibility to be involved. A 24-year-old mother, for instance, said, "*He knew it was his responsibility that was why. He knew that I was not working so he was supposed to take care of everything*".

With regard to the safety of the mother and baby, both mothers and their male partners indicated that male partners were motivated to be involved because they wanted to ensure the safety and survival of the pregnant woman and baby. A 28-year-old mother, for instance, summarised her view by saying, "*He did not want any problems to befall us (pointing to herself and her child) for him to bear the cost*". A male partner also indicated,

> *I saw it as she is someone's daughter so I had to make sure nothing happens to her to be held responsible. Because I know something can go wrong during the delivery. I just needed to make sure that nothing bad happens to them.*
>
> *- Male partner, 46 years*

Regarding nearness to a facility, a participant explained that his involvement was motivated by the fact that the hospital is close to their residence and made it easier for him to be present. The 28-year-old male partner said, "*We are close to the hospital. As you can see, our house is just opposite the hospital and that made it easy for me to monitor everything that was going on throughout the delivery*".

4.5.2. Barriers to Male Partner Involvement in Skilled Birth Care. The major factors which were proffered as barriers hindering male partner involvement in skilled birth care were health facility nonconduciveness, cultural norm for females to handle childbirth issues, and male partner's occupation. Concerning the nonconduciveness of health facilities, some of the male partners argued that a major reason why they were unable to be with their spouses was the fact that they were not allowed by health providers to be present during delivery. The health facilities were also cited as not being conducive for men and hence their unwillingness to involve themselves. A mother, 28 years old, for instance, said, "*At times, the men are not allowed by the health staff to witness the process even though they want to be part*". A 32-year-old male partner also retorted, "*We get ignored when we come with our partners to deliver. The midwives will not allow any man to come near the delivery process. They ask us to stay away*". The health professionals corroborated these views with one of them saying,

> *The delivery room is not suitable for male partners to be present with us. Generally, per our delivery rules, they don't accept men to be in the labour room since other women may be giving birth at the same time and we can't allow the men to be looking at other people's wives. Some of the men know so they would not want to come at all. Our labour room does not allow them to be in. Even the female relatives, in only serious situations such as the woman being "stubborn" that we allow the relatives to come and talk to her.*
>
> *- Health professional, female, 29 years*

Concerning cultural norm of female relatives handling childbirth issues, participants explained that their involvement in the skilled delivery process was perceived negatively due to the cultural norm that issues surrounding delivery and childbirth are the domain of females. Also, only female relatives are expected to be present and playing direct roles such as assisting the partner in labour. The following quotes present their views:

> *We grew up to understand that during labour, men are not to be present. Women are supposed to be the only people observing and assisting the woman in labour. So, it is the mother or mother in-laws, aunties and sisters who help the woman. Ours (men) is to just be patient and be ready to provide any 'manly help' such as carrying her when there is no transport, if the need arises.*
>
> *- Male partner, 36 years*
>
> *Traditionally, men are not supposed to be physically present as that is seen as the role of older women in the family such as the mother and mother in-law and sometimes the pregnant woman's sister. The childbirth issues are seen as ours and the only expectations of men is to give us (the women) money for birth items and payment at the facility.*
>
> *- Mother, 34 years*

A male partner, 36 years, also explained that in some instances, due to this cultural norm, men receive undesirable reactions from their mates and relatives which prevented them from involving themselves even if they want to. He said,

> *When you want to even do something like pack her bag with the items (birth preparedness items) and carry it along while accompanying them, they say*

> *a lot of discouraging statements like 'why do you want to follow? Are you a woman or the midwife?' So, I just let them go".*

Regarding male partner's occupation, most of the participants indicated that the stressful nature of the jobs and the long hours needed by the male partners to put into such works inhibited their ability to get involved in the delivery process. A 28-year-old mother, for instance, said, "*My partner's work could not give him the chance to be with me as I wanted*". A male partner also argued,

> *It is because of my work; being a welder, I couldn't absent myself from work to attend to my wife even though I knew her expected delivery is that week. If it was not my work, I think I would have done more.*
>
> *– Male partner, 32 years*

4.6. Improving the Level of Male Partner Involvement in Skilled Birth Care. The study also asked the participants to proffer suggestions to improve the level of male partner involvement in skilled birth care. Suggestions given included improved partner communication about childbirth and the delivery process, education and counselling by health workers, and institutional change.

The male partners and the mothers generally suggested that education and counselling by health workers and other opinion leaders can improve male partner involvement in skilled birth care. For instance, a 46-year-old male partner said,

> *"The health workers at the health facilities pregnant women attend ANC (antenatal clinic) have to be educating the males. There is the need for education so that men can acknowledge what the partner goes through so that they can support".*
>
> *– Male partner, 46 years*

A mother also added her voice saying,

> *Men need to be educated and counselled for them to know the importance of they getting involved and the fact that we (the women and the unborn child) need them to survive. Most of them don't know why they should be involved more than they are doing. As a matter of fact, they feel like they are doing everything even just provision of money. The health workers can do that for us.*
>
> *– Mother, 28 years*

Some of the mothers suggested that improved communication between couples and respect for male partners by the women will improve male partner involvement in skilled birth care. In arguing for the need to improve couple communication, a mother, 27 years, noted, "*I should be able to tell my husband what I am going through and what is being told at the antenatal so that he can be more participative*".

A 22-year-old mother however, suggesting respect for male partners to improve their involvement, said, "*Women should respect their husbands so that they can support them during delivery*".

Though the health professionals also agreed to the need for education and counselling, they further suggested that health facilities have to change their delivery policies to be more accommodating and friendlier to male partners. One of them noted,

> *Education. I think the health professionals should educate the men especially in the communities. You won't get them anywhere except the communities. Any man who comes with his wife to ANC for instance, that person is seen before the other people. This encourages them so that they don't spend so much time at the facility. It should be re-enforced to encourage them to be involved throughout the pregnancy and delivery process.*
>
> *– Health professional, female, 29 years*

A male partner also said,

> *I would have loved to be with my wife in the room while our baby was coming out so that I can encourage my wife to push. That would have possibly prevented the need for operation (Caesarean section) in the last delivery. But the nurses (midwives) said the facility does not allow men to go into the delivery room. I think the nurses should allow us to if we want.*
>
> *– Male partner, 28 years*

5. Discussion

Male partners in our study did not have adequate knowledge of childbirth and the skilled birth process. This finding is consistent with previous studies by Nanjala and Wamalwa [21], Salam et al. [22], and Tweheyo et al. [16] who found that male partners have limited knowledge of safe motherhood including skilled birth and the delivery process. The finding of this study, however, contradicts those of Katiso and Adinew [23] and Nasreen et al. [24] who argued that male partners are knowledgeable about childbirth and the delivery process. The fact that male partners were not knowledgeable about childbirth and the delivery process in the present study only reinforces the general assumption in the Ghanaian context that males have nothing to concern themselves with when it comes to issues of maternal and child health. Such issues are considered the sole preserve of women and, as such, men have no need to worry themselves about them. A male who involves himself in the delivery process is typically referred to as a weak man as argued by Abass, Sakoalia, and Mensah [25] and Davis et al. [8]. In relation to the conceptual framework, Andersen [26] argued that knowledge is a factor in adopting a health behaviour or utilising a healthcare service. Hence, the lack of adequate knowledge of childbirth and the delivery process observed in this study influences the involvement level of the male partners.

The finding that most of the male partners lacked appropriate knowledge of the possible complications during childbirth and the delivery process confirms the outcome of a previous study conducted by Nanjala and Wamalwa [21] in Western Kenya. Nanjala and Wamalwa in their study argued that male partners had low level of knowledge concerning delivery-related complications. In the present study, however, male partners were not aware of umbilical cord prolapse and amniotic fluid embolism as complications.

Male partners' lack of knowledge about the possible complications arising during childbirth is argued by Rosenstock [17] in the conceptual framework of the study to imply a lack of perceived threat whose existence would have influenced male partners to be involved in skilled birth if they realise that the threat posed by the delivery process to their partners and unborn children was severe. The fact that male partners had low knowledge about possible problems during childbirth can also be attributed to the fact that maternal issues have been considered to be women's domain. Hence, most men do not see the need to seek the prerequisite knowledge as they do not see its usefulness since they have left these matters to the women, as indicated earlier [27, 28].

The meanings of male partner involvement expressed by the participants agree with those found by Olugbenga-Bello et al. [29]. Olugbenga-Bello et al. argued that the men they surveyed perceived involvement in childbirth and skilled birth process as taking care of their spouses and the unborn/newborn child and providing emotional and moral support as well as providing financial support. The views of participants in the present study also conform to the definition that male partner involvement in skilled birth care comprises combined responsibility of male partners through increased awareness and support for their partner's maternal health needs (Waltson, 2005; [6, 7]). These findings are relevant to the propositions by Andersen and Newman [18] and Rosenstock [17] in the conceptual framework that what is considered male involvement is derived from the knowledge and beliefs the participants upheld. Hence, they defined male partner involvement in delivery care in terms of how much they understood childbirth and perceptions about their involvement.

The finding of positive perception among male partners towards skilled birth in the present study is in line with postulations of Mangeni et al. [30] and Yargawa and Leonard-Bee [31] in which the authors realised that their male partner participants generally had positive perception. The findings are, however, in disagreement with that of Wai et al. [32] which stated that male partners do not perceive skilled birth care positively.

Regarding male partners exhibiting positive perceptions towards skilled birth, this may be attributed to the perceived benefits of seeking skilled birth as against home delivery. In the framework underpinning this study, Rosenstock [17] posits that male partners will assume or favour a particular health behaviour, that is, skilled birth, if they perceive some form of benefit or protection from adopting it. And so, it can be adduced that the perceived benefit from skilled birth is the cause of the positive perception male partners have about it.

Concerning positive perception of male partners about their involvement in skilled birth found, this study is consistent with those of Tweheyo et al. [16] and Olugbenga-Bello et al. [29] which observed that male partners have favourable perceptions towards their involvement in skilled birth. The findings support the conceptual framework's perceived susceptibility of partner to delivery complications which may make the male partner perceive supporting her as important. Perceived benefits of male partner involvement and use of skilled birth care are influential in the level of involvement of male partners in the skilled birth process as argued by Rosenstock et al. [33] and this probably informed the perceptions of the male partners towards their involvement in the process.

The level of male partner involvement realised in this study can be linked to their perception and level of knowledge of the process. From the conceptual framework, Andersen [26] argued that the level of male partner involvement is a result of male partners' knowledge about the skilled birth process. Thus, as observed in this study, almost all male partners lacked adequate knowledge of childbirth and the delivery process and this may have accounted for their low involvement as they do not know what is required of them in the process and what they can do to support their partners during the process. Furthermore, Rosenstock [17] argued that male partners' perceptions are influenced by their knowledge of childbirth and the delivery process and possible complications. This is, however, not the case in this study as most male partners had positive perception about skilled birth and their involvement even though they lacked adequate knowledge of childbirth and the delivery process. Low level of male partner involvement observed in this study is consistent with the lack of knowledge of childbirth and the delivery process though not consistent with the positive perception male partners have of skilled birth and their involvement.

The fact that most male partners included in the present study took part in the decision-making process concerning the choice of place of delivery even though they did not participate in other areas which needed their support (such as accompanying the women to the facility for delivery) could be attributed to the traditional role of men, which is to wield the decision-making power of the household as heads [9, 10]. The findings of the present study, where male partners were the ones who mainly took the decision regarding choice of place of delivery by women, are in line with previous findings by Wai et al. [32] and Dickson et al. [5]. The authors in these studies realised that most men were involved in the decision-making regarding the choice of delivery, supporting the argument that men control decision-making in the home including that of the partner's health. Contrary to this finding, however, was a study by Kwambai et al. [34] which argued that men seldom contribute to the decision regarding maternal care including choice of place of delivery.

Our finding regarding some male partners seeing their involvement as a responsibility leading to their involvement is consistent with the study of Vermeulen et al. [35] which proffered that male partner's perceived role is a factor behind their involvement in skilled birth care. Also, Rosenstock [17] in the conceptual framework argued the fact that male partners' role is a direct function of their perception about the delivery process and what they are to do as men and, for that matter, heads of the family.

Concerning distance to health facility being a factor in male partners' involvement, the participants' responses are congruent with the study by Ditekemena et al. [36] which stated that the closer male partners to the delivery facility, the more the willingness to be involved. Also, Andersen and Newman [18] posited that some health-related factors such as availability of space, health provider attitude, distance to facility, and quality of care are influential in male partners' level of involvement as shown in the framework.

Also, cultural norm of childbirth being the domain of women as an inhibiting male partner involvement in skilled birth care supports the findings of Nanjala and Wamalwa [21] and Abass et al. [25]. In their studies, it was shown that existing cultural norms result in undesirable reactions from family and peers of male partners, which precludes them from participating in maternal processes including skilled birth care. This is further explained by the conceptual framework that cultural norms shape the perception of individuals and subsequently engaging in positive health behaviour like male involvement in skilled birth care.

The finding that delivery facilities were not accommodative for male partners as well as them being not allowed to be present with the partner during delivery is consistent with the studies of Ditekemena et al. [36] and Vermeulen et al. [35]. In their studies, it was found that lack of space to accommodate male partners and the feeling of being ignored by health providers when they accompany their partners for delivery contribute to males' perception that they are not welcomed, thus affecting their involvement and reducing their roles to only finance. Also, this finding is consistent with the study of Kululanga et al. [37] which found that the lack of privacy in the labour room stalled birthing women to have a partner or family member present in the labour ward for emotional support.

The findings point to the important roles of partner's education and occupation in influencing their involvement in issues relating to maternal and child health as realised in previous studies [5, 21]. Regarding employment, Nanjala and Wamalwa note that women with male partners who are formally employed are more likely to seek skilled birth than those with partners who are not employed in the formal sector. In relation to the conceptual framework, Andersen and Newman [18] noted that a person's education and occupation make him or her more willing to assume a particular health behaviour. As such, the involvement of the male partner is a correlate to his available time from work, educational level, and even, to some extent, study area.

Regarding the cues to improve male partner involvement in skilled birth, Rosenstock [17] in the conceptual framework argued that the perceived threat of a health condition can be influenced by some activities to improve the knowledge level of the individual. The participants' suggestion that male partners need to be educated on childbirth and delivery complications as well as the roles they need to play is consistent with the argument that knowledge of the risk of negative maternal and child health outcome and the seriousness of these complications if male partners do not get involved [33] is important.

We relied on verbal reports of behaviour in relation to male involvement in skilled birth. This has the tendency for the interviews to overreport good behaviour as participants may want to provide socially desirable responses. Also, recall bias could have been present as pregnancy may not represent as much significance to the male partner as it does to the female. Nevertheless, the study used both partners and, hence, was able to overcome this by cross-validation of the responses provided in both interviews.

6. Conclusion

Male partners' level of involvement resulted more from their sense of responsibility than a general understanding and acceptance of the idea of assisting their partners' maternal health needs. Also, male partners' lack of adequate knowledge of childbirth, the delivery process, and related complications implies that men cannot recognise delivery-related complications and plan together with the partner to seek early medical attention to avert the problem. This will affect the struggle of the country to attain the SDG goal three of reducing maternal and infant mortalities. Stakeholders need to develop a skilled birth policy that encourages male partner presence during labour and delivery as a way of integrating them into the process.

Disclosure

This research, as part of the dissemination of results, was presented as a conference material at the 50th Asia Pacific Academic Consortium for Public Health (APACPH) Conference and can be found in (https://www.researchgate.net/publication/327821576_Male_partner_involvement_in_skilled_delivery_care_at_the_North_Dayi_District_of_Ghana_A_qualitative_study).

Acknowledgments

We acknowledge the chiefs and people of the study communities as well as management of the Anfoega Catholic Hospital for providing us with the needed support during the data collection period upon which the findings of this study were based.

References

[1] D. Osborn, A. Cutter, and F. Ullah, *Universal Sustainable Development Goals: Understanding The Transformational Challenge*

for Developed Countries, Stakeholder Forum, New York, NY, USA, 2015.

[2] World Health Organization (WHO), *Proportion of Births Attended by A Skilled Health Worker: 2008 Updates*, Author, Geneva, Switzerland, 2008.

[3] United Nations Children's Fund (UNICEF), *Delivery Care*, New York, NY, USA, 2017, http://data.unicef.org/topic/maternal-health/delivery-care/.

[4] T. Ensor and S. Cooper, "Overcoming barriers to health service access: Influencing the demand side," *Health Policy and Planning*, vol. 19, no. 2, pp. 69–79, 2004.

[5] K. S. Dickson, K. S. Adde, and H. Amu, "What influences where they give birth? Determinants of place of delivery among women in rural Ghana," *International Journal of Reproductive Medicine*, vol. 1, pp. 1–8, 2016.

[6] A. Kumar, "Role of males in reproductive and sexual health decisions," The Bihar Times (1-4), 2007, http://www.bihartimes.com/articles/anant/roleofmales.html.

[7] F. Ampt, M. M. Mon, K. K. Than et al., "Correlates of male involvement in maternal and newborn health: A cross-sectional study of men in a peri-urban region of Myanmar," *BMC Pregnancy and Childbirth*, vol. 15, no. 122, pp. 1–11, 2015.

[8] J. Davis, S. Luchters, and W. Holmes, *Men And Maternal And Newborn Health: Benefits, Harms, Challenges And Potential Strategies for Engaging Men*, Women's and Children's Health Knowledge Hub, Melbourne, Australia, 2012.

[9] EngenderHealth, *Men as partners*, 2011, http://www.engenderhealth.org/our-work/gender/men-as-partners.php.

[10] B. K. Takyi and F. N.-A. Dodoo, "Gender, lineage, and fertility-related outcomes in Ghana," *Journal of Marriage and Family*, vol. 67, no. 1, pp. 251–257, 2005.

[11] World Health Organization (WHO), *Programme for Male Involvement in Reproductive Health*, Author, Geneva, Switzerland, 2001.

[12] A. Ntabona, *Involving Men in Safe Motherhood: The Issues*, World Health Organization, Washington, DC, USA, 2002.

[13] Ghana Statistical Service (GSS), Ghana Health Service (GHS), and ICF International, *Ghana Demographic and Health Survey*, Authors, Maryland, USA, 2015.

[14] C. Oppong, "Some biosocial aspects of childcare in Ghana: Decades of change," in *Childcare in A Globalizing World: Perspectives from Ghana*, C. Oppong, D. M. Badasu, and K. Wærness, Eds., pp. 38–63, University of Bergen, Bergen, Norway, 2012.

[15] C. Aparajita, "Men in maternal care: Evidence from India," *Journal of Biosocial Science*, vol. 44, no. 2, pp. 129–153, 2012.

[16] R. Tweheyo, J. Konde-Lule, N. M. Tumwesigye, and J. N. Sekandi, "Male partner attendance of skilled antenatal care in peri-urban Gulu district, Northern Uganda," *BMC Pregnancy and Childbirth*, vol. 10, no. 53, pp. 1–9, 2010.

[17] I. M. Rosenstock, "Why people use health services," *Milbank Memorial Fund Quarterly*, vol. 44, no. 3, pp. 94–127, 1966.

[18] R. Andersen and J. F. Newman, "Societal and individual determinants of medical care utilization in the United States," *Milbank Quarterly*, vol. 83, no. 4, 2005.

[19] Ghana Statistical Service (GSS), *2010 Population And Housing Census: District Analytical Report: North Dayi District*, Author, Accra, Ghana, 2014.

[20] R. Kumar, *Research Methodology: A Step-By-Step Guide for Beginners*, Sage Publications, New Delhi, India, 2nd edition, 2005.

[21] M. Nanjala and D. Wamalwa, "Determinants of male partner involvement in promoting deliveries by skilled attendants in Busia, Kenya.," *Global Journal of Health Science*, vol. 4, no. 2, pp. 60–67, 2012.

[22] S. S. Salam, M. J. Leppard, M. Al-Mamun, and H. E. Nasreen, *Men'S Knowledge And Practices of Maternal, Neonatal And Child Health in Rural Bangladesh: Do They Differ from Women?* Research and Evaluation Division, BRAC, Dhaka, Bangladesh, 2012.

[23] N. A. Katiso and Y. M. Adinew, "Male partners' involvement in institutional delivery in rural Ethiopia: Community based survey," *Journal of Women's Health Care*, vol. 4, no. 239, pp. 1–4, 2015.

[24] H. E. Nasreen, M. Leppard, M. Al Mamun et al., "Men's knowledge and awareness of maternal, neonatal and child health care in rural Bangladesh: A comparative cross sectional study," *Reproductive Health*, vol. 9, no. 18, pp. 1–9, 2012.

[25] K. Abass, P. Sakoalia, and C. Mensah, "Socio-cultural practices and male involvement in reducing maternal mortality in rural Ghana: The case of Savelugu/Nanton District of the Northern Region of Ghana," *International Journal of Asian Social Science*, vol. 2, no. 11, pp. 2009–2026, 2009.

[26] R. M. Andersen, "Revisiting the behavioural model and access to medical care: Does it matter?" *Journal of Health and Social Behaviour*, vol. 36, pp. 1–10, 1995.

[27] S. Mullick, B. Kunene, and M. Wanjiru, "Involving men in maternity care: Health service delivery issues," *Agenda Special Focus*, vol. 1, pp. 124–135, 2005.

[28] R. G. Horstman, "Husband involvement in the prevention of maternal ill-health: the determinants of husband domestic support in rural low-land Nepal," in *Proceedings of The Poster Presentation Session at The 2004 Annual Meeting of The Population Association of America*, pp. 1–3, Boston, Mass, USA, 2004.

[29] A. I. Olugbenga-Bello, E. O. Asekun-Olarinmoye, A. O. Adewole, A. A. Adeomi, and S. O. Olarewaju, "Perception, attitude and involvement of men in maternal health care in a Nigerian community," *Journal of Public Health and Epidemiology*, vol. 5, no. 6, pp. 262–270, 2013.

[30] J. N. Mangeni, A. Mwangi, S. Mbugua, and V. Mukthar, *Male Involvement in Maternal Health Care as A Determinant of Utilization of Skilled Birth Attendants in Kenya*, ICF International, Columbia, MD, USA, 2013.

[31] J. Yargawa and J. Leonardi-Bee, "Male involvement and maternal health outcomes: systematic review and meta-analysis," *Journal of Epidemiology and Community Health*, vol. 69, no. 6, pp. 604–612, 2015.

[32] K. M. Wai, A. Shibanuma, N. N. Oo, T. J. Fillman, Y. M. Saw, and M. Jimba, "Are husbands involving in their spouses' utilization of maternal care services?: a cross-sectional study in Yangon, Myanmar," *PLoS ONE*, vol. 10, no. 12, pp. 1–13, 2015.

[33] I. M. Rosenstock, V. Strecher, and M. Becker, "The health belief model and HIV risk behaviour change," in *Preventing AIDS: Theories and Methods of Behavioural Interventions*, R. J. DiClemente and J. L. Peterson, Eds., pp. 5–24, Plenum Press, New York, NY, USA, 1994.

[34] T. K. Kwambai, S. Dellicour, M. Desai et al., "Perspectives of men on antenatal and delivery care service utilisation in rural western Kenya: a qualitative study," *BMC Pregnancy and Childbirth*, vol. 13, no. 134, pp. 1–10, 2013.

[35] E. Vermeulen, A. Solnes Miltenburg, J. Barras, N. Maselle, M. van Elteren, and J. van Roosmalen, "Opportunities for

male involvement during pregnancy in Magu district, rural Tanzania," *BMC Pregnancy and Childbirth*, vol. 16, no. 66, pp. 1–9, 2016.

[36] J. Ditekemena, O. Koole, C. Engmann et al., "Determinants of male involvement in maternal and child health services in sub-Saharan Africa: a review," *Reproductive Health*, vol. 9, no. 32, pp. 1–8, 2012.

[37] L. I. Kululanga, J. Sundby, A. Malata, and E. Chirwa, "Striving to promote male involvement in maternal health care in rural and urban settings in Malawi—a qualitative study," *Reproductive Health*, vol. 8, no. 36, pp. 1–12, 2011.

12

Cervical Cancer Screening: Assessment of Perception and Utilization of Services among Health Workers in Low Resource Setting

C. C. Ifemelumma,[1] C. C. Anikwe ,[1] B. C. Okorochukwu,[2] F. A. Onu,[1] J. A. Obuna,[1] B. N. Ejikeme,[1] and O. P. Ezeonu[1]

[1]*Department of Obstetrics and Gynaecology, Federal Teaching Hospital Abakaliki Ebonyi State, PMB 102 Abakaliki, Ebonyi State, Nigeria*
[2]*Department of Obstetrics and Gynaecology, Federal Medical Centre Owerri, P. O. Box 1010, Owerri, Imo State, Nigeria*

Correspondence should be addressed to C. C. Anikwe; drchideanikwechristian@gmail.com

Academic Editor: Kai-Fai Lee

Background. Cervical cancer is a preventable disease and the most common cancer among women in Nigeria. *Objectives.* To appraise the perception and utilization of cervical cancer screening services among female nurses in Federal Teaching hospital, Abakaliki. *Materials and Methods.* A cross-sectional study was done using semi-structured questionnaires on 408 consenting female nurses. Data was represented using simple percentages, charts, and Chi-square. *Results.* Of the 408 questionnaires shared, 388 were correctly and completely filled and analyzed. The respondents in this study showed good knowledge of cervical cancer as all (388) were aware that cervical cancer is a preventable disease of public health concern. Majority of them, 179 (46.1%) were between 21 and 30 years of age. The most common symptom of cervical cancer identified was postcoital bleeding (57%). Nursing training was the most common (73.5%) source of cervical cancer information. Utilization of cervical cancer screening was poor in this study as only 20.6% of the respondents had ever undergone screening. The most common reason for nonscreening was that they have not thought of it (28.4%). *Conclusion.* Despite the high level of awareness of cervical cancer screening, utilization remains low. There is, therefore, the need for cervical cancer education for the nurses to help improve utilization.

1. Introduction

Cancer of the cervix, a potentially preventable disease [1], is the second most common cancer among women worldwide [2, 3] and the most common malignancy of the female genital tract in the developing countries [4, 5]. Worldwide, cervical cancer accounts for about 500,000 new diagnoses and 273,000 deaths every year, of the new cases 80% occur in the developing countries [2]. About 85% of the 250,000 deaths recorded yearly from cervical cancer occur in developing countries like Nigeria where the majority of cases present in the late stages of the disease [6, 7]. In Nigeria, the national incidence of cancer of the cervix is 250/100,000 [7]. Each year approximately, 10,000 women develop cervical cancer, and about 8,000 women die from cervical cancer in Nigeria [8]. It is worrisome as all sexually active women are at risk for the development of cervical cancer.

Sexually transmitted Human Papilloma Virus (HPV) infection leads to the development of cervical intraepithelial neoplasia and cervical cancer. Women with many sexual partners and those whose partners have had many sexual consorts or have been previously exposed to the virus are most at risk of developing the disease [7]. Early detection and prompt treatment of precancerous conditions provide the best possible protection against cancer [9]. In developed countries with well-established screening programs, the incidences of cervical cancer have been reduced by 70-90%. Sporadic screening is being carried out in Nigeria using opportunist method for those who visit certain clinics. Also, there is no standard policy or protocol for cervical cancer screening in Nigeria [10]. The different methods of cervical cancer screening include Papanicolaou (Pap) smear, visual inspection of the cervix with acetic acid (VIA), HPV DNA test, and colposcopy [11]. Colposcopy is not used as a primary screening test but it is combined with other tests.

The high burden of cervical cancer in developing countries, like Nigeria, is due both to a high prevalence of HPV infection and the lack of effective cervical cancer screening programmes [10]. In cases where effective screening programmes are available, poor knowledge and negative health-seeking behavior of the populace have led to poor utilization of such services [10]. An important strategy towards the reduction of the incidence and mortality associated with cervical cancer is by increasing the screening rate of women that have not screened or those that screen infrequently [12]. Knowledge about cancer of the cervix and its screening is important in screening uptake. Women with low levels of knowledge about cervical cancer and its prevention are less likely to access screening services [3, 7, 9, 13]. Previous studies done among female health workers have shown good knowledge of cervical cancer; however, cervical cancer screening attendance rates are still far from satisfactory in most countries [5, 14, 15]. Nurses play a major role in promoting health care services and in enlightening the public on many health-related issues and their knowledge and attitude on health-related issues are crucial in gaining and promoting patients' uptake of care. They also help to improve women's confidence. This study was embarked upon to fill a knowledge gap since no such has been done in our centre. Our aim is to appraise the perception and utilization of cervical cancer screening services among female nurses in a Federal Teaching Hospital Abakaliki. We specifically assessed the knowledge of the nurses towards cervical cancer, the percentage of female nurses utilizing cervical cancer screening services, and the factors influencing utilization of cervical cancer screening services.

2. Materials and Methods

2.1. Study Area. The study was carried out among female nurses of the Federal Teaching Hospital, Abakaliki. The hospital is a referral tertiary centre and the only teaching hospital in the state. It was formed in 2012 from the merger of the former Ebonyi State Teaching Hospital and the then Federal Medical Centre, Abakaliki. The hospital has an active Well Woman Centre which offers screening for genital tract cancer as one of its activities. There are 1306 female nurses working in Federal Teaching Hospital, Abakaliki (FETHA), in all departments.

2.2. Study Design. This was a descriptive cross-sectional study.

2.3. Sample Size. The sample size (N_0) was calculated using

$$N_o = \frac{Z^2 pq}{e^2} \tag{1}$$

where Z^2 is a constant = 1.96.

e: the desired level of precision also known as sampling error: 5%.

p: prevalence of utilization of cervical cancer screening services from similar study[9] = 0.35.

q: 1-p.

$$N_o = \frac{(1.96)^2 \times 0.35 \times 0.65}{(0.05)^2} = 349.58 \tag{2}$$

Attrition rate of 20% was added to the sample size, i.e., 350 + 70 = 420. Therefore the sample size of 420 was used.

2.4. Sample Technique and Data Collection. Data were collected using self-administered semistructured questionnaire. The questionnaire had 3 parts; the first part assessed the sociodemographic characteristics of the respondents while the other 2 parts assessed their perception and utilization of cervical cancer screening, respectively. Proportionate and systematic sampling techniques were employed. Six (6) clinical departments, namely, Obstetrics and Gynecology, Family Medicine, Internal Medicine, General Surgery, Ophthalmology, and Paediatrics, were selected by balloting from the total number of the 13 clinical departments in the facility. A proportionate allocation of the 420 questionnaires to the female nurses in the respective departments was done based on the total number of female nurses in each of the selected departments; i.e., 1 questionnaire was allotted for every 2 nurses in each of the respective department. This resulted in 112, 49, 60, 78, 41, and 80 questionnaires allotted to Obstetrics and Gynecology, Family Medicine, Internal Medicine, General Surgery, Ophthalmology, and Paediatrics Departments, respectively. The allotted questionnaires were then shared randomly, using a systematic sampling method using the nurses on the departmental duty register as the sampling frame. Care was taken to avoid readministering the questionnaire to those that had previously been administered. This was done by simply asking if they had previously answered to this particular questionnaire. The purpose of the study was explained and consent obtained. Five (5) medical students were trained to administer the questionnaires. The questionnaires were retrieved from each respondent immediately after completion and they were reviewed for completeness. The male nurses were exempted.

2.5. Data Analysis. The data obtained were analyzed using IBM SPSS Statistics version 20 (IBM Corp., Armonk, NY, USA). The data obtained were reclassified for easy analysis, age-grouped into ≤ 40 years and > 40 years, marital status into married and unmarried, parity into ≤ 4 and > 4, and duration of service into < 5 years and ≥ 5 years. The results were presented in frequency tables, charts, and Chi-square contingency tables.

2.6. Ethical Consideration. Permission to carry out this research was sought and obtained from the Research and Ethics Committee of the Federal Teaching Hospital Abakaliki. The ethical approval number is FETHA/REC VOL 1 /2014/189.

TABLE 1: Sociodemographic characteristics of study population.

VARIABLE	FREQUENCY	PERCENTAGE
Age (years)		
21-30	179	46.1
31-40	163	42
41-50	38	9.8
51-60	8	2.1
≥60	-	-
Total	388	100
Marital status		
Married	209	53.9
Single	106	41.2
Divorced	-	-
Widowed	15	3.9
Separated	4	1
Total	388	100
Ethnicity		
Igbo	350	90.2
Yoruba	15	3.9
Hausa	4	1
Others	19	4.9
Total	388	100
Religion		
Christianity	384	99
Islam	4	1
Traditional	-	-
Total	388	100
Parity		
Nullipara	179	46.1
1-4	190	49
≥5	19	4.9
Total	388	100
Duration of practice (years)		
<5	183	47.2
5-10	152	39.2
>10	53	13.6
Total	388	100

3. Results

In this study, 388 out of 420 questionnaires were correctly completed and returned which gave a retrieval rate of 92.4%. As in Table 1, the majority of the respondents, 179 (46.1%), were between 21 and 30 years of age and the fewest, 8 (2.1%), were between ages of 51 to 60 years. Of the respondents, 209 (53.9%) were married, while 160 (41.2%) were single. Most of (190, 46.1%) the respondents belong to Para 1-4. Nurses with less than 5 years of working experience made up the largest proportion (47.2%).

From Table 2, the respondents in this study showed good knowledge of cervical cancer as all were aware that cervical cancer is a preventable disease of public health concern. The most common symptom of cancer of the cervix identified was posted coital bleeding (57.7%). The majority (72.4%) of the respondents knew that history of Human Papilloma Virus (HPV) infection is a risk factor although only 86.2% (335) correctly identified HPV as the primary cause of cervical cancer (Figure 2). Less than 10% identified poor hygiene and alcohol intake, respectively, as risk factors for cancer of the cervix. Most of the respondents (89.2%) identified Pap smear as a screening modality, while only 74.5% of the respondents were aware of the HPV vaccine. Two hundred and thirty-two (59.8%) of the respondents perceived being above 21 years of age or sexually active for the last 3 years (whichever is earlier) as an indication to be screened for cancer cervix.

In Figure 1, nursing training is the commonest source of information about cervical cancer.

Figure 3 shows the study population knowledge of cervical cancer screening frequency. It depicts poor knowledge

TABLE 2: Knowledge of cervical cancer and screening.

VARIABLES	FREQUENCY	PERCENTAGE
Symptoms		
No symptoms	99	25.5
Foul Offensive vaginal discharge	190	49
Irregular vaginal bleeding	167	43
Postcoital vaginal bleeding	224	57.7
Fever	38	9.8
Pelvic pain	106	27.3
Weight loss	76	19.6
Risk factors		
Sexual intercourse < 16 years	209	53.9
Multiple sexual partners	277	71.4
Smoking	53	13.7
History of HPV infection	281	72.4
Use of IUCD	34	8.8
Impaired immunity	42	10.8
Poor hygiene	30	7.7
Alcohol use	23	5.9
Screening modalities		
Pap smear	346	89.2
VIA	160	41.2
Cervical biopsy	179	46.1
HPVDNA test	99	25.5
Colposcopy	53	13.7
Who should be screened		
Above 21 years/sexually active	232	59.8
Married women only	4	1
Women above 30 years	152	39.2
If cervical changes are found early are they curable		
Yes	288	74.2
No	27	6.9
Not aware	23	5.9

Multiple answers allowed.

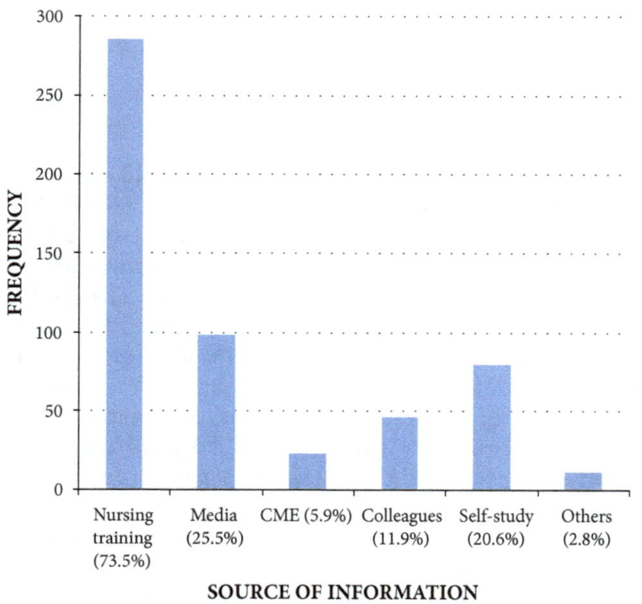

FIGURE 1: Nurses' sources of cervical cancer information. CME: continuing medical education.

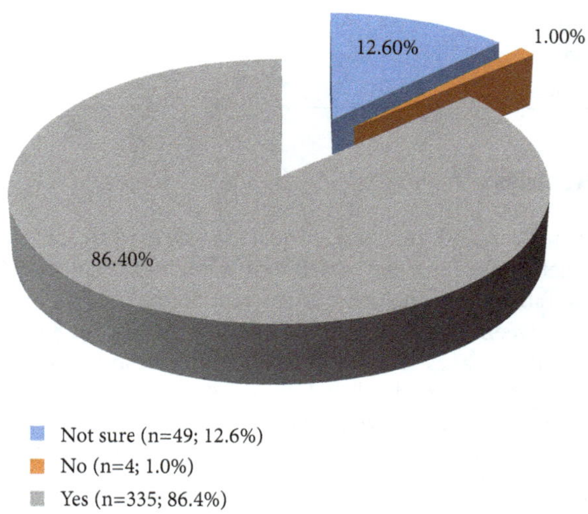

FIGURE 2: HPV as primary cause of cancer of the cervix.

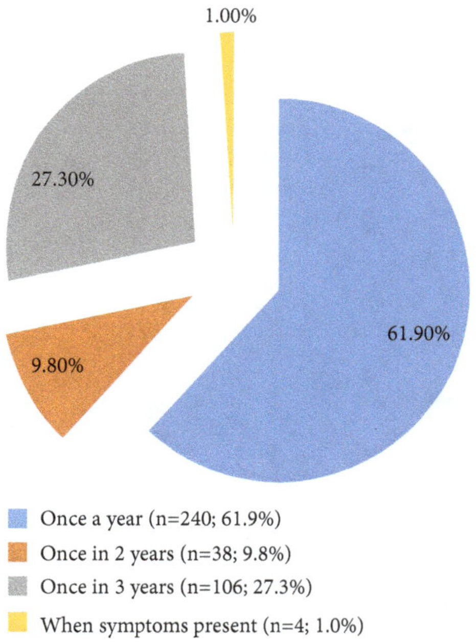

FIGURE 3: Frequency of cervical cancer screening.

as only 27.3% (106) of the respondents are aware that the screening frequency is once in 3 years.

Table 3 shows that only 20.6% of the respondents had ever undergone screening for cervical cancer. The most common reason for nonscreening was that they had not thought of it (28.4%) and 10.8% ascribe their nonscreening to the fear of the result. Among the 80 (20.6%) respondents that had ever been screened, 68 (85%) of them had been screened once while 12 (15%) had been screened twice.

Table 4 shows that majority 327 (84.3%) of the respondents were aware of a cervical cancer screening centre. Of these respondents, 168 (43.3%) do not routinely recommend cervical screening to others; majority 76.8% of them had no reason for not recommending the screening while 7.1% considered the procedure being painful as their reason

The result in Table 5 showed a significant association between age, marital status, duration of practice, and parity with the utilization of cervical cancer screening services by the respondents.

A cross-tabulation done using duration of practice, respondent age, marital status, and parity as dependent variables and having being screened of cervical cancer as independent variable shows that being 40 years or less (OR 1.18 95% CI 1.12–1.23), parity (OR 1.07 95% CI 1.04–1.10), married (OR 2.08 95% CI 1.85–2.34), and duration of practice of less than five (5) years (OR 2.99 95% CI 2.55-3.50) is associated with increased chances of being screened for cervical cancer among our respondents.

4. Discussion

Cervical cancer is largely a preventable disease [1, 16]. An important strategy towards the reduction of its burden in a developing country is by early diagnosis and management of the premalignant lesions of the disease; this would be achieved via screening of women at risk. The current study evaluated the perception and utilization of cervical cancer screening services among female nurses in Federal Teaching Hospital, Abakaliki. The respondents in our study had a good knowledge of cervical cancer, as all of them correctly identified cervical cancer as a preventable disease and the majority of them noted HPV as the primary cause. The high knowledge of cervical cancer found in this study is not surprising considering the profession of the respondents, as they are expected to be more knowledgeable than other women in the community. This is consistent with the previous studies done on this subject [4, 9]. Most of the respondent in our study acquired their knowledge about the disease from their training although mass media, self-study, and colleagues constituted other common sources of information. This is similar to the study done in Tanzania [17] and Lagos, Nigeria [4]. The most common symptom of cervical cancer identified in this study was postcoital vaginal bleeding (57.7%). Barely half of the respondents identified offensive vaginal discharge as a symptom of cervical cancer, while less than half knew that pelvic pain and irregular vaginal bleeding could be caused by cervical cancer. This finding is in tandem with the work of Urasa et al. [17] in Tanzania and which might be attributed to the nature of training given to our nurses which does not go in-depth in discussing the pathology of diseases.

Many nurses in this study had inadequate knowledge of risk factors for cervical cancer, as only 13.7% and 10.8% knew that smoking and impaired immunity, respectively, are risk factors. Low knowledge of association of smoking with cervical cancer is not surprising as smoking is not a common practice among Nigerian women but poor knowledge of the link between impaired immunity and cervical cancer is not encouraging in view of the evidence linking cervical cancer with HIV. Some of the respondents even had the erroneous belief that IUCD, poor hygiene, and alcohol could result in cervical cancer. This finding is similar to the findings in studies done in Tanzania [17, 18] and Lagos, Nigeria [4].

Development of any national cervical cancer prevention and control programme is pivotal in reducing morbidity and mortality associated with cervical cancer in sub-Saharan Africa [16] but this is still a distant dream in Nigeria [5]. It was therefore not surprising that only about one-quarter of the respondents knew the cervical cancer screening interval. The commonest known screening modality in this study was Pap smear (89.2%). Less than half of the respondents recognized VIA, cervical biopsy, HPV DNA testing, and colposcopy (13.7%) as screening modalities for cervical cancer. This finding is similar to the study done in Lagos, Nigeria [4], where colposcopy was the least recognized form of screening for cervical cancer. This low knowledge of other methods calls for more awareness campaign on screening modalities for cervical cancer so as to give people more knowledge of the disease.

The utilization of cervical cancer screening services in this study was poor; only 20.6% had undergone screening. The commonest reason given for this was that they had never thought of it. Other reasons given included not being sexually active, no time, and the fear of the result. This

TABLE 3: Utilization of cervical cancer screening.

	FREQUENCY	PERCENTAGE
SCREENING		
Yes	80	20.6
No	308	79.4
REASON FOR NOT SCREENING		
No time	50	12.9
Fear of result	42	10.8
Procedure being cumbersome	15	3.9
Not sexually active	50	12.9
Cost	0	0
Not thought of it	110	28.4
Lack of awareness of test	11	2.8
Don't know where a test is done	15	3.9
Others	30	7.7

TABLE 4: Nurses' attitude towards recommendation for cervical cancer screening.

	Frequency	Percentage
Do not routinely recommend		
Screening		
No	168	43.3
Yes	220	56.7
Reasons for not recommending screening		
Procedure is painful	12	7.1
Females 21 years old are safe	8	4.8
The test could be dangerous and Risky	4	2.4
No reason	129	76.8
Others	19	11.3
Awareness of cancer screening center	327	84.3

Multiple answers allowed.

TABLE 5: Association between sociodemographic variables and utilization of cervical cancer screening services.

Variables	Total number	Have been screened		Chi-square	Df	P value
		Yes	No			
Age						
≤40	342	80	262	13.56	1	0.001*
>40	46	0	46			
Marital status						
Married	228	80	148	70.72	1	0.001*
Unmarried	160	0	160			
Religion						
Christianity	384	80	304	1.86	1	0.424**
Islam	4	0	4			
Parity						
≤4	369	80	289	9.03	1	0.013**
]=>4	19	0	19			
Duration of practice						
<5	183	80	103	111.90	1	0.001*
≥5	205	0	205			

*Pearson Chi-square. **Likelihood ratio.

study further revealed that there is a significant association between some sociodemographic factors like the age of respondents, marital status, parity, and duration of practice with the utilization of cervical cancer screening services. This is similar to the finding by Awodele [4]. It might be explained by the fact that nearly half of the respondents were less than 30 years and had practiced for 5 years or less and therefore being young may perceive themselves as not susceptible to the development of precancerous/cancerous lesion and are therefore not bothered about such issues and hence not likely to use the service. These findings were slightly different from the study in Nnewi, Nigeria [5], where majority gave no reason for not testing; and of those that had reasons, the commonest were the fear of the result and not being susceptible to cervical cancer. These reasons need to be addressed in an intervention programme targeting this category of health workers, considering their number and the influence they have in the community. Institutional-based workshop and training on cervical cancer can be of enormous help in improving utilization of cervical cancer screening.

In conclusion, it is evident from this study that despite the high level of awareness of cervical cancer screening, utilization among nurses remains low. We, therefore, recommend that there is a need for the nurses to be actively involved in the cancer screening units and possibly undergo rotation through the unit to help douse the fear and uncertainties associated with the cervical cancer screening process. Cervical cancer screening education programmes need to be carried out among health care professionals at all levels, especially among nurses. The continuing education based programme provides an opportunity for doing this, especially as nurses constitute one of the most authoritative sources of information on health matters for the general populace, especially for women. As they become informed, they should be motivated to practice what they teach and lead by example. The adoption of cervical cancer screening as a preemployment test may also be considered.

Consent

Consent was obtained prior to administration of the questionnaire- consent form signed by the respondent.

Disclosure

Funding is borne by the authors.

Authors' Contributions

C. C. Anikwe and C. C. Ifemelumma participated in the study design, data collection/analysis, and interpretation of finding and drafting of the manuscript. J. A. Obuna and B. N. Ejikeme participated in the interpretation of findings and data analysis. F. A. Onu and B. C. Okorochukwu participated in study design, interpretation of findings, and drafting of the manuscript. O. P. Ezeonu conceptualized the study and participated in the interpretation of finding. All the authors approved the manuscript.

Acknowledgments

We want to appreciate the medical students that helped in the administration of the questionnaire and also the respondents without whom the study would not have been possible.

References

[1] I. O. G. Owoeye and I. A. Ibrahim, "Knowledge and attitude towards cervical cancer screening among female students and staff in a tertiary institution in the Niger Delta," *International Journal of Medicine and Biomedical Research*, vol. 2, no. 1, pp. 48–56, 2013.

[2] M. I. Shafi, "Premalignant and malignant diseases of the cervix," in *Dewhurst's Textbook of Obstetrics and Gynecology*, D. K. Edmonds, Ed., vol. 56, pp. 747–759, Wiley-Blackwell, London, UK, 8th edition, 2012.

[3] B. U. Ezem, "Awareness and uptake of cervical cancer screening in Owerri, South-Eastern Nigeria," *Annals of African Medicine*, vol. 6, no. 3, pp. 94–98, 2007.

[4] O. Awodele, A. A. A. Adeyomoye, D. F. Awodele, V. Kwashi, I. O. Awodele, and D. C. Dolapo, "A study on cervical cancer screening amongst nurses in Lagos University Teaching Hospital, Lagos, Nigeria," *Journal of Cancer Education*, vol. 26, no. 3, pp. 497–504, 2011.

[5] G. O. Udigwe, "Knowledge, attitude and practice of cervical cancer screening (pap smear) among female nurses in Nnewi, South Eastern Nigeria.," *Nigerian Journal of Clinical Practice*, vol. 9, no. 1, pp. 40–43, 2006.

[6] R. I. Anorlu, "Cervical cancer: the sub-Saharan African perspective," *Reproductive Health Matters*, vol. 16, no. 32, pp. 41–49, 2008.

[7] J. N. Eze, O. U. Umeora, J. A. Obuna, V. E. Egwuatu, and B. N. Ejikeme, "Cervical cancer awareness and cervical screening uptake at the Mater Misericordiae Hospital, Afikpo, Southeast Nigeria," *Annals of African Medicine*, vol. 11, no. 4, pp. 238–243, 2012.

[8] L. Airede, J. Onakewhor, M. Aziken, A. Ande, and J. Aligbe, "Carcinoma of the Uterine Cervix in Nigerian women: the Need to adopt a national prevention strategy," *Sahel Medical Journal*, vol. 11, no. 1, pp. 1–11, 2008.

[9] O. S. Arulogun and O. O. Maxwell, "Perception and utilization of cervical cancer screening services among female nurses in University College Hospital, Ibadan, Nigeria," *Pan African Medical Journal*, vol. 11, article 69, 2012.

[10] C. M. Ndikom and B. A. Ofi, "Awareness, perception and factors affecting utilization of cervical cancer screening services among women in Ibadan, Nigeria: a qualitative study," *Reproductive Health*, vol. 9, article 11, 2012.

[11] F. Ali, R. Kuelker, and B. Wassie, "Understanding cervical cancer in the context of developing countries," *Annals of Tropical Medicine and Public Health*, vol. 5, no. 1, pp. 3–15, 2012.

[12] C. C. Dim, "Towards improving cervical cancer screening in Nigeria: A review of the basics of cervical neoplasm and cytology," *Nigerian Journal of Clinical Practice*, vol. 15, no. 3, pp. 247–252, 2012.

[13] C. M. Nwozor and A. L. Oragudosi, "Awareness and Uptake of Cervical Cancer Screening among Women in Onitsha, South-East, Nigeria," *Greener Journal of Medical Sciences*, vol. 3, no. 8, pp. 283–288, 2013.

[14] M. O. Oche, A. U. Kaoje, G. Gana et al., "Cancer of the cervix and cervical screening: Current knowledge, attitude,

and practices of female health workers in Sokoto, Nigeria," *International Journal of Medicine and Medical Sciences*, vol. 5, no. 4, pp. 184–190, 2013.

[15] E. I. Nwobodo and S. A. Malami, "Knowledge and practice of cervical screening among female health workers in Sokoto, North Western Nigeria.," *Nigerian Postgraduate Medical Journal*, vol. 12, no. 4, pp. 255–257, 2005.

[16] World Health Organization (WHO), *Comprehensive Cervical Cancer Control: A guide to essential practice*, 2nd edition, 2014, http://apps.who.int/iris/bitstream/handle/10665/144785/9789241548953_eng.pdf.

[17] M. Urasa and E. Darj, "Knowledge of cervical cancer and screening practices of nurses at a regional hospital in Tanzania," *African Health Sciences*, vol. 11, no. 1, pp. 48–57, 2011.

[18] A. Goyel, G. Vaishnav, A. Shrivastava et al., "Knowledge, attitude practices about cervical cancer and screening among nursing staff in a tertiary hospital," *International Journal of Medical Science and Public Health*, vol. 2, no. 2, pp. 249–253, 2013.

13

Factors Associated with Utilization of Complete Postnatal Care Service in Baglung Municipality, Nepal

Sita Chhetri,[1] Rajani Shah,[2] and Laxmi Rajbanshi[3]

[1]*Charak Hospital Nursing College, Pokhara, Kaski, Nepal*
[2]*Nepal Public Health Foundation, Kathmandu, Nepal*
[3]*Teaching Hospital, Chitwan Medical College, Bharatpur, Nepal*

Correspondence should be addressed to Rajani Shah; rajani_shah89@yahoo.com

Academic Editor: Robert Gaspar

Background. Postnatal period is six weeks after birth. It is critical but is the most neglected period. A large proportion of maternal and neonatal deaths occur during 48 hours following childbirth. The utilization of the recommended three postnatal checkups within seven days after delivery, which plays a vital role in preventing maternal and neonatal deaths, is low in Nepal. *Objective.* This study is aimed at identifying the factors associated with the utilization of complete postnatal care (PNC) among mothers. *Method.* A cross-sectional study was carried out among 318 mothers in wards 1, 2, 3, and 4 of Baglung municipality, Nepal. Data was collected by semi-structured interviews. Descriptive analysis and comparison of characteristics of women/families with complete vs. partial postnatal checkups using multivariable logistic regression were done. *Results.* Among 314 respondents receiving at least one PNC, 78% had partial and 22% had complete PNC. Relatively advantaged caste/ethnicity-Brahman/Chhetri (aOR = 3.18, 95% CI: 1.24-8.12) and Janajati (aOR = 2.87, 95% CI: 1.09-7.53) - compared to Dalits, husbands working as a job holder in Nepal (aOR = 3.49, 95% CI: 1.50-8.13), and delivery in a private hospital (aOR = 11.4, 95% CI: 5.40-24.2) were associated with having complete PNC. *Conclusion.* Although PNC attendance at least once was high, utilization of complete PNC was low. More focus to mothers from disadvantaged caste/ethnicity, those whose husbands are in foreign employment, and improvement in quality of care in government health facilities may increase the use of complete PNC.

1. Introduction

A large proportion of maternal and neonatal deaths occur during 48 hours following childbirth. Almost all (99%) newborn and maternal deaths happen in developing countries. Globally, there were an estimated 303000 maternal deaths from complications related to pregnancy and childbirth in 2015 [1]. South Asia and Sub-Saharan Africa shared the highest proportion [2]. The first week of birth accounts for the highest number of the deaths [3]. In Nepal, maternal mortality ratio stands at 239 per 100000 live births, while neonatal mortality rate is 33 per 1000 live births [4]. Sustainable development goal aims at reducing the MMR to less than 70 per 100000 live births, reducing preventable deaths of newborn to less than 1%, and providing postnatal care (PNC) for 90 percent of mothers by 2030 [5].

Postnatal period is up to six weeks after childbirth. The major purposes of PNC are to maintain and promote the health of the woman and her baby. It is generally the most neglected period in developing countries. Mothers and newborn babies do not receive PNC from a skilled health care provider during the first few days after delivery [6]. The national essential maternal and neonatal health care service package for Nepal recommends three PNC for all women, whether delivered at home or at health facility: first PNC within 24 hours, second and third ones on the third and seventh day, respectively [7].

Nepal Demographic and Health Survey 2016 showed that only 57% of mothers received a PNC within two days of delivery [4]. According to the Department of Health Services Nepal, the proportion of mothers having three PNC visits as per protocol stands at 11% in Baglung district, compared to

18% at the national level [8]. The national figure even declined to 16% in 2018 from 19% in 2017. The low utilization of the service has been attributed to cultural and geographical factors as well as perceived low importance of care during the postpartum period [9]. Utilization of maternal health services is a complex phenomenon influenced by many factors. Sociodemographic factors such as age, education, wealth index, ethnicity, culture, decision making power, religion and service delivery environment are important determinants for the use of maternal health services [10, 11].

Although information on the use of PNC in Nepal is available [11–14], there is very little information about the use of the service according to protocol [9]. Hence, this study assessed the magnitude of and factors associated with the utilization of complete PNC service.

2. Methods

2.1. Study Area. Baglung district which represents a typical hilly district of Nepal and that has low utilization of PNC service was chosen [8]. It has population of 270000. The center of the district, i.e., Baglung municipality, is about 275 kilometer west of Kathmandu, the capital of Nepal, and is connected to Nepal's one of the biggest cities, Pokhara. According to district population profile 2017, the total population of Baglung municipality is 63511, with 1495 children of age 0-11 months [15]. Out of 14 wards of the municipality, ward numbers 1, 2, 3, and 4 are city areas of the municipality and are connected to one government hospital and two private hospitals located at headquarter of the municipality by concrete road. It takes less than 30 minutes to reach the hospitals by walking from wards 1, 2, and 4, whereas 10 to 60 minutes is needed from ward number 3 as it stretches from the market area to its outskirts.

2.2. Study Design and Population. A community based cross-sectional study was conducted among mothers residing in the selected wards of the municipality who gave birth a week before data collection to the last 12 months.

2.3. Sample. Sample size of the study was calculated by using the population proportion formula taking into account the proportion of women using PNC service $(p) = 50\%$ [16, 17], 95% confidence level, and margin of error $(d) = 5.8\%$.

$$\text{Sample size } (n) = \frac{Z^2pq}{d^2} = \frac{(1.96 \times 1.96)(0.05) \times (0.05)}{(0.58)^2} 285.49 \quad (1)$$

Considering a non-response rate of 10%, the final sample size of the study was 317.21. Hence, a total of 318 respondents were included in the study.

2.4. Sampling. Baglung municipality, the only municipality of the district, was purposively selected as the study aimed at assessing the use of PNC service in an urban setting where the service is relatively more accessible. Four connected wards, namely, ward numbers 1 to 4, were also purposively selected being the market area and its surrounding. All the mothers who had given birth one week prior to data collection for the past 12 months and residing in the selected wards of ward numbers 1, 2, and 3 and some mothers of ward number 4 were interviewed by house screening.

2.5. Data Collection and Procedure. Data was collected from 25th June to 25thJuly 2017 by face-to-face interview using a pretested [18] semi-structured questionnaire in Nepali language. The questionnaire included questions on use of PNC service, socio-demographic variables (age, education and occupation of respondents, caste/ethnicity, annual family income, and occupation of husbands), obstetrical variables (parity, antenatal care (ANC), place of delivery, duration of hospital stay, and complication during delivery), and awareness of PNC service. The number of mothers was identified from the registry of female community health volunteers of the respective wards and immunization registry of the local health facility. Then, house-to-house visit was done for data collection. Data was collected by the first author. The collected data was edited on the same day throughout the data collection period.

2.6. Variables

2.6.1. Dependent Variable. The dependent variable was the 'utilization of complete PNC.'

2.6.2. Independent Variables. Independent variables include socio-demographic characteristics, ANC visit, type of facility used for childbirth, complication during childbirth, duration of hospital stay, and awareness of PNC services.

2.7. Operational Definition

2.7.1. Utilization of Complete PNC. Utilization of complete PNC refers to at least three PNC within seven days after delivery. It was classified into two categories based on frequency and timing of postnatal checkup: 'partial' means one and/or two PNC within 24 hours and on third day following delivery, respectively, while 'complete' means three PNC with at least the third one on the seventh day following delivery.

(1) Caste/Ethnicity. 'Brahman/Chhetri' (so-called upper caste group), 'Janajati', and 'Dalits' [19]

(2) Education. Education was measured in terms of the ability to read and write and level of education completed. The four categories included 'no schooling,' 'basic education' (completion of any of the grades from 1 to 8), 'secondary education' (completion of any of 9 to 12 grades), and 'higher education' (bachelor's degree or higher) [20]

(3) Economic Status. Total yearly income of the household in Nepalese rupee (NPR) was classified into three categories: 'less than 250000,' '250000-600000,' and 'more than 600000' [21, 22]

(4) Parity. The parity of the recent birth was categorized as 'one' and 'two or more' for further analysis. Type

of Family. The type of family was categorized as 'nuclear' and 'joint'

(5) Number of ANC Visit. The number of ANC visit a respondent had during her last pregnancy was counted. The responses were grouped as 'no visit,' 'less than 4 visits,' and '4 or more visits'

(6) Childbirth Complication. Complication that arose during last childbirth. It was categorized as 'yes' and 'no'

(7) Type of Health Facility Used for Childbirth. 'Government facility' and 'private facility'

(8) Duration of Hospital Stay after Delivery. The duration of hospital stay after delivery was categorized as '6 hours or less,' '7 to 24 hours,' and 'more than 24 hours' [3, 7, 23].

(9) Awareness of PNC Services. It refers to information regarding meaning of postnatal period, timing and frequency of PNC visit, recommended health care provider for PNC, types of PNC services, and danger signs that may arise during postnatal period. It was classified into two categories based on the mean score: 'good awareness' (mean ≥ 5.50) and 'poor awareness' (mean < 5.50)

2.8. Data Processing and Analysis. Collected data were checked daily for completeness, consistency, and accuracy. The data were coded and then entered in data entry software EpiData 3.1 [24] and analyzed in the software Statistical Package for the Social Sciences version 18 [25]. Descriptive and inferential statistics were used for data analysis. As descriptive statistics, frequency, percentage, mean and standard deviation were used. In inferential statistics, chi-square test was applied to find out the association between level of utilization of PNC and independent variables. The variables that showed significant association at 5% level of significance were further analyzed to estimate unadjusted and then adjusted odds ratio (aOR) using multivariable logistic regression [26] to determine the factors associated with the utilization of complete PNC and their strength of association.

2.9. Ethics and Consent to Participate. Ethical approval was obtained from Chitwan Medical College-Institutional Review Committee. Permission to carry out the study was taken from municipality office of Baglung. Verbal informed consent was obtained from each respondent by clarifying the purpose of the study prior to the data collection. Confidentiality was maintained by not disclosing the information to anyone else and using it for research purpose only. Respondents' dignity was maintained by giving the right to reject or discontinue from the study at any time without any penalty.

3. Results

3.1. Sociodemographic Characteristics of the Respondents. Among 318 total respondents, 39% were in the age group 20-24 years. Regarding caste/ethnicity, about 47% were Brahman/Chhetri. Around 91% of the respondents belonged to the Hindu by religion. About two-thirds (63.7%) of the respondents had secondary level schooling. With regard to occupation, more than half (55.2%) of the respondents were involved in household work. Regarding the type of family, 54% of the respondents belonged to a nuclear family. More than one-third (35.6%) of the respondents stated that the annual income of their family was 250000 to 600000 NPR. About 31% of the husbands were involved in foreign employment. Nearly half (48.7%) of the respondents had given birth for the first time (Table 1).

3.2. Obstetrical Characteristics of the Respondents. Nearly all (99.4%) of the respondents had ANC checkup during last pregnancy. Of these, around 88% had four or more ANC. Regarding the place of delivery, almost all (98.7%) of the respondents had their last delivery in a health facility, while 84% of these used government hospitals for delivery. Around three-quarters (74.8%) of the mothers delivered by spontaneous vaginal delivery, while about 22% of the respondents had caesarean section. Slightly more than two-thirds (67.2%) of the births were assisted by a staff nurse/auxiliary nurse midwife (ANM). Regarding duration of hospital stay after delivery, 50% of the respondents stayed for seven to 24 hours. About 19% of the mothers had complication during the last childbirth. Half of the respondents (50.6%) had poor level of awareness on PNC services (Table 2).

3.3. Utilization of PNC. Of the total respondents, almost all (98.7%) had PNC. Among them, 78% had partial utilization (1-2 visit), while 22% had complete PNC. About 62% of the respondents received the PNC from nurses, and 85% of the respondents received the service from government hospital (Table 3).

3.4. Factors Associated with Utilization of Complete PNC. Caste/ethnicity, occupation of respondent's husband, type of health facility used for delivery, complication during delivery, duration of hospital stay after delivery, and awareness level on PNC service were found to be significantly associated with the utilization of complete PNC (Table 4).

3.5. Odds Ratio of Factors Associated with Use of Complete PNC. In multivariable logistic regression analysis, only caste/ethnicity, occupation of respondent's husband, and type of health facility where delivery happened were significantly associated with the utilization of complete PNC. The mothers who belonged to Brahman/Chhetri (aOR = 3.18, 95% CI: 1.24-8.12) and Janajati (aOR = 2.87, 95% CI: 1.09-7.53) caste/ethnicity were more likely to have complete PNC as compared to Dalits. Similarly, respondents whose husbands were job holders within the country were more likely (aOR = 3.49, 95% CI: 1.50-8.13) to get complete PNC as compared to those whose husbands were in foreign employment. Respondents who delivered their last child at a private hospital had higher likelihood (aOR=11.4, 95% CI: 5.40-24.2) of having complete PNC compared to those who delivered in a government hospital (Table 5).

TABLE 1: Sociodemographic characteristics of respondents ($n = 318$).

Variables	Frequency	Percentage
Age of mothers (in years)		
Less than 20	26	8.2
20 to 24	124	39.0
25-29	120	37.7
30 and above	48	15.1
Ethnicity		
Brahman/Chhetri	148	46.5
Janajati	95	29.9
Dalits	75	23.6
Religion		
Hindu	290	91.2
Non-Hindu*	28	8.8
Maternal education		
No schooling	13	4.1
Basic education	49	15.4
Secondary education	189	59.4
Higher education	67	21.1
Maternal occupation		
Household work	167	52.5
Farmer	55	17.3
Service	48	15.1
Business	34	10.7
Labour	14	4.4
Type of family		
Nuclear	173	54.4
Joint	145	45.6
Annual family income (in NPR)		
Less than 250000	120	37.7
250000 to 600000	113	35.6
More than 600000	85	26.7
Occupation of respondent's husband		
Foreign employment	98	30.8
Business	83	26.1
Service (job holder)	81	25.5
Labour	56	17.6
Parity		
One	155	48.7
Two or more	163	51.25

*Buddhist, Christian, and Islam.

TABLE 2: Obstetrical characteristics of respondents ($n = 318$).

Variables	Frequency	Percentage
Had ANC during last pregnancy		
Yes	316	99.4
No	2	0.6
Number of ANC visit ($n = 316$)		
<4 times	37	11.7
≥4 times	279	88.3
Place of delivery of last child		
At health facility	314	98.7
At home	4	1.3
Type of health facility used for delivery ($n = 314$)		
Government hospital	265	84.4
Private hospital	49	15.6
Type of delivery		
Spontaneous vaginal delivery	238	74.8
Assisted vaginal delivery	11	3.5
Caesarean section	69	21.7
Birth attendant at hospital		
Doctor	103	32.8
Staff nurse/ANM	211	67.2
Birth attendant at home ($n = 4$)		
Relative/friend	2	50.0
Staff nurse	1	25.0
No one	1	25.0
Duration of hospital stay after delivery ($n = 314$)		
≤6 hrs.	65	20.7
7-24 hrs.	157	50.0
>24 hrs.	92	29.3
Had complication during childbirth		
Yes	60	18.9
No	258	81.1
Type of the complications** ($n = 60$)		
Prolonged labour	29	48.4
Severe vaginal bleeding	18	30.0
Meconium stained liquor	12	20.0
Retained placenta	5	8.3
Raised blood pressure	5	8.3
Level of awareness on PNC services		
Poor awareness (<5.50)	161	50.6
Good awareness (≥5.50)	157	49.4

**Multiple responses.

4. Discussion

The study showed that about 99% of the respondents had utilized PNC service at least once, 34.7% had received two PNC, and only 21.7% of them had received the service three times within seven days following delivery. A similar study carried out in India found that 36.6% of the respondents had received one postnatal checkup, 18.5% received two, and 14.7% had three postnatal checkups [27]. Likewise, a study conducted in Ethiopia revealed that 57.4% of the mothers had one PNC, 40.4% had two PNC, and 2.2% had three or more PNC [28]. The difference in the proportions in the present and the previous studies may be attributed to the study setting and study population. Regarding the level of the utilization of PNC, 78% of the respondents had partial (1 to 2 times) utilization, while only 22% of the respondents had utilized complete PNC. A national figure showed that

Table 3: Utilization of PNC.

Variables	Frequency	Percentage
Received PNC ($n = 318$)		
Yes	314	98.7
No	4	1.3
Frequency of PNC ($n = 314$)		
Once	205	65.3
Two times	40	12.7
Three times	69	22.0
Level of utilization of PNC		
Partial	245	78.0
Complete	69	22.0
PNC provided by		
Doctors	108	34.3
Staff nurse/ANM	194	61.9
Health assistant	12	3.8
Place for PNC		
Government hospital	268	85.4
Private hospital/clinic	46	14.6

in Nepal 19% of women had PNC checkup as per protocol [9]. Similarly, a study conducted in Myanmar demonstrated that the prevalence of the utilization of complete PNC was 25.2% [29].

In the present study, respondents who belonged to Brahman/Chhetri (aOR = 4.33, 95% CI: 1.59-11.80) and Janajati (aOR = 4.06, 95% CI: 1.44-11.4) caste/ethnicity were more likely to have complete PNC as compared to Dalits. Consistently, a study conducted in Nepal showed that the Tamang ethnic group was less likely to have had PNC than Brahman/Chhetri (aOR = 0.15, 95% CI: 0.05-0.44) [11]. Similarly, another study in Nepal revealed that women from Janajati were less likely to utilize the maternal services (aOR = 0.75) than women from Brahman/Chhetri [12]. A systematic review and meta-analysis on inequities in the utilization of PNC in the low- and middle-income countries concluded that the use of PNC varies significantly by socioeconomic status of people [30]. The differences in the service utilization might be explained by the differentials in socioeconomic status reflected in the hierarchy of caste/ethnicity persistent in Nepal [31].

The respondents whose husbands were job holders in Nepal were more likely (aOR = 3.6, 95% CI: 1.54-8.66) to have complete PNC as compared to the respondents whose husbands were in foreign employment. Another study in Nepal revealed that mothers whose husbands were involved in the technical field (aOR = 1.7, 95% CI: 1.35-2.17) and labour (aOR = 1.3, 95% CI: 1.10-1.77) were more likely to receive PNC than the respondents whose husbands were involved in agriculture [14]. Another study supports the findings of the current study that women whose husbands were employees of the government or private sectors (aOR = 2.60, 95% CI=1.21-5.98) tended to be more likely to use PNC service than women whose husbands were involved in agriculture and/or labour work [32]. In the current study, however, the

Table 4: Factors associated with the utilization of complete PNC.

Variables	Utilization of PNC services Fully utilized, N. (%)	Partial utilized, N. (%)	p value
Age groups (in years)			
Less than 30	58 (21.8)	270 (78.2)	0.846
30 and above	11 (22.1)	37 (77.1)	
Ethnicity			
Janajati	23 (24.7)	70 (75.3)	**0.029**
Brahman/Chhetri	38 (32.3)	109 (74.1)	
Dalits	8 (10.8)	66 (89.2)	
Education status			
No schooling	3(23)	10 (77)	
Basic education	8 (17)	38 (83)	0.668
Secondary education	40 (21)	148(79)	
Higher education	18 (27)	49 (73)	
Occupation of respondents			
Household work	38 (23.0)	127(77.0)	
Farmer	10 (18.9)	43 (81.1)	
Service	11 (22.9)	37 (77.1)	0.907
Business	8 (23.5)	26 (76.5)	
Labour	2 (14.3)	12 (85.7)	
Occupation of respondents' husband			
Service	26 (32.9)	53 (67.1)	
Business	18 (21.7)	65 (78.3)	
Labour	9 (16.7)	45 (83.3)	**0.042**
Foreign employment	16 (16.3)	82 (83.7)	
Annual family income (in NPR)			
Less than250000	24 (20.5)	93 (79.5)	
250000 to 600000	35 (22.2)	123(77.8)	0.797
More than 600000	10 (25.6)	29 (74.4)	
Parity			
One	36 (23.2)	119(76.8)	0.597
More than one	33 (20.8)	126 (79.2)	
Number of ANC visit			
<4 times	4 (11.1)	32 (28.1)	0.101
≥4 times	65 (23.4)	213 (76.6)	
Type of facility used for delivery			
Government hospital	38 (14.3)	227 (85.7)	**<0.001**
Private hospital	31 (63.3)	18 (36.7)	
Had complication during childbirth			
Yes	19 (31.7)	41 (68.3)	**0.044**
No	50 (22.6)	204 (80.3)	
Awareness level on PNC services			
Poor	27 (17.2)	130 (82.8)	**0.041**
Good	42 (26.8)	115 (73.2)	

Table 5: Odds ratio of factors associated with use of complete PNC.

Variables	Unadjusted OR (95% CI)	Adjusted OR (95% CI)	Adjusted p value
Occupation of respondents' husbands			
Service (job holder)	2.51 (1.23-5.12)	**3.49 (1.50-8.13)**	0.004
Business	1.41 (0.67-2.99)	1.69 (0.71-4.00)	0.229
Labour	1.02 (0.41-2.50)	2.11 (0.72-6.18)	0.171
Foreign employment	1	1	
Type of facility used for delivery			
Government hospital	1	1	
Private hospital	10.2 (5.23-20.2)	**11.4 (5.40-24.2)**	<0.001
Caste/ethnicity			
Janajati	2.71 (1.13-6.48)	**2.87 (1.09-7.53)**	0.031
Brahman/Chhetri	2.87 (1.26-6.54)	**3.18 (1.24-8.12)**	0.016
Dalits	1	1	
Awareness level on PNC			
Poor	1	1	
Good	1.75 (1.02-3.03)	1.34 (0.71-2.54)	0.362
Complication during childbirth			
Yes	1.89 (1.01-3.53)	1.25 (0.58-2.67)	0.561
No	1	1	

1 indicates reference category.

husbands were not involved in agriculture but were in foreign employment along with in business, labour, and service. This could be because of the urban setting of the study. Involvement of male is necessary for improved maternal health outcomes in developing countries [33]. Husbands have an important role in the maternity care of their wives [34]. A study conducted in Myanmar revealed that male involvement is more likely (aOR, 2.19; 95% CI, and 1.02-4.69) to result in having complete PNC [29]. In Nepal, husbands' involvement in maternal health care is in giving advice, supporting with household work, and arranging money and transportation for the delivery in a health facility [34]. In addition, the husbands may be the one to accompany wives to health facilities [35]. A husband accompanying his wife is associated with higher likelihood of using PNC from a trained service provider [36]. The involvement of the husband is influenced by his availability, cultural beliefs, and traditions [35].

The present study depicted that respondents who delivered their last child at a private hospital were more likely (aOR = 11.9, 95% CI: 5.52-25.7) to have complete PNC as compared to those who delivered in a government hospital. This finding is supported by the study conducted in Palestine (aOR = 1.8, 95% CI: 1.0-3.4) that women who delivered at a private hospital had a higher likelihood to have PNC [37]. Consistent results were observed in a study in Zambia where women giving birth at a private hospital/clinic had higher odds (aOR 10.08 95% CI 3.35–30.35) of having PNC than at a government hospital (aOR 7.24, 95% CI 4.92–11.84) or government health center/clinic (aOR 7.15 95% CI 4.79–10.66) [38]. PNC counseling and provision of appointment are associated with a higher likelihood of using PNC service [28]. Timeliness and hospitality to patients are greater in private facilities than in public [39]. Women preferred private facilities for maternal health services because of longer consultation time, better interpersonal and communication skills of health care providers, better treatment, more advanced equipment and devices, availability of female obstetricians, and more flexible appointment times [40]. Women who delivered at health facilities rated private facilities to be of higher quality in terms of amenities and interpersonal aspects than public ones [41]. Consistently, interpersonal process was also found of better quality in private health facilities by the women attending health facilities for family planning service [42]. Public facilities are generally used due to financial and physical accessibility [43].

5. Strengths and Limitations of the Study

There was a possibility of recall bias as the mothers were asked about the utilization of the service received within last one year prior to the data collection. The findings may not be generalizable in all places as the sample was restricted to four wards of the municipality. Some risk factors have not been measured in this study such as neonatal complication and sociocultural practices during puerperium. However, the study has some strengths as well. The study identifies the status of the utilization of complete PNC in which very limited information is available in community-based studies in Nepal. Secondly, the study shows the status of the utilization of PNC in an urban setting where almost all mothers had institutional delivery, unlike in previous studies of Nepal.

6. Conclusion

The utilization of complete PNC is low, although having at least one PNC was high, despite the availability of and accessibility to the service. Caste/ethnicity, occupation of respondents' husband, and type of health facility used for delivery were found to have influenced the utilization. Uptake of complete PNC service may increase by raising awareness on the importance and schedule of PNC. PNC services should be focused on the mothers who belong to a disadvantaged caste/ethnicity and whose husbands are in foreign employment. Involvement of husbands in maternity care, including in PNC service utilization, should be promoted. In addition, improving the quality of the service, particularly in government health facilities, such as interpersonal aspects, timely service, and amenities, may increase the use of PNC service. Implementation research to explore feasibility and sustainability of providing complete PNC by a health worker such as ANM by home visits is needed considering difficult geography and fragile condition of the mother and newborn to travel to a health facility for second and third PNC.

Abbreviations

ANC: Antenatal care
ANM: Auxiliary nurse midwife
aOR: Adjusted odds ratio
CI: Confidence interval
NPR: Nepalese rupees
PNC: Postnatal care.

Consent

Informed verbal consent was obtained from each respondent. Confidentiality of information and privacy were maintained.

Authors' Contributions

SC conceptualized the design of the study, prepared tools, collected and analyzed data, interpreted results, and drafted the manuscript. RS contributed to the conceptualization and design of the analysis, interpreted data, reviewed literature, and contributed extensively to the drafting of the manuscript. LR supported in the conceptualization of the study, data analysis and interpretation, and provided feedback throughout the research. All authors have read and approved the final version of the manuscript.

Acknowledgments

The authors would like to thank the faculty of nursing department, Chitwan Medical College, as well as the Baglung municipality for their support during the study period.

References

[1] World Health Organization, UNICEF, *Trends in maternal mortality: 1990-2015: estimates from WHO, UNICEF, UNFPA, World Bank Group and the United Nations Population Division*, World Health Organization, 2015.

[2] E. Sines, U. Syed, S. Wall, and H. Worley, "Postnatal care: a critical opportunity to save mothers and newborns," in *Policy Perspectives on Newborn Health*, pp. 1–7, Population Reference Bureau, 2007.

[3] World Health Organization, *WHO recommendations on postnatal care of the mother and newborn*, World Health Organization, 2014.

[4] Ministry of Health, New ERA, ORC Macro, *Nepal demographicand health survey 2016*, Family health division, Ministry of Health; New ERA; ORC Macro, Calverton, Maryland, 2017.

[5] National Planning Commission, "Sustainable development goals, 2016-2030, National (preliminary) report," Nepal Government of Nepal, National Planning Commission, Kathmandu, 2015.

[6] World Health Organization, *WHO technical consultation on postpartum and postnatal care*, World Health Organization, Geneva, 2010.

[7] Ministry of Health and Population, *National medical standard for reproductive health. Volume III: maternal and neonatal care*, Ministry of health and population, Family health division, Nepal, 2009.

[8] Department of Health Services, *Annual report 2015/2016*, Department of Health Services, Ministry of Health and Population, Government of Nepal, Kathmandu, Nepal, 2017.

[9] Department of Health Services, *Annual report 2017/2018*, Department of Health Services, Ministry of Health and Population, Government of Nepal, Kathmandu, Nepal, 2019.

[10] A. Singh, S. S. Padmadas, U. S. Mishra, S. Pallikadavath, F. A. Johnson, and Z. Matthews, "Socio-economic inequalities in the use of postnatal care in India," *PLoS One*, vol. 7, no. 5, article e37037, 2012.

[11] S. Dhakal, G. N. Chapman, P. P. Simkhada, E. R. Van Teijlingen, J. Stephens, and A. E. Raja, "Utilisation of postnatal care among rural women in Nepal," *BMC Pregnancy and Childbirth*, vol. 7, no. 1, p. 19, 2007.

[12] R. Adhikari, "Effect of Women's autonomy on maternal health service utilization in Nepal: a cross sectional study," *BMC Women's Health*, vol. 16, no. 1, p. 26, 2016.

[13] M. Paudel, V. Khanal, B. Acharya, and M. Adhikari, "Determinants of postnatal service utilization in a Western District of Nepal: community based Cross Sectional study," *Journal of Womens Health Care*, vol. 2, no. 3, p. 2167, 2013.

[14] V. Khanal, M. Adhikari, R. Karkee, and T. Gavidia, "Factors associated with the utilisation of postnatal care services among the mothers of Nepal: analysis of Nepal demographic and health survey 2011," *BMC Women's Health*, vol. 14, no. 1, p. 19, 2014.

[15] District Public Health Office, *District population profile 2017*, Nepal, DPHO, Baglung, 2017.

[16] L. Naing, T. Winn, and B. Rusli, "Practical issues in calculating the sample size for prevalence studies," *Archives of Orofacial Sciences*, vol. 1, pp. 9–14, 2006.

[17] R. Arya, B. Antonisamy, and S. Kumar, "Sample size estimation in prevalence studies," *The Indian Journal of Pediatrics*, vol. 79, no. 11, pp. 1482–1488, 2012.

[18] E. van Teijlingen and V. Hundley, "Pilot studies in family planning and reproductive health care," *Journal of Family Planning and Reproductive Health Care*, vol. 31, no. 3, pp. 219–221, 2005.

[19] J. P. Pandey, M. R. Dhakal, S. Karki, P. Poudel, and M. S. Pradhan, *Maternal and Child Health in Nepal: The Effects of Caste, Ethnicity, and Regional Identity:Further Analysis of the 2011 Nepal Demographic and Health Survey.Kathmandu: Calverton,*

Nepal Ministry of Health and Population, New ERA, and ICF International, Maryland, USA, 2013.

[20] National Institute for Research and Training, *Nepal education sector analysis*, National Institute for Research and Training (NIRT), Kathmandu, Nepal, 2017, Vii..

[21] A. A. Rurangirwa, I. Mogren, L. Nyirazinyoye, J. Ntaganira, and G. Krantz, "Determinants of poor utilization of antenatal care services among recently delivered women in Rwanda; a population-based study," *BMC Pregnancy and Childbirth*, vol. 17, no. 1, p. 142, 2017.

[22] S. Pandey and S. Karki, "Socio-economic and demographic determinants of antenatal care services utilization in Central Nepal," *International Journal of MCH and AIDS*, vol. 2, no. 2, pp. 212–219, 2014.

[23] O. M. Campbell, L. Cegolon, D. Macleod, and L. Benova, "Length of stay after childbirth in 92 countries and associated factors in 30 Low- and middle-income countries: compilation of reported data and a cross-sectional analysis from nationally representative surveys," *PLoS Medicine*, vol. 13, no. 3, article e1001972, 2016.

[24] J. M. Lauristen and M. Bruus, *Epi Tour: An Introduction to Validated Data Entry and Documentation of Data by Use of EpiData*, The Epidata Association, Odense Denmark, 2008.

[25] M. Norusis, *SPSS 16.0 Statistical Procedures Companion*, Prentice Hall Press, 2008.

[26] C.-Y. J. Peng, K. L. Lee, and G. M. Ingersoll, "An introduction to logistic Regression analysis and reporting," *The Journal of Educational Research*, vol. 96, no. 1, pp. 3–14, 2010.

[27] A. Sharma, P. S. Thakur, P. K. Kasar, R. Tiwari, and R. Sharma, "Utilization of post natal care in tribal area of Madhya Pradesh, India: a community based cross-sectional study," *International Journal of Medical Science and Public Health.*, vol. 3, no. 10, pp. 1266–1272, 2014.

[28] S. Berhanu Sr., Y. Asefa, and B. W. Giru, "Prevalence of postnatal care utilization and associated factors among women who gave birth and attending immunization clinic in selected government health centers in Addis Ababa, Ethiopia, 2016," *Prevalence*, vol. 26, 2016.

[29] A. S. Mon, M. K. Phyu, W. Thinkhamrop, and B. Thinkhamrop, *Utilization of full postnatal care services among rural Myanmar women and its determinants: a cross-sectional study*, F1000Research, 2018.

[30] É. V. Langlois, M. Miszkurka, M. V. Zunzunegui, A. Ghaffar, D. Ziegler, and I. Karp, "Inequities in postnatal care in low- and middle-income countries: a systematic review and meta-analysis," *Bulletin of the World Health Organization*, vol. 93, no. 4, pp. 259–270, 2015.

[31] L. Bennett, "Gender, caste and ethnic exclusion in Nepal," in *Following the policy process from analysis to action*, World Bank, Washington, DC, 2005.

[32] R. Khadka, S. A. Hong, and B. O. Thepthien, "Postnatal care service utilization and its determinants in Ramechhap district, Nepal: a community-based cross-sectional study," *Journal of Public Health and Development*, vol. 15, no. 3, pp. 1–6, 2017.

[33] J. Yargawa and J. Leonardi-Bee, "Male involvement and maternal health outcomes: systematic review and meta-analysis," *Journal of Epidemiology and Community Health*, vol. 69, no. 6, pp. 604–612, 2015.

[34] D. K. Thapa and A. Niehof, "Women's autonomy and husbands' involvement in maternal health care in Nepal," *Social Science & Medicine*, vol. 93, pp. 1 10, 2013.

[35] S. Lewis, A. Lee, and P. Simkhada, "The role of husbands in maternal health and safe childbirth in rural Nepal: a qualitative study," *BMC Pregnancy and Childbirth*, vol. 15, no. 1, p. 162, 2015.

[36] A. E. Rahman, J. Perkins, S. Islam et al., "Knowledge and involvement of husbands in maternal and newborn health in rural Bangladesh," *BMC Pregnancy and Childbirth*, vol. 18, no. 1, p. 247, 2018.

[37] E. Dhaher, R. T. Mikolajczyk, A. E. Maxwell, and A. Krämer, "Factors associated with lack of postnatal care among Palestinian women: a cross-sectional study of three clinics in the West Bank," *BMC Pregnancy and Childbirth*, vol. 8, no. 1, p. 26, 2008.

[38] C. Chungu, M. Makasa, M. Chola, and C. N. Jacobs, "Place of delivery associated with postnatal care utilization among childbearing women in Zambia," *Frontiers in Public Health*, vol. 6, p. 94, 2018.

[39] S. Basu, J. Andrews, S. Kishore, R. Panjabi, and D. Stuckler, "Comparative performance of private and public healthcare systems in low-and middle-income countries: a systematic review," *PLoS Medicine*, vol. 9, no. 6, article e1001244, 2012.

[40] M. S. Alyahya, Y. S. Khader, A. Batieha, and M. Asad, "The quality of maternal-fetal and newborn care services in Jordan: a qualitative focus group study," *BMC Health Services Research*, vol. 19, no. 1, p. 425, 2019.

[41] R. Karkee, A. H. Lee, and P. K. Pokharel, "Women's perception of quality of maternity services: a longitudinal survey in Nepal," *BMC Pregnancy and Childbirth*, vol. 14, no. 1, p. 45, 2014.

[42] P. L. Hutchinson, M. Do, and S. Agha, "Measuring client satisfaction and the quality of family planning services: a comparative analysis of public and private health facilities in Tanzania, Kenya and Ghana," *BMC Health Services Research*, vol. 11, no. 1, p. 203, 2011.

[43] R. Karkee and J. Kadariya, "Choice of health-care facility after introduction of free essential health services in Nepal," *WHO South-East Asia Journal of Public Health*, vol. 2, no. 2, pp. 96–100, 2013.

14

Diagnosis and Treatment in a Tertiary Hospital of a Series of Complex Genital Malformations Corresponding to Double Uterus with Obstructed Hemivagina and Ipsilateral Renal Agenesis

Júlia Kefalás Troncon,[1] Júlio César Rosa-e-Silva,[2] Rayssa Miranda,[3] Francisco José Candido-dos-Reis,[2] Omero Benedicto Poli-Neto,[4] and Antônio Alberto Nogueira[5]

[1] *MSc in Obstetrics and Gynecology, Department of Obstetrics and Gynecology, Ribeirão Preto Medical School, University of São Paulo, Ribeirão Preto, SP, Brazil*
[2] *Associate Professor, Department of Obstetrics and Gynecology, Ribeirão Preto Medical School, University of São Paulo, Ribeirão Preto (SP), Brazil*
[3] *Undergraduate student, Ribeirão Preto Medical School, University of São Paulo, Ribeirão Preto, SP, Brazil*
[4] *Associate Professor, Department of Obstetrics and Gynecology, Ribeirão Preto Medical School, University of São Paulo, Ribeirão Preto, SP, Brazil*
[5] *PhD, Professor, Department of Obstetrics and Gynecology, Ribeirão Preto Medical School, University of São Paulo, Ribeirão Preto, SP, Brazil*

Correspondence should be addressed to Júlio César Rosa-e-Silva; juliocesarrosaesilva@gmail.com

Academic Editor: Hind A. Beydoun

Aim. To evaluate the clinical features, diagnostic routine, treatment, and prognosis of patients with double uterus with obstructed hemivagina and ipsilateral renal agenesis at a University Hospital. *Methods*. A retrospective study analyzing the medical charts of outpatients with similar complex genital malformations seen at the University Hospital of the Ribeirão Preto Medical School from 1994 to 2015. *Results*. Fourteen patients were included in this retrospective study, all presenting with double uterus with obstructed hemivagina and ipsilateral renal agenesis. The main symptom was dysmenorrhea occurring shortly after menarche, and pelvic ultrasound was the examination of choice. The treatment consisted of resection of the vaginal septum, complemented by an abdominal approach in 5 cases. Complications of the syndrome observed in this case series included severe endometriosis, pelvic abscess, need for hysterectomy, and salpingectomy. *Conclusions*. Severe dysmenorrhea shortly after menarche is a typical symptom of this kind of malformation, even though the diagnosis of patients who present with fistulization of the vaginal septum can be delayed due to milder clinical features. Pelvic ultrasound can be considered the first-choice examination in diagnostic routine. Relief of pain and prevention of complications can be achieved successfully in most cases by resection of the vaginal septum.

1. Introduction

The presence of double uterus with obstructed hemivagina and ipsilateral renal agenesis, also referred to as Herlyn-Werner-Wünderlich (HWW) syndrome, or OHVIRA syndrome, is a type of complex anomaly associated with changes in the fusion of the müllerian ducts, with different degrees of uterine duplicity (class III of Buttran and Gibbons) [1, 2], in addition to obstruction of the hemivagina and ipsilateral renal agenesis [3], corresponding to a concomitant Wolffian abnormality. This malformation more frequently courses with a uterus didelphys with partial vaginal duplication forming a transverse septum and obstruction of menstrual flow in this hemivagina associated with the ipsilateral renal agenesis.

However, it may also be associated with a bicornuate bicollis uterus or a septate uterus with septation extending to the cervix and the vagina or also with unilateral cervical atresia [4]. Whatever the type of malformation, in all cases there is obstruction of the unilateral hemivagina and ipsilateral renal agenesis, so that the condition is also known as obstructed hemivagina and ipsilateral renal agenesis (OHVIRA).

Müllerian malformations are frequently associated with urinary malformations due to the intimate relationship between the müllerian ducts and the Wolff ducts during the embryonic period. If the Wolff duct fails to develop on one side, with the consequent occurrence of renal agenesis, the ipsilateral müllerian duct will develop in a more lateralized manner, thus impairing its fusion with the contralateral müllerian duct. In addition, the malformed hemivagina will not join the urogenital sinus in an appropriate manner, resulting in obstruction [3, 4]. Therefore, apparently this malformation results from anomalies of both Müllerian and Wolffian (or mesonephric) origin. That is, renal agenesis and disruption of vaginal development occur if the mesonephric ducts do not play their proper role. Concomitantly, the induction of the Müllerian by the mesonephric ducts is also disrupted, resulting in nonabsorption defects as the uterine duplicate [5, 6].

The real prevalence of this anomaly is difficult to measure since in general the diagnosis is not made during a clinical gynecological examination but rather during some surgical procedure or by imaging evaluation. The prevalence is higher among groups with a specific condition such as infertility or endometriosis than among unselected populations. However, the estimated incidence is 0.1 to 0.8% and the condition is usually discovered after menarche by causing progressive dysmenorrhea due to the presence of the transverse vaginal septum which prevents blood flow through the vaginal canal, causing the formation of hematocolpos [7–9]. In view of the accumulation of menstrual blood that is not discharged due to the septum, at diagnosis the condition may also appear as a pelvic mass. In addition, due to the obstruction of menstrual flow that potentially intensifies tubal reflux, the patient may develop the more severe forms of endometriosis. In cases of hematocolpos fistulization through the vaginal septum, the complaint may be fetid leukorrhea [3, 10]. Asymptomatic or barely symptomatic cases are associated with the form of anomaly that involves communication between the two uterine horns or an incomplete transverse septum. The condition is also associated with signs and symptoms of infertility, although pregnancy can occur in the normal uterine horn and in the previously obstructed horn after surgical intervention.

The objective of the present study was to analyze the clinical signs and symptoms, the procedures used at diagnosis and the short- and long-term prognosis of patients with this type of malformation seen in our service that could be compatible with the also called Herlyn-Werner-Wünderlich (HWWS) or OHVIRA Syndrome.

2. Methods

This was a retrospective study based on the survey of the medical records of patients seen from 1994 to 2015 at the Human Reproduction, Gynecological Endoscopy and Children's and Pubertal Outpatient Clinics of the Department of Gynecology and Obstetrics of FMRP-USP with a diagnosis of double uterus with obstructed hemivagina and ipsilateral renal agenesis, according to diagnostic criteria established in the scientific literature [1–4].

Date and age at first visit, symptoms, clinical examination, subsidiary exams, treatment instituted, associated pregnancies, and their results were obtained from the medical records.

3. Results

The data of 14 patients seen at the service during the follow-up period and fulfilling the diagnostic criteria of this kind of malformation were obtained from the medical records. Data regarding age and clinical signs and symptoms at the time of diagnosis, type of anatomical malformation, treatment, and the occurrence or absence of pregnancy during follow-up are presented in Table 1.

Most of the patients analyzed sought gynecological care a short time after menarche. Most patients had dysmenorrhea as the main clinical manifestation. In the initial approach, ultrasound was the examination of choice and was performed in almost all cases.

Regarding treatment, in addition to exeresis of the vaginal septum, 6 patients required a joint abdominal approach. Three patients underwent salpingectomy due to large tubal dilation associated with hematosalpinxs. One patient underwent hysterectomy three months after the septum exeresis due to infectious complications, one underwent salpingectomy and oophorectomy due to tube ovarian abscess, and one patient was submitted to salpingectomy due to pyosalpinx associated with rudimentary horn exeresis.

We observed not infrequent complications associated with this entity, among them 2 cases of severe endometriosis, 2 cases of abscess, 1 case of hysterectomy, and 4 cases requiring salpingectomy. In these cases the complications were not associated with age, the duration of symptoms, or type of surgical approach. Only 3 of the 14 patients studied reported pregnancy during a ten-year follow-up. But it is important to emphasize that conservative treatment with exclusive vaginal septum exeresis is the preferred treatment.

4. Discussion

The main symptom detected among the patients was dysmenorrhea and pelvic pain due to the presence of an obstructed hemivagina that resulted in the accumulation of metabolized blood, causing hematocolpos, hematometra, and hematosalpinx. Dysmenorrhea was reported to be moderate to intense and the patients with a less symptomatic condition had communication between the uterine horns or an incomplete or fistulized vaginal septum. In one of the most extensive reviews of published cases, 94% of the patients complained about dysmenorrhea, 14% about vaginal discharge, and 2% about an acute abdomen [4].

The gynecological examination and investigation confirmed the diagnosis of uterus didelphys, transverse vaginal septum, and ipsilateral renal agenesis with hematocolpos,

TABLE 1: Description of the 14 cases of diagnosed HWWS.

Case	Age at 1st visit	Clinical signs and symptoms	Diagnosis	Treatment	Pregnancy
1	11	Progressively worsening dysmenorrhea persisting after the end of the menstrual flow	Uterus didelphys, complete transverse vaginal septum, R renal agenesis, R hematometra	Exeresis of the vaginal septum with discharge of chocolate brown blood	G1P1A0 (preterm pregnancy at 17 years)
2	13	Irregular cycles accompanied by dysmenorrhea since menarche	Uterus didelphys, complete transverse vaginal septum, R renal agenesis, R hematocolpos	Exeresis of the vaginal septum and drainage of hematocolpos	G0
3	24	Purulent and constant vaginal secretion	Uterus didelphys, transverse vaginal septum, R renal agenesis, purulent secretion	Resection of the transverse vaginal septum on the right and abscess drainage	G0
4	14	Irregular cycles with severe dysmenorrhea and difficulty urinating	Uterus didelphys, transverse vaginal septum, L renal agenesis, L hematometra	Resection of the vaginal septum, drainage of hematometra and L salpingectomy	G0
5	23	Daily bleeding associated with chronic pelvic pain of moderate intensity and dysmenorrhea	Uterus didelphys, transverse vaginal septum, L renal agenesis hematometra	Resection of the vaginal septum, drainage of hematometra and L salpingectomy	G0
6	13	Progressive dysmenorrhea since menarche	Uterus didelphys, transverse vaginal septum, R renal agenesis, hematocolpos (dilated cervix, body and right uterine tube)	Opening of the vaginal septum, drainage of hematocolpos and total abdominal hysterectomy 3 months after septum exeresis	G0
7	11	Progressively worsening dysmenorrhea persisting after the end of the menstrual flow	Uterus didelphys, transverse vaginal septum, L renal agenesis, hematocolpos, hematosalpinx	Exeresis of the vaginal septum, drainage of hematocolpos and salpingectomy	G0
8	12	Continuous pain in the hypogastrium arising with the menstrual flow	Uterus didelphys, transverse vaginal septum, L renal agenesis, hematocolpos	Exeresis of the vaginal septum, drainage of hematocolpos, oophorectomy and salpingectomy	G0
9	13	Progressive dysmenorrhea	Uterus didelphys, transverse vaginal septum, R renal agenesis, hydrosalpinx	Exeresis of R rudimentary horn and pyosalpinx	G0
10	13	Extensive vaginal bleeding and pelvic pain in inguinal regions	Uterus didelphys, transverse vaginal septum, R renal and ureteral agenesis	Exeresis of the vaginal septum	G0
11	29	Constant and progressive pain in a hypogastric region during the perimenstrual period	Uterus didelphys, transverse vaginal septum, R renal agenesis, hematocolpos, pelvic endometriosis	Exeresis of the vaginal septum and drainage of hematocolpos	G1P1A0 (cesarean delivery of a preterm liveborn at 35 weeks)
12	13	Increased menstrual flow since menarche	Uterus didelphys, transverse vaginal septum, L renal agenesis, presence of purulent content	Exeresis of the vaginal septum	G0
13	16	Vaginal discharge, blood clots after menstruation and intense menstrual cramps	Uterus didelphys, transverse vaginal septum, R renal agenesis, R hydrosalpinx	Exeresis of the vaginal septum	G4P3A1
14	21	Progressive dysmenorrhea and severe pelvic endometriosis	Uterus didelphys, transverse vaginal septum, R renal agenesis	Exeresis of the vaginal septum	G0

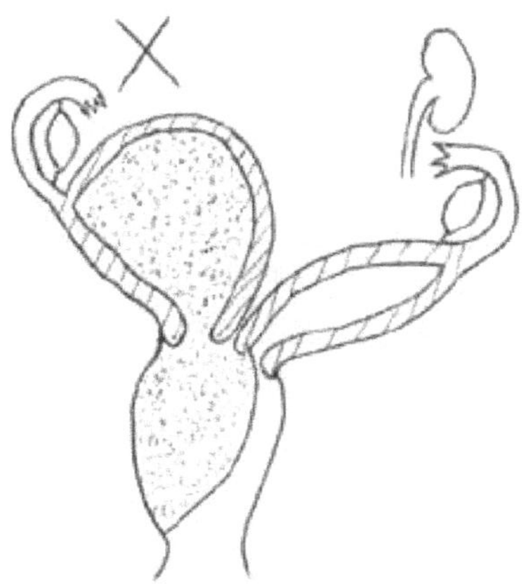

Figure 1: Genital malformation with uterus didelphys and right renal agenesis characteristic of the syndrome.

representing the most common form of the so-called Herlyn-Werner-Wünderlich syndrome. The exam most frequently used and most efficient for the diagnosis of the reproductive apparatus was ultrasound, applied to 13 of the 14 patients. The only exception was a patient who exhibited an infectious complication with purulent secretion through the vagina. In the present series, contrast radiography was used to confirm renal agenesis. Diagnostic hysteroscopy with vaginoscopy and diagnostic laparoscopy were used in the more complex cases. Magnetic resonance was carried out in 4 patients but did not modify the diagnosis or the management in this case series. Ultrasound is the first line examination for the complementary evaluation of these patients, with the primary condition being dysmenorrhea. The magnetic resonance can be considered as second-line examination because of the cost-effectiveness; however in cases of complex müllerian malformations it can be extremely helpful [11].

The literature has extensively reported and confirmed the use of imaging methods such as ultrasound and magnetic resonance for the diagnosis of both müllerian and urinary tract malformations [3, 10], and laparoscopy continues to play an important role on the diagnosis of pelvic diseases and on the identification of complications such as endometriosis or pelvic abscesses.

Complicated evolution of the cases was due to either infection or endometriosis. Both occur in consequence of the existing obstruction to the menstrual flow: in the first case, when this accumulation of menstrual blood becomes infected and in the case of endometriosis due to menstrual blood reflux into the abdominal cavity.

Patient treatment consisted of exeresis of the vaginal septum and drainage of hematocolpos, with consequent relief of symptoms. This approach is resolutive for cases of classical presentation as illustrated in Figure 1. Abdominal surgical intervention is usually unnecessary and, if indicated, is preferentially performed by the laparoscopic route. Other possible anatomical variations may require an individualized therapeutic approach. The primary objective of treatment, which involved relief of symptoms and the prevention of complications, was achieved. Resolution of symptoms occurred in most patients with the removal of the vaginal septum and three patients became pregnant without the need for additional treatment.

5. Conclusion

The main clinical manifestation observed in the patients was progressive dysmenorrhea after menarche. However, the diagnosis of patients with fistulization of the vaginal septum or communication between the uterine horns was delayed since their dysmenorrhea was less severe.

Although this is a rare condition, a high index of suspicion can lead to early diagnosis and timely intervention. It is also important to remember that, whenever malformation of müllerian ducts is diagnosed, it is essential to check for the associated renal malformations once they often coexist.

Acknowledgments

This work was supported by the National Council for Scientific and Technological Development (CNPq).

References

[1] V. C. Buttram Jr. and W. E. Gibbons, "Müllerian anomalies: a proposed classification. (An analysis of 144 cases)," *Fertility and Sterility*, vol. 32, no. 1, pp. 40–46, 1979.

[2] P. Acién, M. Acién, and M. Sánchez-Ferrer, "Complex malformations of the female genital tract. New types and revision of classification," *Human Reproduction*, vol. 19, no. 10, pp. 2377–2384, 2004.

[3] R. Bhoil, A. Ahluwalia, and N. Chauhan, "Herlyn werner wunderlich syndrome with hematocolpos: An unusual case report of full diagnostic approach and treatment," *International Journal of Fertility & Sterility*, vol. 10, no. 1, pp. 136–140, 2016.

[4] L. Fedele, F. Motta, G. Frontino, E. Restelli, and S. Bianchi, "Double uterus with obstructed hemivagina and ipsilateral renal agenesis: Pelvic anatomic variants in 87 cases," *Human Reproduction*, vol. 28, no. 6, pp. 1580–1583, 2013.

[5] P. Acién and M. I. Acién, "The history of female genital tract malformation classifications and proposal of an updated system†," *Human Reproduction Update*, vol. 17, no. 5, pp. 693–705, 2011.

[6] M. L. Sánchez-Ferrer, M. I. Acién, F. Sánchez del Campo, M. J. Mayol-Belda, and P. Acién, "Experimental contributions to the study of the embryology of the vagina," *Human Reproduction*, vol. 21, no. 6, pp. 1623–1628, 2006.

[7] R. Rana, S. Pasrija, and M. Puri, "Herlyn-Werner-Wunderlich syndrome with pregnancy: A rare presentation," *Congenital Anomalies*, vol. 48, no. 3, pp. 142-143, 2008.

[8] A. Sarac and M. K. Demir, "Herlyn-Werner-Wunderlich syndrome: A rare cause of infertility (2009: 2b)," *European Radiology*, vol. 19, no. 5, pp. 1306–1308, 2009.

[9] C. Simon, L. Martinez, F. Pardo, M. Tortajada, and A. Pellicer, "Mullerian defects in women with normal reproductive outcome," *Fertility and Sterility*, vol. 56, no. 6, pp. 1192-1193, 1991.

[10] C. Orazi, M. C. Lucchetti, P. M. S. Schingo, P. Marchetti, and F. Ferro, "Herlyn-Werner-Wunderlich syndrome: Uterus didelphys, blind hemivagina and ipsilateral renal agenesis. Sonographic and MR findings in 11 cases," *Pediatric Radiology*, vol. 37, no. 7, pp. 657–665, 2007.

[11] S. M. Khaladkar, V. Kamal, A. Kamal, and S. K. Kondapavuluri, "The Herlyn-Werner-Wunderlich syndrome - A case report with radiological review," *Polish Journal of Radiology*, vol. 81, pp. 395–400, 2016.

15

Antenatal Care Attendance and Factors Influenced Birth Weight of Babies Born between June 2017 and May 2018 in the Wa East District, Ghana

Prince Kubi Appiah [1,2] **Mohammed Bukari,** [3] **Simon Nidoolah Yiri-Erong,** [4] **Kwabena Owusu,** [5] **George Borogyante Atanga,** [6] **Stephen Nimirkpen,** [7] **Blaise Bagyliku Kuubabongnaa,** [3] **and Martin Adjuik** [8]

[1] *Department of Family and Community Health, School of Public Health, University of Health and Allied Sciences, Ho, Ghana*
[2] *Department of Medical Law and Ethics, Asian Institute for Bioethics and Health Law, College of Medicine, Yonsei University, Seoul, Republic of Korea*
[3] *Health Information Unit, District Health Administration, Ghana Health Service, Wa East District, Upper West Region, Ghana*
[4] *Department of Public Health and Community Medicine, Institute of Medicine, University of Gothenburg, Sweden*
[5] *Health Information Unit, District Health Administration, Ghana Health Service, Wa West District, Upper West Region, Ghana*
[6] *Health Information Unit, District Health Administration, Ghana Health Service, Sissaala West District, Upper West Region, Ghana*
[7] *Health Information Unit, Municipal Health Administration, Ghana Health Service, Lawra Municipal, Upper West Region, Ghana*
[8] *Department of Epidemiology and Biostatistics, School of Public Health, University of Health and Allied Sciences, Ho, Ghana*

Correspondence should be addressed to Prince Kubi Appiah; appiahkubiprince23@yahoo.com

Academic Editor: Robert Gaspar

Background. In sub-Saharan Africa, there is high coverage of the recommended four or more times antenatal care (ANC) visits during pregnancy without complications; notwithstanding this achievement, the negative birth outcomes related to childbirth such as low birth weights and stillbirths are still high despite the increased access to antenatal services. Hence, the study assessed the association between antenatal attendance and birth weight in the Wa East District. *Method.* The cross-sectional study design was used with a semistructured questionnaire to collect data from mothers who delivered within a one-year period through a review of antenatal and birth records from health facilities where the women delivered and interviewed. The chi-squared test and univariate and multivariate logistic regression were performed to establish the association between normal birth weight and ANC services the woman received and other predictor variables, and p value < 0.05 was considered a significant association between dependent and independent variables. *Result.* The study involved 233 women. About 62.2% attended ANC clinics 4+ times before giving birth, 70.0% did not received the minimum ANC services required for every pregnant woman, 0.9% of pregnancies resulted in stillbirth, and 24.5% of babies born had a birth weight < 2.5 kg. Women marital status (legally married) [AOR: 2.05, 95% CI: 1.33-6.89, $p = 0.044$], religion (Islam) [AOR: 0.33, 95% CI: 0.08-0.39, $p = 0.013$], and educational level (SHS/tertiary) [AOR: 4.27, 95% CI: 0.08-0.88, $p = 0.031$] were the background characteristics associated with normal birth weight (2.5-40 kg). Also, women who had their urine tested at the ANC clinics [AOR: 6.59, 95% CI: 8.48–15.07, $p < 0.001$] and women who received a long-lasting insecticide-treated net [AOR: 2.17, 95% CI: 0.03-0.92, $p = 0.039$] from the ANC clinic were associated with normal birth weight. *Conclusion.* Notwithstanding the benefits of antenatal care services, only 62.2% of pregnant women attended 4 or more ANC visits before giving birth, while 70% did not received the services they need. These might have influence the 24.5% of babies born with a low birth weight. Therefore, there is a need for special attention from all stakeholders to reverse the trend.

1. Introduction

Antenatal care (ANC) is a fundamental component of routine maternal and child health services and provides opportunities for many different services to be offered to pregnant mothers with the aim of screening and detecting danger signs early and providing the necessary timely interventions. The goal of antenatal care is to reduce maternal and child mortality and morbidity; for example, the roll-out of antimalarial drugs and antiretroviral therapy for maternal HIV/AIDS are services offered at antenatal care sessions to reduce maternal and child morbidity and mortality [1]. Therefore, frequent visits to the ANC clinic are crucial in realizing the full benefits of ANC services. Antenatal services such as tetanus toxoid-diphtheria vaccination, IPTp for malaria control, and HIV prevention of mother-to-child transmission (PMTCT) depend on several visits and the trimester in which they occur to be effective [2].

Pregnant women stand a greater risk of losing their lives or their babies if proper care and attention are not given to them during antenatal care until delivery. Globally, in 2015, the maternal mortality ratio was estimated to be around 216 per 100,000 live births and occurring mostly in low-resource settings [3] due to pregnancy-related causes [4] while skilled attendance at birth coverage in 2013 was estimated to have reached 73%; however, more than 40% of births in WHO Africa Region were not attended to by a skilled health personnel [5]. Also, globally, an estimated 5.9 million children in less than 5 years lost their lives in 2015, with neonatal and under-five mortality rates of 19 per 1,000 live births and 42.5 per 1,000 live births, respectively, occurring; however, the highest mortality occurred in sub-Saharan Africa, where antenatal care (4+ visits) in 2015 was 55% [6]. It is also known that good quality of care at childbirth can produce a triple effect on any investment made, saves mothers and newborns, and prevents stillbirths and low birth weights. Therefore, the provision of effective care for all women and babies during birth in health facilities could prevent about 113,000 maternal deaths; 531,000 stillbirths; and 1.3 million neonatal deaths that occurred annually by 2020 [6]. Yet, about half of the under-five deaths are caused by malaria, tetanus, measles, sepsis, pneumonia, and AIDS which are directly associated with the lack or insufficient antenatal care services [7].

In Ghana, the maternal mortality ratio is estimated at 310/100,000 live births, while neonatal and infant mortality rates were 25/1,000 and 37/1,000 pregnancies [8], respectively. Also, the Ghana Demographic and Health Survey estimates ANC coverage at 97.3%, ANC 4+ visits at 82.9%, and low birth weight at 9.5% [9]. In particular, the Wa East District has seen some improvement over the years in ANC coverage from 84.6% in 2017 to 85.8% in 2019, while ANC 4+ visits increased from 70.7% in 2017 to 71.9% in 2019. With the consistent increase of ANC coverage and significant coverage of the 4th visit, it was expected that the negative birth outcomes such as stillbirths and low birth weights would have been reduced to the minimum levels. But, the district recorded an increase in the low birth weight rate from 6.2% in 2017 to 7.5% in 2019, which could be a contributory factor to neonatal deaths and increased in stillbirths from 5 per 1,000 pregnancies in 2017 to 15 per 1,000 pregnancies in 2019 [10]. Although the district is yet to fall above the national ANC coverage (80%) and ANC 4+ visits (78%) targets, the increase in stillbirth and low birth weight rates amidst the increased ANC coverage and ANC 4+ visits suggests an investigation; hence, the study examined the association between antenatal care attendance and birth outcomes among mothers who delivered from June 2017 to May 2018 in the Wa East District.

2. Materials and Methods

2.1. Study Site. The Wa East District is a complete rural district with 145 communities. Currently, the district has an estimated population of about 87,182 with a 3.9% fertility rate. There are 9 health centres, a health post/clinic, and 28 functional community-based health planning and service (CHPS) facilities in the district rendering health services to the people. Although there are no hospitals and polyclinics in the district, the health centres there possess the needed resources and the potentials to render the basic emergency obstetrics and newborn care (EmONC) services to whoever needs these services [10].

2.2. Study Population. The study population includes women aged 15 to 45 years, who attended ANC clinics and delivered in health facilities in the district between June 2017 and May 2018. However, women who went through a caesarean section before delivery were excluded from the study because a study has shown that babies delivered through a caesarean section may gain more weight due to the fluids given to the mother before and during surgery [11]. Also, women with missing ANC and delivery data from health facility records, health professionals, and foreign nationals were excluded from the study.

2.3. Study Design. A descriptive cross-sectional design was employed to collect the study data at one point in time. The study involved reviewing individual records of women who gave birth at a health facility between June 2017 and May 2018 and interviewed the women for additional information. Variables that data were collected in the facility include parity, number of ANC visits made before delivery, birth weight of the child, still/live birth, and a minimum amount of ANC services received by mothers before delivery. Data collected from the mothers directly include the mothers' demographic data and counselling information given to mothers during ANC visits. Mothers' ANC booklets were referred to as where necessary to ascertain the needed information.

2.4. Sample Size. The sample size of two hundred and thirty-three (233) participants involved in the study was determined using the Cochran formulated formula for cross-sectional population-based studies: $n = z^2 \times p(q)/d^2$ [12], where n was the sample size to be determined, z was the z -score of the area under the standard normal curve corresponding to the desired confidence level of 95% (1.96), p was the prevalence of low birth weight of 16.5% (0.165) in the population [13], q was 1-p, and d was the 5% (0.005) acceptable margin of error. Considering a 10% nonresponse rate for the 212 participants, the sample size, finally became 233 participants. This was to ensure that the estimated prevalence fell within ±5% of the true population coverage, with a probability of 95%.

2.5. Sampling Method. Nine health centres were providing basic emergency obstetrics and newborn care (EmONC) services in the district. Hence, we purposively selected all the nine health centres for the study, and a probability proportionate to the size sampling method was used to allocate the sample size to each health centre based on the total deliveries conducted between 1st June 2017 and 31st May 2018. After getting the sample size for the health centres, the number of deliveries registered in each health centre's delivery register became a sample frame, and a systematic sampling method was used to select the number of women allocated to the health centre. The selected women were traced to their homes using the contact information in their health records.

2.6. Data Collection Tools and Procedure. A semistructured questionnaire was used for data collection, and pretesting of the tool was done using five (5) women who were not part of the study participants to ensure that it addressed all the objectives without ambiguity. Four nurses who were familiar with ANC activities and services were recruited from outside the study area, and were trained to collect data for the study, and were persons who understood the local dialect and could explain the questionnaire to the understanding of the study participants using the three main languages in the area, namely, Dagaare, Sisaali, and Chakali. The participants were interviewed, and their ANC and delivery records were reviewed. Information collected includes age, educational level, religion, parity, gestational age at first ANC visit, number of ANC visits, child's birth weight, livebirth, stillbirth, and counselling during ANC visits.

2.7. Data Analysis. The analytical software STATA version 13.1 was used for data analysis, and frequencies and proportions were used to report on ANC attendance, minimum ANC services received, and other variables. The minimum ANC service received was determined using the following fourteen services provided to pregnant women during an antenatal care visit: measured weight, height, blood pressure, and hemoglobin level; assessed gestational age; performed urine, syphilis, and PMTCT tests; gave iron-folic acid supplementation, tetanus-diphtheria injection, sulphadoxine-pyrimethamine (SP) tablets, and LLIN; and counselled on nutrition and family planning services. Mothers who received 13 or less of these services were classified as getting below the minimum requirements. The chi-squared and logistics regression tests were performed to determine the association between independent and dependent variables. The p value < 0.05 was considered statistically significant.

3. Results

3.1. Background Characteristics of Participants. A total of 233 women who attended ANC clinics and delivered in health facilities in the district were interviewed and health records reviewed with more than half 148 (63.5%) of them being within the ages of 20 to 34 years and a mean age of 27 years ± 7.0 standard deviation. Majority 215 (92.3%) of them were legally married and as high as 113 (48.5%) of the women have no formal education while only 17 (7.3%) have secondary and tertiary education. More than half 149 (64.0%) of them were farmers, and 53 (22.7%) were unemployed. Islamic religion 167 (71.7%) was the major form of religious expression in the district. About 56 (24.0%) of the women had delivered four or more children before the current child, while 99 (42.5%) and 78 (33.5%) of the women had delivered 1 and 2-3 times before the current child they have (Table 1).

3.2. Antenatal Services Women Received. About 145 (62.2%) of the women attended four or more ANC clinics for care while 12 (5.2%) went to ANC clinics only once. All the women had their weight and height measured, and blood pressure checked. Also, about 229 (98.3%) received iron-folic supplementation of which 84 (36.7%) and 100 (43.7%) had it four and five or more times, respectively, 161 (69.1%) were given sulphadoxine-pyrimethamine (SP) tablets out of which 107 (66.5%) got it twice, 202 (86.7) got tetanus-diphtheria vaccination, and 171 (73.4%) received a long-lasting insecticide-treated net (LLITN). Again, 230 (98.7%) were tested against PMTCT, 204 (87.6%) had their urine tested and 228 (97.9%) tested for syphilis, and 222 (95.3%) had their hemoglobin levels checked, while 231 (99.1%) had gestational age checked, and 223 (95.7%) and 230 (98.7%) received counselling on family planning and nutrition, respectively. Generally, only 30.0% of the women received all the 14 minimum services required (Table 2).

3.3. Pregnancy Outcome and Birth Weight. About 2 (0.9%) out of the 233 pregnancies resulted in stillbirth (Figure 1(a)), while 57 (24.5%) of the babies born had birth weight below 2.5 kg (abnormal) (Figure 1(b)).

3.4. Associations between Background Characteristics and Normal Birth Weight. The chi-squared analysis showed significant associations between birth weight and marital status ($p = 0.04$), religion ($p = 0.016$), and educational level ($p = 0.003$) of the women. To further confirm the associations, bivariate logistic analysis was performed, and it was confirmed and showed associations between normal birth weight and legally married women [COR: 2.71, 95% CI: 1.01-7.24, $p = 0.047$], women who were Muslims [COR: 0.39, 95% CI: 0.18-0.85, $p = 0.018$], and women who have attained secondary/tertiary education [COR: 3.15, 95% CI: 0.04-0.61, $p = 0.008$]. The associations indicated that married women were 2.7 times more likely to give birth to children with a normal birth weight than women who were in cohabitation relationships, women who were Muslims were 61% less likely to deliver babies with a normal birth weight than those who were Christians, while women with secondary/tertiary education were about 3.2 times more likely to give birth to children with a normal birth weight than women with no education.

Furthermore, when variables that were having associations with normal birth weight from the bivariate analysis

Table 1: Background characteristics of participants.

Variable		Frequency	Percentage
Age group (years)	<20	41	17.6
	20-34	148	63.5
	≥35	44	18.9
Marital status	Legally married	215	92.3
	Cohabitation	18	7.7
Religion	Christianity	66	28.3
	Islam	167	71.7
Occupation	Unemployed	53	22.7
	Farmer	149	64.0
	Trader	31	13.3
Educational level	No education	113	48.5
	Primary/JHS	103	44.2
	SHS/tertiary	17	7.3
Parity	0-1	99	42.5
	2-3	78	33.5
	4+	56	24.0

were tested for confounding effects using multiple logistic regression analysis, it was further confirmed that women who are legally married [AOR: 2.05, 95% CI: 1.33-6.89, $p = 0.044$], women who were Muslims [AOR: 0.33, 95% CI: 0.08-0.39, $p = 0.013$], and women who have attained secondary/tertiary education [AOR: 4.27, 95% CI: 0.08-0.88, $p = 0.031$] were associated with normal birth weight. This also indicated that legally married women were about 2.1 times more likely to give birth to children with a normal birth weight than women who are in cohabitation relationships, women who were Muslims were 67% less likely to deliver babies with a normal birth weight than those who were Christians, while women who have attained secondary/tertiary education were 4.3 times more likely to give birth to babies with a normal birth weight than women who had no education (Table 3).

3.5. Associations between Antenatal Services the Woman Received and Normal Birth Weight. Again, chi-squared analysis showed significant associations between the birth weight and checking of hemoglobin levels ($p = 0.002$), urine test ($p = 0.000$), times sulphadoxine-pyrimethamine (SP) tablets received ($p = 0.018$), syphilis test ($p = 0.003$), LLITN distribution ($p = 0.002$), counsel on FP ($p = 0.008$), counsel on nutrition ($p = 0.013$), and birth outcome ($p = 0.013$).

To further confirmed the associations, a bivariate logistic analysis was performed, and this confirmed and showed associations between a normal birth weight and women who had their hemoglobin levels tested [COR: 6.02, 95% CI: 1.69-21.39, $p = 0.006$], women who had their urine tested [COR: 15.18, 95% CI: 6.23-8.28, $p < 0.001$], women who received SP tablets 2 times [COR: 1.37, 95% CI: 0.16-0.86, $p = 0.021$], women who were tested for syphilis [COR: 3.21, 95% CI: 1.45-2.73, $p = 0.022$], women who received LLITN [COR: 3.26, 95% CI: 0.11-0.65, $p = 0.004$], and women who were counselled on FP [COR: 5.06, 95% CI: 1.37-8.62, $p = 0.015$]. The associations indicated that women who had their hemoglobin levels checked were 6 times more likely to give birth to children with a normal birth weight than women whose hemoglobin levels were not tested, women who had their urine tested were 15.2 times more likely to deliver babies with a normal birth weight than those without urine test, women who received SP tablets 2 times were about 1.4 times more likely to give birth to children with a normal birth weight than women who received SP once, women who were tested for syphilis were 3.2 times more likely to give birth to babies with a normal birth weight than those who were not tested, and women who received LLITN were also 3.3 times more likely to deliver babies with a normal birth weight than those who were not given, while women who were counseled on FP were 5.1 times more likely to deliver children with a normal birth weight than those who were not counseled.

Additionally, when variables that were having associations with normal birth weight from the bivariate analysis were tested for confounding effects using multiple logistic regression analysis, it was confirmed that women who had their urine tested [AOR: 6.59, 95% CI: 8.48–15.07, $p < 0.001$] and women who received LLITN [AOR: 2.17, 95% CI: 0.03-0.92, $p = 0.039$] were associated with normal birth weight. This indicated that women who had their urine tested and women who received LLITN were 6.6 and 2.2 times more likely to give birth to babies with a normal birth weight than women whose urine were not tested and those who did not receive LLITN, respectively (Table 4).

4. Discussion

Almost half (48.5%) of the mothers in Wa East District never went to school. Meanwhile, decreasing levels of education has been linked to lower birth weight [14]. Again, maternal educational level is known to influence child health as well as reducing unhealthy behaviours, including smoking [15, 16]. Mothers who are employed and work characteristics have been associated with reduced low birth weight [17], yet the present study showed that 22.7% of mothers are unemployed. Another study in Nigeria also indicated that higher maternal education and occupation were associated with higher mean birth weights and showed that low birth weight was higher among mothers in the lower social class compared with mothers in the upper social class [18]. About 7.7% of mothers in the current study were involved in cohabiting relationships. Meanwhile, a study has shown that mothers who were not married are associated with an increased risk of low birth weight [19]. Though a study has shown that advancing in maternal age enhances birth weight by influencing foetal growth, 17.6% of mothers in the present study were below 20 years of age [20].

Globally, pregnant women are to make at least four or more antenatal care visits from skilled personnel before giving birth [21]. However, only 62.2% of mothers in the present study made four or more ANC visits, which is far below the 80% target set for all districts to achieve and Ghana's demographics and health survey [9, 22]. Contrary, the Nigeria and

TABLE 2: Antenatal services women received.

Variable		Frequency	Percentage
	0-1	12	5.2
Number of ANC visits	2-3	76	32.6
	4+	145	62.2
Gestational age determined	No	2	0.9
	Yes	231	99.1
Height taken	No	0	0.0
	Yes	233	100.0
PMTCT tested	No	3	1.3
	Yes	230	98.7
Iron-folic acid supplementation given	No	4	1.7
	Yes	229	98.3
	1-2	45	19.6
Times folic acid received ($n = 229$)	3-4	100	43.7
	5+	84	36.7
Hemoglobin level checked	No	11	4.7
	Yes	222	95.3
Urine tested	No	29	12.4
	Yes	204	87.6
Tetanus-toxoid vaccination received	No	31	13.3
	Yes	202	86.7
Weight taken	No	0	0.0
	Yes	233	100.0
SP tablets received	No	72	30.9
	Yes	161	69.1
Times SP tablets received ($n = 161$)	1	54	33.5
	2	107	66.5
Syphilis tested	No	5	2.1
	Yes	228	97.9
LLITN received	No	62	26.6
	Yes	171	73.4
Counselled on FP	No	10	4.3
	Yes	223	95.7
Counselled on nutrition	No	3	1.3
	Yes	230	98.7
Blood pressure checked	No	0	0.0
	Yes	233	100.0
Received minimum ANC service	No	163	70.0
	Yes	70	30.0

Eastern Sudan studies reported lower proportions (54% and 11%, respectively) [23, 24]. Admittedly, a cross-sectional study in Kumasi, Ghana, indicated the lack of ANC attendance to the fact that mothers were not sick and so there was no need to visit ANC clinics or hospitals, as well as cultural beliefs [25]. These could also be the reasons why mothers in the Wa East District were not attending ANC clinics, although why mothers were not attending ANC clinics were not captured in the present study. The minimum ANC package in the study refers to the 14 services outlined in Table 2 in Results of the paper which are provided for pregnant mothers at the ANC clinic. However, the study revealed that only 30% of the mothers received all ANC services required. Partly, the pregnant women who were unable to attend the recommended four or more visits could not have received all services. Again, in a rural district such as Wa East, where there are no laboratory facilities, services such as urine test and hemoglobin checks are not readily offered. Therefore, pregnant women are usually requested to visit another district for these services to be rendered. As a result, some mothers find it inconvenient and may not adhere to the referral and hence did not receive all the services that every

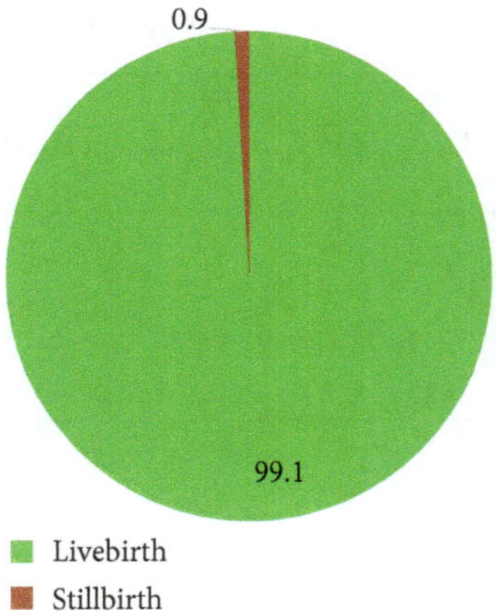

(a) Pregnancy outcome

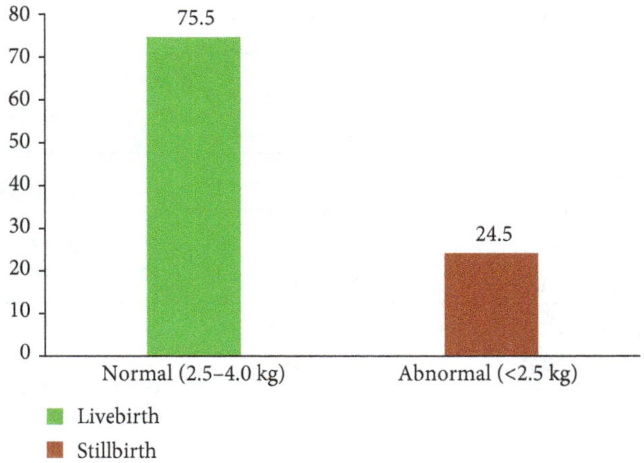

(b) Birth weight of children

FIGURE 1: (a) Pregnancy outcome. (b) Birth weight of children.

TABLE 3: Associations between background characteristics and a normal birth weight.

Variable	Birth weight: Normal (2.5-4.0 kg) $n = 176$ (%)	Birth weight: Abnormal (<2.5 kg) $n = 57$ (%)	Pearson chi²: Chi²	Pearson chi²: p value	COR (95% CI); p value	AOR (95% CI); p value
Age group (years)						
<20	33 (80.5)	8 (19.5)			1	
20-34	112 (75.7)	36 (24.3)	1.160	0.560	0.75 (0.32-1.78); 0.520	
≥35	31 (70.5)	13 (29.5)			0.58 (0.21-1.58); 0.287	
Marital status						
Cohabitation	10 (55.6)	8 (44.4)	4.215	0.040	1	1
Legal married	166 (77.2)	49 (22.8)			2.71 (1.01-7.24); 0.047	2.05 (1.33-6.89); 0.044
Religion						
Christianity	57 (86.4)	9 (13.6)	5.842	0.016	1	1
Islam	119 (71.3)	48 (28.7)			0.39 (0.18-0.85); 0.018	0.33 (0.08-0.39); 0.013
Occupation						
Farmer	115 (77.2)	34 (22.8)			1	
Trader	23 (74.2)	8 (25.8)	0.671	0.715	0.85 (0.35-2.07); 0.721	
Unemployed	38 (71.7)	15 (28.3)			0.75 (0.37-1.52); 0.425	
Educational level						
No education	84 (74.3)	29 (25.7)			1	1
Primary/JHS	82 (79.6)	21 (20.4)	11.919	0.003	1.35 (0.71-2.55); 0.359	1.20 (0.12-2.14); 0.876
SHS/tertiary	10 (58.8)	7 (41.2)			3.15 (0.04-0.61); 0.008	4.27 (0.08-0.88); 0.031
Parity						
0-1	78 (78.8)	21 (21.2)			1	
2-3	55 (70.5)	23 (29.5)	1.6789	0.432	0.64 (0.33-1.28); 0.208	
4+	43 (76.8)	13 (23.2)			0.89 (0.41-1.95); 0.772	

pregnant woman is required. Also, shortages of logistics, such as iron-folic acid tablets, long-lasting insecticide-treated nets, sulphadoxine-pyrimethamine tablets, and HIV and syphilis test kits, mean that mothers who attended ANC clinics at the times of shortages were denied such services. Hence, most pregnant women did not receive ANC services required. Nonetheless, a comparative cross-sectional study in northern Ghana made a similar finding and indicated that only 34.6% of mothers received adequate ANC care services [26]. Again, a study conducted in Bangladesh reported a lower proportion (22%) of mothers who received all the prescribed ANC services [27]. The Bangladesh study also revealed that mothers who received the minimum ANC service were about 2.4 times more likely to give birth to children with a normal birth

TABLE 4: Associations between antenatal services woman received and normal birth weight.

Variable	Birth weight: Normal (2.5-4.0 kg) $n = 176$ (%)	Birth weight: Abnormal (<2.5 kg) $n = 57$ (%)	Pearson chi^2: Chi^2	Pearson chi^2: p value	COR (95% CI); p value	AOR (95% CI); p value
Number of ANC visits						
0-1	11 (91.7)	1 (8.3)			1	
2-3	61 (80.3)	15 (19.7)	4.255	0.235	0.31 (0.04-2.69); 0.288	
4+	104 (71.7)	41 (28.3)			0.23 (0.03-1.84); 0.167	
Gestational age determined						
Yes	176 (76.2)	55 (23.8)	3.101	0.078		
No	0 (0.0)	2 (100)			Omitted	
PMTCT tested						
Yes	176 (76.5)	54 (23.5)	3.214	0.073		
No	0 (0.0)	3 (100)			Omitted	
Iron-folic acid supplementation given						
Yes	172 (75.1)	57 (24.9)	1.318	0.251		
No	4 (100)	0 (0.0)			Omitted	
Times folic acid received ($n = 229$)						
1-2	39 (86.7)	6 (13.3)			1	
3-4	74 (74.0)	26 (26.0)	3.209	0.201	0.47 (0.18-1.26); 0.133	
5+	60 (71.4)	24 (28.6)			0.42 (0.16-1.12); 0.082	
Hemoglobin level checked						
No	4 (36.4)	7 (63.6)	9.587	0.002	1	1
Yes	172 (77.5)	50 (22.5)			6.02 (1.69–2.14); 0.006	0.15 (0.01-2.27); 0.17
Urine tested						
No	7 (24.1)	22 (75.9)	47.353	<0.001	1	1
Yes	169 (82.8)	35 (17.2)			5.18 (6.23-8.28); <0.001	6.59 (8.48-15.07); <0.001
Tetanus-toxoid vaccination received						
No	23 (74.2)	8 (25.8)	0.082	0.775	1	
Yes	153 (75.7)	49 (24.3)			1.14 (0.48-2.71); 0.775	
SP tablets received						
No	59 (81.9)	13 (18.1)	2.315	0.128	1	
Yes	117 (72.7)	44 (27.3)			0.59 (0.29-1.17); 0.131	
Times SP tablets received ($n = 161$)						
1	45 (83.3)	9 (16.7)	5.597	0.018	1	1
2	72 (66.7)	35 (33.3)			1.37 (0.16-0.86); 0.021	1.34 (0.10-1.12); 0.077
Syphilis tested						
No	1 (20.0)	4 (80.0)	8.529	0.003	1	1
Yes	175 (76.8)	53 (23.2)			3.21 (1.45-2.73); 0.022	1.27 (0.05-1.45); 0.885
LLITN received						
No	55 (88.7)	7 (11.3)	9.245	0.002	1	1
Yes	121 (70.8)	50 (29.2)			3.26 (0.11-0.65); 0.004	2.17 (0.03-0.92); 0.039
Counselled on FP						
No	4 (40.0)	6 (60.0)	7.140	0.008	1	1
Yes	172 (77.1)	51 (22.9)			5.06 (1.37-8.62); 0.015	3.13 (0.33-1.37); 0.331
Counselled on nutrition						
No	0 (0.0)	3 (100)	6.194	0.013		

Table 4: Continued.

Variable	Birth weight Normal (2.5-4.0 kg) $n = 176$ (%)	Birth weight Abnormal (<2.5 kg) $n = 57$ (%)	Pearson chi^2 Chi^2	Pearson chi^2 p value	COR (95% CI); p value	AOR (95% CI); p value
Yes	176 (76.5)	54 (23.5)			Omitted	
Birth outcome						
Still birth	0 (0.0)	2 (100)	6.229	0.013		
Live birth	176 (76.2)	55 (23.8)			Omitted	
Received minimum ANC service						
No	116 (73.4)	42 (26.6)	2.391	0.122	1	
Yes	58 (82.9)	12 (17.1)			1.75 (0.86-3.58); 0.125	

weight (2.5–4.0 kg) compared with those who received fewer services. This finding was not surprising, because mothers who attend ANC sessions and receive all services required and put the pieces of advice into practice have more chance of delivering healthy babies [28].

Approximately 24.5% of babies born between June 2017 and May 2018 were below the normal birth weight (<2.5 kg). In contrary, the Nigerian studies and the Ethiopian study reported prevalence (6.3%, 10.2%, and 17.1%) of a low birth weight, which are lower than what the present study reported [29–31]. Meanwhile, low-birth-weight children are known to suffer from lack of proper physical growth and mental development, are susceptible to infections and physical handicaps, and are prone to emotional disorders [32]. About 1% of pregnancies in the Wa East District resulted in a stillbirth. This disagrees with a study carried out in the Hohoe Municipality in Ghana, which reported a high prevalence of stillbirth [33] and the study among the ethnically diverse population in the United Kingdom [34].

Religion was found to be associated with birth weight in the present study and agrees with a study in India [35], and in Africa, the tradition of selection and preference of nutritionally poor food items during pregnancy is deep-rooted in communities and may be due to religious practices that affect maternal healthcare-seeking behaviour and nutrition [36]. Again, another study has shown that maternal religious attendance has a protective effect against low birth weight [37]. Maternal marital status was also found to be associated with normal birth weight in the present study and agrees with the Nigerian studies [29, 30]. However, mothers who are not married are known to have a higher risk of delivering low-birth-weight children [19]. The present study also indicated that mothers who have attained higher education were more likely to give birth to babies with a normal birth weight compared with mothers who have attained lower education or did not go to school. This educational finding concurs with Tayie and Lartey's study, which reported that pregnant women with higher educational attainment turn to seek early care and that those who seek early care are likely to give birth to children with a normal birth weight (2.5-4.0 kg) than women with no education [38]. Meanwhile, maternal education has an influence on negative health behaviours, which in turn impact child health outcomes [15, 16].

Mothers who had their urine tested were found to be associated with given birth to a child with a normal birth weight, and a study has shown that mothers who had their urinary metabolites measured at the end of the first trimester are associated with an increased risk of negative birth outcomes [39]. Also, mothers who were given LLITN to help protect them from mosquitoes' bite and prevent malaria were significantly associated with a normal birth weight, with a study indicating reduce birth weight among mothers who has malaria during pregnancy [40]. These services are part of the minimum services all pregnant women were supposed to receive from ANC facilities visited. A study has shown that mothers who did not go for antenatal care and for that reason could not receive services required were associated with low birth weight and other birth outcomes [41]. All efforts should be instituted to ensure pregnant mothers receive all required services because these services are essential to ensure both the mother and child's life are saved.

5. Conclusion

Notwithstanding the benefits of antenatal care services, only 62.2% of pregnant women attended 4 or more ANC visits and 70% of the mothers did not receive all ANC services required. Also, 24.5% and 0.9% of pregnancies resulted in low birth weights and stillbirths, respectively. Normal birth weight is significantly associated with maternal religion, educational attainment, marital status, mothers who received long-lasting insecticide-treated nets, and those who had their urine tested. Inconsistency in logistics and medical supply to health facilities in the district should be addressed to ensure mothers who attend ANC clinics can receive all services required. Again, the rate of low-birth-weight children is very high. Therefore, there is a need for special attention from all stakeholders to reverse the trend.

5.1. Recommendations. The district health administration and other stakeholders in health should enhance education on the importance of antenatal care services including the necessity for early antenatal care and male involvement in women's health. The health authorities should institute supply-chain management systems to prevent logistics and medicine shortages. Again, there should be a study to ascertain the actual cause of the low birth weight in the district.

Abbreviations

ANC:	Antenatal care
IPTp:	Intermittent preventive treatment in pregnancy
HIV/AIDS:	Human immunodeficiency virus/acquired immune deficiency syndrome
PMTCT:	Prevention of mother-to-child transmission
WHO:	World Health Organization
CHPS:	Community-based health planning and services
EmONC:	Basic emergency obstetrics and newborn care
SP:	Sulphadoxine-pyrimethamine
LLITN:	Long-lasting insecticide-treated net
JHS:	Junior secondary school
SHS:	Senior secondary school
FP:	Family planning
COR:	Crude odds ratio
AOR:	Adjusted odds ratio.

Consent

Informed consent for voluntary participation was obtained from the study subjects.

Authors' Contributions

PKA, MB, and MA had extensive contribution to the conception and acquisition of data of this research. PKA, MB, MA, SNY, KO, GBA, and SN had considerable contribution to the design, analysis data, and interpretation of the findings. All authors critically revised the paper for important intellectual contents. All authors read and approved the final manuscript.

Acknowledgments

The authors express their appreciations to the Wa East District Director of Health Service for granting us the permission to carry out the study and also to all the heads of ANC and delivery facilities within the district where the study was conducted.

References

[1] O. M. R. Campbell, W. J. Graham, and on behalf of The Lancet Maternal Survival Series steering group, "Strategies for reducing maternal mortality: getting on with what works," *The Lancet*, vol. 368, no. 9543, pp. 1284–1299, 2006.

[2] O. Lincetto, S. Mothebesoane-Anoh, P. Gomez, and S. Munjanja, "Antenatal care," *Opportunities for Africa's newborns: Practical data, policy and programmatic support for newborn care in Africa*, pp. 55–62, 2006.

[3] World Health Organization, World Bank, and United Nations Population Fund & United Nations Children's Fund, *Trends in Maternal Mortality: 1990-2015: Estimates from WHO, UNICEF, UNFPA, World Bank Group and the United Nations Population Division*, World Health Organization, 2015, https://apps.who.int/iris/handle/10665/194254.

[4] J. E. Lawn, S. Cousens, J. Zupan, and for the Lancet Neonatal Survival Steering Team, "4 million neonatal deaths: when? Where? Why?," *The Lancet*, vol. 365, no. 9462, pp. 891–900, 2005.

[5] World Health Organization, *Tracking Universal Health Coverage: First Global Monitoring Report*, World Health Organization, 2015, https://www.who.int/health_financing/documents/tracking-uhc/en/.

[6] World Health Organization, *World Health Statistics 2016: Monitoring Health for the SDGs Sustainable Development Goals*, World Health Organization, 2016, https://www.who.int/gho/publications/world_health_statistics/2016/en/.

[7] Unicef, "Committing to child survival: a promise renewed," 2014, http://files.unicef.org/publications/files/APR_2014_web_15Sept14.pdf.

[8] Ghana Statistical Service (GSS), Ghana Health Service (GHS), and ICF, *Ghana maternal health survey 2017: key findings*, GSS, GHS, and ICF, Rockville, MD, USA, 2018.

[9] Ghana Statistical Service (GSS), Ghana Health Service (GHS), and ICF International, *Ghana demographic and health survey 2014*, GSS, GHS, and ICF International, Rockville, MD, USA, 2015.

[10] GHS Annual Report, "Ghana Health Service: Wa East Annual Report," 2019, unpublished.

[11] E. F. C. Murta, G. C. Freire, D. C. Fabri, and R. H. Fabri, "Could elective cesarean sections influence the birth weight of full-term infants?," *Sao Paulo Medical Journal*, vol. 124, no. 6, pp. 313–315, 2006.

[12] G. W. Snedecor and W. G. Cochran, *Statistical Methods*, Iowa State Univ. Press Iowa, Ames, 8th edition, 1989.

[13] I. K. Ndu, B. O. Edelu, S. N. Uwaezuoke et al., "Maternal risk factors associated with low birth weight neonates: a multi-centre, cross-sectional study in a developing country," *Journal of Neonatal Biology*, vol. 101, 2015.

[14] H. Cammu, G. Martens, and M. J. N. C. Keirse, "Mothers' level of education and childbirth interventions: a population-based study in Flanders, Northern Belgium," *Birth*, vol. 38, no. 3, pp. 191–199, 2011.

[15] P. M. Güneş, "The role of maternal education in child health: evidence from a compulsory schooling law," *Economics of Education Review*, vol. 47, pp. 1–16, 2015.

[16] H. Jürges, S. Reinhold, and M. Salm, "Does schooling affect health behavior? Evidence from the educational expansion in Western Germany," *Economics of Education Review*, vol. 30, no. 5, pp. 862–872, 2011.

[17] J. D. Meyer, N. Warren, and S. Reisine, "Racial and ethnic disparities in low birth weight delivery associated with maternal occupational characteristics," *American Journal of Industrial Medicine*, vol. 53, no. 2, pp. 153–162, 2010.

[18] O. A. Kehinde, O. F. Njokanma, and D. M. Olanrewaju, "Parental socioeconomic status and birth weight distribution of Nigerian term newborn babies," *Nigerian Journal of Paediatrics*, vol. 40, no. 3, pp. 299–302, 2013.

[19] P. S. Shah, J. Zao, and S. Ali, "Maternal marital status and birth outcomes: a systematic review and meta-analyses," *Maternal and Child Health Journal*, vol. 15, no. 7, pp. 1097–1109, 2011.

[20] S. MacLeod and J. L. Kiely, "The effects of maternal age and parity on birthweight: a population-based study in New York

City," *International Journal of Gynecology & Obstetrics*, vol. 26, no. 1, pp. 11–19, 1988.

[21] WHO Reproductive Health Library, "WHO recommendation on group antenatal care," in *The WHO reproductive health library*, World Health Organization, Geneva, 2016, https://extranet.who.int/rhl/topics/improving-health-system-performance/implementation-strategies/who-recommendation-group-antenatal-care.

[22] GHS, "Ghana Health Service guidelines for performance review and reporting by Budget and Management Centers 2016-2019," 2016, unpublished.

[23] T. Dahiru and O. M. Oche, "Determinants of antenatal care, institutional delivery and postnatal care services utilization in Nigeria," *Pan African Medical Journal*, vol. 21, no. 1, 2015.

[24] A. A. A. Ali, M. M. Osman, A. O. Abbaker, and I. Adam, "Use of antenatal care services in Kassala, eastern Sudan," *BMC Pregnancy and Childbirth*, vol. 10, no. 1, p. 67, 2010.

[25] N. N. Asundep, A. P. Carson, C. A. Turpin et al., "Determinants of access to antenatal care and birth outcomes in Kumasi, Ghana," *Journal of Epidemiology and Global Health*, vol. 3, no. 4, pp. 279–288, 2013.

[26] M. Saaka, K. Emmanuel, and I. Farruza, *Adequacy of prenatal care utilization and its effect on postpartum infant feeding behaviors in Northern Ghana*, SciMedCentral, 2016, http://hdl.handle.net/123456789/1403.

[27] M. M. Islam and M. S. Masud, "Determinants of frequency and contents of antenatal care visits in Bangladesh: assessing the extent of compliance with the WHO recommendations," *PLoS One*, vol. 13, no. 9, article e0204752, 2018.

[28] H. Zhou, A. Wang, X. Huang et al., "Quality antenatal care protects against low birth weight in 42 poor counties of Western China," *PloS one*, vol. 14, no. 1, article e0210393, 2019.

[29] H. B. Oladeinde, O. B. Oladeinde, R. Omoregie, and A. A. Onifade, "Prevalence and determinants of low birth weight: the situation in a traditional birth home in Benin City, Nigeria," *African Health Sciences*, vol. 15, no. 4, pp. 1123–1129, 2016.

[30] B. O. Olusanya and G. E. Ofovwe, "Predictors of preterm births and low birthweight in an inner-city hospital in sub-Saharan Africa," *Maternal and Child Health Journal*, vol. 14, no. 6, pp. 978–986, 2010.

[31] B. M. Zeleke, M. Zelalem, and N. Mohammed, "Incidence and correlates of low birth weight at a referral hospital in Northwest Ethiopia," *Pan African Medical Journal*, vol. 12, no. 1, 2012.

[32] C. M. Drillien, "Growth and development in a group of children of very low birth weight," *Archives of Disease in Childhood*, vol. 33, no. 167, pp. 10–18, 1958.

[33] F. Agbozo, A. Abubakari, J. Der, and A. Jahn, "Prevalence of low birth weight, macrosomia and stillbirth and their relationship to associated maternal risk factors in Hohoe Municipality, Ghana," *Midwifery*, vol. 40, pp. 200–206, 2016.

[34] N. Penn, E. Oteng-Ntim, and P. Doyle, "PPO. 34 The role of ethnicity in determining the prevalence of stillbirth in an ethnically-diverse UK population," *Archives of Disease in Childhood-Fetal and Neonatal Edition*, vol. 99, article A161, Supplement 1, 2014.

[35] P. S. Thomre, A. L. Borle, J. D. Naik, and S. S. Rajderkar, "Maternal risk factors determining birth weight of newborns: a tertiary care hospital based study," *International Journal of Recent Trends in Science and Technology*, vol. 5, no. 1, pp. 3–8, 2012.

[36] M. Gebremedhin, F. Ambaw, E. Admassu, and H. Berhane, "Maternal associated factors of low birth weight: a hospital based cross-sectional mixed study in Tigray, Northern Ethiopia," *BMC Pregnancy and Childbirth*, vol. 15, no. 1, p. 222, 2015.

[37] A. M. Burdette, J. Weeks, T. D. Hill, and I. W. Eberstein, "Maternal religious attendance and low birth weight," *Social Science & Medicine*, vol. 74, no. 12, pp. 1961–1967, 2012.

[38] F. A. Tayie and A. Lartey, "Antenatal care and pregnancy outcome in Ghana, the importance of women\'s education," *African Journal of Food, Agriculture, Nutrition and Development*, vol. 8, no. 3, pp. 291–303, 2008.

[39] L. Maitre, E. Fthenou, T. Athersuch et al., "Urinary metabolic profiles in early pregnancy are associated with preterm birth and fetal growth restriction in the Rhea mother–child cohort study," *BMC Medicine*, vol. 12, no. 1, p. 110, 2014.

[40] P. De Beaudrap, E. Turyakira, L. J. White et al., "Impact of malaria during pregnancy on pregnancy outcomes in a Ugandan prospectivecohort with intensive malaria screening and prompt treatment," *Malaria Journal*, vol. 12, no. 1, p. 139, 2013.

[41] N. Assefa, Y. Berhane, and A. Worku, "Wealth status, mid upper arm circumference (MUAC) and antenatal care (ANC) are determinants for low birth weight in Kersa, Ethiopia," *PLoS One*, vol. 7, no. 6, article e39957, 2012.

16

Substance Use among Homeless Reproductive Age People in Southern Ethiopia

Negash Wakgari, [1] Terefe Woyo, [2] Emnet Kebede, [2] Hirut Gemeda, [2] Wakgari Binu, [3] and Gonfa Moti [4]

[1] *Department of Midwifery, Ambo University, Ambo, Ethiopia*
[2] *Department of Midwifery, Hawassa University, Hawassa, Ethiopia*
[3] *School of Public Health, Wolaita Soddo University, Wolaita, Ethiopia*
[4] *Ambo University Referral Hospital, Ambo, Ethiopia*

Correspondence should be addressed to Negash Wakgari; negashwakgari@yahoo.com

Academic Editor: Vikas Roy

Introduction. Substance use by homeless reproductive age people may result to anxiety, involvement of risky sexual behaviors, and increasing the likelihood of unwanted pregnancy and sexually transmitted diseases (STDs). Therefore, this study assessed the magnitude of alcohol use, sexual intercourse after alcohol use, and its associated factors among homeless reproductive age people in southern Ethiopia. *Methods.* Community-based cross-sectional study design was conducted among homeless reproductive age people. The snowball sampling technique was used to recruit 842 participants. Pretested and structured interviewer-administered questionnaire was used to collect the data. Data were entered into Epidata version 3.1 and exported to SPSS version 23 for analysis. Binary logistic regression was used to determine the association of independent variables with the outcome variables. Odds ratio with their 95% confidence interval and P value was used to identify the significant variables. *Results.* More than half 423 (53.2%) of the respondents had taken a drink that contains alcohol in the last one year of the study period. Out of 324 khat chewers, 190 (58.64%) had sex after chewing khat. More than one-thirds, 323(38.4%) homeless people were smoking cigarette during the study period. Factors associated with alcohol use were age 19-25 years (AOR: 0.49; CI: 0.34, 0.72), ≥26 years (AOR: 0.40; CI: 0.25, 0.65), level of education (AOR: 0.61; CI: 0.39, 0.94), place of residence: major urban (AOR: 0.31; CI: 0.18, 0.51), small town (AOR: 0.38; CI: 0.23, 0.63), ever heard about STDs (AOR: 0.14; CI: 0.07, 027), and being a cigarette smoker (AOR: 2.67; CI: 1.94, 3.71). *Conclusions.* In this study, significant percentage of respondents had taken a drink that contains alcohol. Age, level of education, place of residence, ever heard about STDs, and smoking cigarette were variables significantly associated with alcohol use. Awareness creation on the effect and outcome of substance use is recommended.

1. Introduction

The health effect of substance use among the general population is well documented [1–5]. A multiple use of substances such as tobacco, alcohol, marijuana, and khat is reported [2, 5]. Despite the awareness of its ill effect on the health, the severity of alcohol consumption among adolescents is highly prevalent [3, 6–9]. This would be much more problematic among homeless people due to their lifestyle and economic dependency [6, 10–13].

People who sleep on streets, main roads, railway terminals, bus stations, parks, religious centers, construction sites, and other public places are defined as homeless people [14]. Alcohol consumption by the street-dwelling population may result to anxiety, depression, stressful life events, relative abstinence, and low self-esteem [15, 16]. It may also lead the street-dwelling reproductive age group [15-49 years] to the involvement of risky sexual behaviors and increasing the likelihood of unwanted pregnancy, STDs, and its consequence [6, 17, 18]. In addition, sexual intercourse after alcohol use is linked to inconsistent condom use, commercial sex, and rape [19, 20]. Moreover, both executing a crime and being a victim of an offence are also associated with alcohol use [21].

The proportion of alcohol use and its associated factors varies from region to region based on the context and sociodemographic characteristics of the street-dwelling people. For instance, previous studies reported 38% in Texas [10], 40% in Toronto [22], 35% in Egypt [23], 63.5% in Democratic Republic of Congo [24], and 64% alcohol use among street-dwelling people in Addis Ababa, Ethiopia [18].

Factors such as gender, age, duration of stay on the street, and peer influence were reported in previous studies as the major triggers for substance use [12, 13, 18, 24–29]. Though there are some studies conducted on substance abuse, risky sexual behavior, sexual, and reproductive health status of street children and youths [17, 18], none of them focused specifically on alcohol consumption, sexual intercourse after alcohol use, and its associated factors among homeless reproductive age people [15-49 years] in the study setting. Similarly, few of the previous studies done in the study area were focused on homeless women and children [30–33] and fail to notice sexual intercourse after alcohol use among both sexes in small towns of Ethiopia considering the differences in sociodemographic characteristics, culture, and awareness about the substances uses across the country. Therefore, this study assessed the magnitude of alcohol use, sexual intercourse after alcohol use, and its associated factors among homeless reproductive age people in southern Ethiopia.

2. Materials and Methods

2.1. Study Setting, Design, and Population. Community-based cross-sectional study design was conducted among homeless reproductive age people in southern Ethiopia. Hawassa; Arba Minch, Soddo, Dilla, Hosanna, Durame, Jinka, Werabe, Welkite, Segen, Yergalem, Bench, Tercha, Masha, and Mizan Aman are major cities in the southern Ethiopia. All homeless reproductive age people [15-49 years] in the selected cities in the southern Ethiopia were considered as the study population.

2.2. Sample Size Determination and Sampling Procedure. The sample size was determined by using single population proportion formula the following assumptions: 95% confidence level, 5% margin of error, and taking 50% proportions (p).

$$n = \frac{(z_{\alpha/2})^2 * p(1-q)}{d^2}. \quad (1)$$

Thus, the calculated sample size became 845 by considering two design effects due to the multistage nature of the study and 10% nonresponse.

Selecting seven cities: Arba Minch, Dilla, Durame, Hawassa, Mizan Aman, Soddo, and Yergalem among fourteen major cities in the southern Ethiopia lottery method was employed. To estimate number of street reproductive age groups in each selected city and the venues they frequently used for the purpose of survival work, an individual was assigned by an authorized person from the social and labor affair office. In addition, information regarding number of street-dwelling people in each city was requested from all concerned stakeholders. Finally, 845 samples were allocated proportionally to each selected cities. By using an individual who assigned by an authorized person, the first study respondent was identified. Then, the snowball sampling technique was used to recruit the representative sample [34].

2.3. Data Collection Tools and Procedure. Pretested and structured interviewer-administered questionnaire was used to collect the data. Data collection tool was adapted from the previous studies [1, 3, 6, 9–11, 16–18] and modified to fit the local context. The questionnaire designed to assess sociodemographic characteristics, alcohol use, and factors associated with alcohol use and sex after alcohol consumption. The pretest was conducted among 5% of street-dwelling people in nonselected cities. The result of the pretest used to modify the instrument. Four BSc midwives with previous experience on the data collection used as data collectors, and MSc holders were employed as supervisors.

2.4. Data Quality Control. The quality of the data was maintained by pretesting the tool and giving training for the data collectors and supervisors before the actual data collection. Every day after data collection, data reviewed and checked for completeness, accuracy, and clarity by the supervisors, and the necessary feedback was offered to data collectors. Data cleanup and crosschecking was done before analysis. To verify the internal consistency of the instrument, Cronbach's alpha analysis of alcohol use and sex after alcohol consumption-related questionnaire parts were done with the value of 0.81 which mean that the instrument items have good internal consistency.

2.5. Data Management and Analysis. The data were checked manually for completeness, coded, and entered into Epidata version 3.1 and exported to SPSS version 23.0 for analysis. Binary logistic regression was used to determine the association of independent variables with the outcome variables. Odds ratio with their 95% confidence interval and P value was used to identify the significant variables. The variables with P value less than or equal to 0.05 were considered as significant.

2.6. Operational Definition. Substance use: any substance that is taken into the living organism that may modify one or more of its function. In this study, the concept of substance use includes alcoholic drinks, tobacco, khat, and marijuana.

Alcohol use: street-dwelling people used alcoholic drinks such as beer and local alcohols [Tella and Xeji] during the previous one year of study either always, every day, or at least once a week reportedly were considered as alcohol use, while those who were not used at all and using less than once peer week were taken as not utilizing [29].

Sexual intercourse after taking alcohol: those respondents who had sexual intercourse after taking alcohols such as beer and local alcohols [Xeji and Tella] reportedly within one year prior to the study.

2.7. Ethical Consideration. Ethical approval was obtained from Hawassa University, College of Medicine and Health Sciences Ethical Review Board. Next, official letters were submitted to Regional Health Bureau. Letter of permission was obtained from Regional Health Bureau to Respective Zonal Health Department, Woreda Health Office, and City Administration. Furthermore, a written consent was obtained from Social and Labor Affairs Office. The written and verbal consent was obtained from each study subject prior to the data collection process proceeded. For those who were less than 18 years, written informed consent was obtained from their parent or guardian prior to the data collection process which was also approved by ethical review board [34].

3. Results

3.1. Sociodemographic Characteristics. A total of 842 street-dwelling people were included in the study with a response of 99. 6%. More than half 503 (59.7%) of them were males (Table 1).

3.2. Substance Use among Street Dwellers. More than half 423 (53.2%) of the respondents had taken a drink that contains alcohol (tella, tegi, areke, and beer) in the last one year of the study period. More than half, 265 (59%), of substance users ever had sex after taking alcohol in the last one year. Similarly, among the 324 khat chewers, 190 (58.64%) of the respondents ever had sex after chewing khat in the last one year (Table 2).

3.3. Alcohol Use and Cigarette Smoking. During the last 12 months of the study, 309 (36.7%) of the respondents had taken a drink that contains alcohol [CI: 35.5-39.7]. About 116 (13.8%) were drinking almost every day, and 193 (22.9%) drink at least once a week during the last one year. Regarding the frequency of alcohol use within the last 30 days of the study period, 155 (18.4%) of them did not remember, and 99 (11.8%) were taken every day reportedly.

More than one-third, 323(38.4%), of the street-dwelling people were smoking cigarette during the study period. Among the smokers, 114 (17.1%) were smoking every day, while 179 (21.3%) of them were smoking some days.

3.4. Factors Associated with Alcohol Use. Bivariate analysis factors found to be significantly associated with alcohol use were age, level of education, marital status, prior place of residence, and type of street, duration of stay on the street, ever heard about STDs, and being cigarette smokers. However, age, level of education, prior place of residence, ever heard about STDs, and being cigarette smokers were variables remain to be significantly associated with alcohol use in multivariate analyses. Accordingly, those who aged 19-25 and ≥26 years were about 51% (AOR: 0.49; CI: 0.34, 0.72) and 60% (AOR: 0.40; CI: 0.25, 0.65) less likely to use alcohol compared to those who were 15-18 years, respectively. Literate street-dwelling people were about 39% (AOR: 0.61; CI: 0.39, 0.94) less likely to use alcohol than those who were illiterate. In addition, those who were living in the major urban and small town prior to joining street life were about 69% (AOR: 0.31; CI: 0.18, 0.51) and 62% (AOR: 0.38; CI: 0.23,

TABLE 1: Sociodemographic characteristics of street dwellers in Southern Ethiopia, 2019 ($n = 842$).

Variables	Frequency	Percent
Gender		
Male	503	59.7
Female	339	40.3
Age in years		
15-18 years	246	29.3
19-25	407	48.3
≥26 years	189	22.4
Marital status		
Single/not ever married	521	61.9
Married	233	27.7
Divorced/separated	73	8.7
Widowed	15	1.8
Educational status		
Illiterate	187	22.2
Elementary	542	64.4
High school	102	12.1
College and above	11	1.3
Schooling status		
In school	97	11.5
Out of school	745	88.5
With whom currently living		
Alone	257	30.5
Peers	382	45.4
Boyfriend/girlfriend	135	16.0
Parents	50	5.9
Relatives	18	2.1
Place of current residence		
Hawassa	281	33.4
Soddo	165	19.6
Dilla	138	16.4
Arba Minch	117	13.9
Mizan Aman	108	12.8
Yergalem	20	2.4
Durame	13	1.5
Place of residence prior to starting street life		
Major urban town	313	37.2
Small town	369	43.8
Rural area	160	19.0
Type of street		
Street "on"	274	32.5
Street "off"	568	67.5
Duration of stay on the street		
< 5 years	621	73.8
5-10 years	168	20.0
> 10 years	36	4.3
Could not estimate	17	2.0
Daily income in birr		
5-20	136	16.2
21-50	518	61.5
≥ 51	654	77.7

Table 2: Substance abuse among street dwellers in Southern Ethiopia, 2019.

Variables	Frequency	Percent
A frequency of the drink contains alcohol use in the last 30 days ($n = 842$)		
Every day(30 days)	99	11.8
None in the last 30 days	56	6.7
Not sure/do not remember	155	18.4
A frequency of the drink contains alcohol use one year prior to the study ($n = 423$)		
Almost every day	116	13.8
At least once a week	193	22.9
Less than once a week	80	9.5
Not sure/do not remember	34	4.0
Sex after taking alcohol one year prior to the study		
Yes	265	31.5
No	155	18.4
Not sure/I do not know	1	0.1
Ever chewed khat one year prior to the study		
Yes	324	38.5
No	518	61.5
A frequency of chewing khat 30 days prior to the study		
Every day (30 days)	229	27.2
None in the last 30 days	36	4.3
Not sure/do not remember	59	7.0
Ever had sex after chewing khat		
Yes	190	22.6
No	127	15.1
Not sure/do not remember	1	0.1
A frequencies of smoking cigarette		
Every day	114	17.1
Some day	179	21.3
Not all	519	61.6

0.63) less likely to use alcohol than those who were living in the rural area before joining street life, respectively. Likewise, those who ever heard about STDs were 86% (AOR: 0.14; CI: 0.07, 027) less likely use alcohol than their counterpart. Further, being a cigarette smoker were about 3 times (AOR: 2.67; CI: 1.94, 3.71) more likelihood of alcohol use compared to nonsmoker (Table 3).

3.5. Sexual Intercourse after Alcohol Use and Associated Factors. Out of the total 266 (62.9%) had sexual intercourse after taking alcohol within the last one year of the study period [CI: 58.2-67.4]. Bivariate analysis variables such as gender, age, educational status, type of street, history of rape, ever tested for HIV, and ever heard about STDs were significantly associated with having sexual intercourse after alcohol use. However, gender, educational status, history of rape, and ever heard about STDs were significantly associated with having sexual intercourse after alcohol use in multivariate analysis. Those who were females were about 80% (AOR: 0.20; CI: 0.12, 0.36) less likely to have sexual intercourse following alcohol consumption compared to those who were male. In addition, those who literate were also about 75% (AOR: 0.25; CI: 0.12, 0.51) less likely to have sexual intercourse following alcohol use compared to those who were illiterate. Furthermore, those who had a history of rape in the last one year of the study were about 5 times (AOR: 4.95; CI: 1.67, 14.65) more likely to have sexual intercourse following alcohol use than their counterpart. Those who ever heard about STDs were about 78% (AOR: 0.22; CI: 0.70, 0.68) less likely to have sexual intercourse following alcohol use than their counterpart (Table 4).

4. Discussion

During the last 12 months of the study period, 309 (36.7%) of the respondents had taken a drink that contains alcohol [CI: 34.8-40.7]. This finding is in line with the studies conducted in Texas (38%) [10], Toronto (40%) [22], and Egypt (35%) [23]. The present result is lower than the studies conducted in Los Angeles (30.8%) [19], Democratic Republic of Congo (63.5%) [24], and Ethiopia (64%) [18]; however, it is higher than the studies done in Ghana (12%) [6]. This discrepancy might be due to the difference in sociodemographic characteristics of the study respondents, sample size, and measurement tool. For instance, the study of Ghana was conducted among 227 street connected youths, and daily reported alcohol use was considered. In this study, those respondents reported used alcohol every day and at least once a week were considered as an alcohol user. This finding indicates the desire of an intervention on how to minimize substance misuses and its consequences among homeless people in the urban of Ethiopia.

In the present study, as the age increases, the consumption of alcohol decreases. This is in line with the previous study conducted in Ghana [6]. It could also be explained by the possible commencement of alcohol in early age which is viewed as a normal to create enjoyable physical and psychological environment [35]. In addition, literate street-dwelling people had also a less likelihood of alcohol use than those who were illiterate. This concept is also supported by the previous study done in Korea [36]. This might be due to the fact that being literate may increase a likelihood of awareness about the consequence of alcohol consumption. Another possible explanation is in the present study that more than two-thirds 655(77.8%) of the respondents had either elementary, high school, or college and above.

Place of residence prior to join street life was also significantly associated with alcohol use. Those who were living in the major urban and small town prior to join street life had less likelihood of alcohol use compared to those were living in the rural area. This might be due to the fact that those who joined street life from the towns might have awareness about the effect of alcohol use on health and sexual behaviors compared to those who joined street life from rural area.

On the other hand, ever heard about STDs was positively associated with alcohol use compared to their counterpart. This might be due to the impact of the shared information,

Table 3: Bivariate and multivariate analyses of factors associated with alcohol use among homeless reproductive age people in southern Ethiopia, 2019 ($n = 842$).

Variables	Alcohol use		OR (95% CI)	
	Yes	No	COR (95% CI)	AOR (95% CI)
Age in years				
15-18	71	175	1	1
19-25	153	254	0.67 (0.48, 0.95)	0.49 (0.34, 0.72)
26 and more	85	104	0.49 (0.33, 0.74)	0.40 (0.25, 0.65)
Educational status				
Illiterate	43	144	1	
Literate	266	389	0.48 (0.33, 0.70)	0.61 (0.39, 0.94)
Marital status				
Single	207	314	1	1
Married	60	173	1.90 (1.13, 2.68)	2.29 (0.82, 2.43)
Divorced	42	46	0.72 (0.46, 1.14)	1.22(0.73, 2.03)
Place of residence prior to joining street life				
Major urban town	136	177	0.31 (0.19, 0.49)	0.31 (0.18, 0.51)
Small town	142	227	0.38 (0.25, 0.59)	0.38 (0.23, 0.63)
Rural area	31	129	1	1
Type of street				
Street “on” [return to home at the night]	90	184	1.28 (0.95, 1.74)	1.27 (0.92, 1.77)
Street “off”[sleep on the street]	219	349	1	1
Duration of stay on the street				
< 5 years	194	427	2.66 (1.21, 4.36)	2.37 (0.89, 3.46)
5-10 years	86	82	1.15 (0.62, 2.14)	1.42 (0.73, 2.74)
> 10 years	29	24	1	1
Ever heard about STDs				
Yes	299	431	0.14 (0.07, 0.27)	0 0.14 (0.07, 027)
No	10	102	1	1
Cigarette smokers				
Yes	161	162	2.49 (1.87, 3.33)	2.67 (1.94, 3.71)
No	148	371	1	1

and there might also an opportunity to hear about the health consequence of alcohol use. Moreover, being a cigarette smoker had also a more likelihood of alcohol use than non-smoker. As evident in the previous studies, this is might be due to the intercorrelation between cigarette smoking and alcohol use [37, 38]. This finding is also in line with the previous study conducted among adolescents in Ethiopia [1].

Being a female had a less likelihood to practice sexual intercourse after alcohol use compared to those who were male. This might be due to the fear of sexual assault following alcohol consumption consequently resulted to unwanted pregnancy and its consequence. As evidenced by the previous study, females had a more likelihood of practicing safe sex than males [39] which could be achieved by avoiding sexual intercourse after alcohol use. The other possible explanations are because being a female is a protective factor of substance use [40].

Literate street-dwelling people had a less likelihood of sexual intercourse after alcohol use than those who were illiterate. This might be due to the fact that those who were literate can easily understand the adverse outcomes of sexual intercourse such as unwanted pregnancy and STDs. On the other hand, having history of rape prior to the study had a more likelihood of sexual intercourse after alcohol use than the counterpart. Even though there is no clear mechanism for the causality, this might be due to the unpleasant life events and psychological problems they faced during sexual assault which could made them to drink alcohol more and prone to sexual intercourse after consuming alcohol [41–43].

Moreover, the respondents who ever heard about STDs had also a less likelihood of having sexual intercourse after alcohol use than the counterpart. This might be due to the impact of the information gained about STDs and a fear of undesired sexual intercourse following alcohol use.

5. Limitations of the Study

Due to the nature of the study design, causality cannot be concluded. Moreover, as in all self-reported studies, we cannot rule out social desirability bias to sensitive questions, which might have introduced biases of unknown magnitude and direction.

Table 4: Bivariate and multivariate analyses of factors associated with sexual intercourse after alcohol use among homeless reproductive age people in southern Ethiopia, 2019 ($n = 842$).

Variables	Sexual intercourse after alcohol use		OR (95% CI)	
	Yes	No	COR (95% CI)	AOR (95% CI)
Gender				
Male	126	129	1	1
Female	140	28	0.19 (0.12, 0.31)	0.20 (0.12, 0.36)
Age in years				
15-18	48	37	1.04 (0.59, 1.82)	1.06 (0.56, 1.98)
19-25	148	68	0.62 (0.39, 0. 98)	0.77 (0.46, 1.29)
26 and more	70	52	1	1
Educational status				
Illiterate	26	28	1	1
Literate	240	129	0.49 (0. 28, 0.89)	0.25 (0.12, 0.51)
Type of street				
*Street "on"	70	52	1.39(0.90, 2.13)	1.70 (0.68, 2.78)
**Street "off"	196	105	1	
Rape in the last 1 year				
Yes	61	4	11.38 (4.05, 31.98)	4.95 (1.67, 14.65)
No	205	153	1	1
Ever heard about STDs				
Yes	261	144	0.21 (0.07, 0.61)	0.22 (0.70, 0.68)
No	5	13	1	
Ever tested for HIV				
Yes	218	105	2.25 (1.43, 3.55)	1.37 (0.83, 2.26)
No	48	52	1	

* = Stay on the street at the day time and return to home at the night for sleep; ** = Stay on the street both during the day and night time.

6. Conclusions

In this study, significant percentage of respondents had taken a drink that contains alcohol one year prior to the study. Age, level of education, prior place of residence, ever heard about STDs, and being cigarette smokers were variables significantly associated with alcohol use. Furthermore, gender, educational status, history of rape, and ever heard about STDs were also significantly associated with having sexual intercourse after alcohol use. Awareness creation on the effect and outcome of substance use is recommended.

Abbreviations

STDs: Sexually transmitted diseases.

Disclosure

The funding body has no role in the design of the study and collection, analysis, and interpretation of data and in writing the manuscript.

Acknowledgments

We are grateful to the Social and Labor Affair office staff at the southern nation, nationality, and people region for assisting us during data collection. This study was supported by the Center for International Reproductive Health Training at the University of Michigan (CIRHT-UM).

References

[1] S. Getachew, S. Lewis, J. Britton, W. Deressa, and A. W. Fogarty, "Prevalence and risk factors for initiating tobacco and alcohol consumption in adolescents living in urban and rural Ethiopia," *Public Health*, vol. 174, pp. 118–126, 2019.

[2] V. Benegal, M. Sathyaprakash, and D. Nagaraja, *Alcohol Misuse in the Andaman and Nicobar Islands*, Report on project commissioned by the Indian Council of Medical Research and funded by Action Aid, India, 2008.

[3] M. Sharma and M. Chaudhary, "A study of drugs and substance abuse among adolescents of slum dwellers," *International Journal of Indian Psychology*, vol. 3, no. 4, pp. 21–27, 2016.

[4] J. Jacobus, L. M. Squeglia, S. Bava, and S. F. Tapert, "White matter characterization of adolescent binge drinking with

and without co-occurring marijuana use: a 3-year investigation," *Psychiatry Research*, vol. 214, no. 3, pp. 374–381, 2013.

[5] G. Battistella, E. Fornari, J. M. Annoni et al., "Long-term effects of cannabis on brain structure," *Neuropsychopharmacology*, vol. 39, no. 9, pp. 2041–2048, 2014.

[6] K. O. Asante, A. Meyer-Weitz, and I. Petersen, "Substance use and risky sexual behaviours among street connected children and youth in Accra, Ghana," *Substance Abuse Treatment, Prevention, and Policy*, vol. 9, no. 1, p. 45, 2014.

[7] B. Lioul and H. Jemal, "Does exposure to sexually explicit films predict sexual activity of the in-school youth? Evidence from Addis Ababa high schools," *Ethiopian Journal of Health Development*, vol. 23, pp. 183–189, 2005.

[8] J. Francis, H. Grosskurth, J. Changalucha, S. H. Kapiga, and H. A. Weiss, "Systematic review and meta-analysis: prevalence of alcohol use among young people in eastern Africa," *Tropical Medicine & International Health*, vol. 19, no. 4, pp. 476–488, 2014.

[9] G. Tesfaye, A. Derese, and M. T. Hambisa, "Substance use and associated factors among university students in Ethiopia: a cross-sectional study," *Journal of Addiction*, vol. 2014, Article ID 969837, 8 pages, 2014.

[10] D. M. S. Maria, S. C. Narendorf, and M. B. Cross, "Prevalence and correlates of substance use in homeless youth and young adults," *Journal of Addictions Nursing*, vol. 29, no. 1, pp. 23–31, 2018.

[11] N. E. Walls and S. Bell, "Correlates of engaging in survival sex among homeless youth and young adults," *Journal of Sex Research*, vol. 48, no. 5, pp. 423–436, 2011.

[12] K. J. Hodgson, K. H. Shelton, M. B. van den Bree, and F. J. Los, "Psychopathology in young people experiencing homelessness: a systematic review," *American Journal of Public Health*, vol. 103, no. 6, pp. e24–e37, 2013.

[13] S. E. Hadland, B. D. Marshall, T. Kerr, R. Zhang, J. S. Montaner, and E. Wood, "A comparison of drug use and risk behavior profiles among younger and older street youth," *Substance Use & Misuse*, vol. 46, no. 12, pp. 1486–1494, 2011.

[14] WHO, *Understanding sexual and reproductive health including HIV/AIDS and STDs among street children*, WHO, Geneva, Switzerland, 2000.

[15] S. Chaudhury, S. K. Das, and B. Ukil, "Psychological assessment of alcoholism in males," *Indian Journal of Psychiatry*, vol. 48, no. 2, pp. 114–117, 2006.

[16] D. R. Siri Gowri, L. N. Suman, S. L. Rao, and P. Murthy, "A study of executive functions in alcohol dependent individuals: association of age, education and duration of drinking," *Indian Journal of Clinical Psychology*, vol. 35, pp. 14–23, 2008.

[17] N. Tadesse, T. Awoke Ayele, Z. Birhanu Mengesha, and K. Addis Alene, "High prevalence of HIV/AIDS risky sexual behaviors among street youth in Gondar town: a community based cross sectional study," *BMC Research Notes*, vol. 6, no. 1, p. 234, 2013.

[18] D. Habtamu and A. Adamu, "Assessment of sexual and reproductive health status of street children in Addis Ababa," *Journal of Sexually Transmitted Diseases*, vol. 2013, 20 pages, 2013.

[19] J. S. Tucker, G. W. Ryan, D. Golinelli et al., "Substance use and other risk factors for unprotected sex: results from an event-based study of homeless youth," *AIDS and Behaviour*, vol. 16, no. 6, pp. 1699–1707, 2012.

[20] J. A. Heerde, K. E. Scholes-Balog, and S. A. Hemphill, "Associations between youth homelessness, sexual offenses, sexual victimization, and sexual risk behaviors: a systematic literature review," *Archives of Sexual Behavior*, vol. 44, no. 1, pp. 181–212, 2015.

[21] J. A. Heerde and S. A. Hemphill, "Sexual risk behaviors, sexual offenses, and sexual victimization among homeless youth: a systematic review of associations with substance use," *Trauma, Violence & Abuse*, vol. 17, no. 5, pp. 468–489, 2016.

[22] M. N. Grinman, S. Chiu, D. A. Redelmeier et al., "Drug problems among homeless individuals in Toronto, Canada: prevalence, drugs of choice, and relation to health status," *BMC Public Health*, vol. 10, no. 1, 2010.

[23] K. H. Nada and E. D. A. Suliman, "Violence, abuse, alcohol and drug use, and sexual behaviors in street children of greater Cairo and Alexandria, Egypt," *AIDS*, vol. 24, Suppl 2, pp. S39–S44, 2010.

[24] P. K. Kayembe, M. A. Mapatano, A. B. Fatuma et al., "Knowledge of HIV, sexual behavior and correlates of risky sex among street children in Kinshasa, democratic republic of Congo," *East African Journal of Public Health*, vol. 5, no. 3, pp. 186–192, 2008.

[25] K. Ahamad, K. DeBeck, C. Feng, T. Sakakibara, T. Kerr, and E. Wood, "Gender influences on initiation of injecting drug use," *The American Journal of Drug and Alcohol Abuse*, vol. 40, no. 2, pp. 151–156, 2014.

[26] D. Hathazi, S. E. Lankenau, B. Sanders, and J. Jackson Bloom, "Pregnancy and sexual health among homeless young injection drug users," *Journal of Adolescence*, vol. 32, no. 2, pp. 339–355, 2009.

[27] L. Embleton, D. Ayuku, L. Atwoli, R. Vreeman, and P. Braitstein, "Knowledge, attitudes, and substance use practices among street children in western Kenya," *Substance Use & Misuse*, vol. 47, no. 11, pp. 1234–1247, 2012.

[28] D. Rosenthal, S. Mallett, N. Milburn, and M. J. Rotheram-Borus, "Drug use among homeless young people in Los Angeles and Melbourne," *The Journal of Adolescent Health*, vol. 43, no. 3, pp. 296–305, 2008.

[29] R. Gomez, S. J. Thompson, and A. N. Barczyk, "Factors associated with substance use among homeless young adults," *Substance Abuse*, vol. 31, no. 1, pp. 24–34, 2010.

[30] K. Haile, H. Umer, G. Ayano, E. Fejo, and T. Fanta, "A qualitative exploration of substance misuse among homeless women in Addis Ababa, Ethiopia," *BMC Psychiatry*, vol. 20, no. 1, p. 204, 2020.

[31] K. Haile, H. Umer, T. Fanta et al., "Pathways through homelessness among women in Addis Ababa, Ethiopia: A qualitative study," *PLoS ONE*, vol. 15, no. 9, article e0238571, 2020.

[32] M. Ayenew, T. Kabeta, and K. Woldemichael, "Prevalence and factors associated with substance use among street children in Jimma town, Oromiya national regional state, Ethiopia: a community based cross-sectional study," *Substance Abuse Treatment, Prevention, and Policy*, vol. 15, no. 1, p. 61, 2020.

[33] M. Kassa, G. Buruh, S. Berhe, A. Aregay, and H. Berhe, "Prevalence and determinants of substance abuse among street children in Mekelle city, Tigray, Ethiopia," *Journal of Bio Innovation*, vol. 3, no. 6, pp. 269–282, 2014.

[34] N. Wakgari, T. Woyo, E. Kebede, H. Gemeda, and S. Gebremedhin, "Sexually transmitted disease among street dwellers in southern Ethiopia: a mixed methods study design," *BMC Public Health*, vol. 20, no. 1, p. 434, 2020.

[35] S. Kingston, M. Rose, J. Cohen-Serrins, and E. Knight, "A qualitative study of the context of child and adolescent substance use initiation and patterns of use in the first year for early and Later initiators," *PLoS ONE*, vol. 12, no. 1, article e0170794, 2017.

[36] S. Park and Y. Kim, "Prevalence, correlates, and associated psychological problems of substance use in Korean adolescents," *BMC Public Health*, vol. 16, no. 1, p. 79, 2015.

[37] B. F. Grant, D. S. Hasin, S. P. Chou, F. S. Stinson, and D. A. Dawson, "Nicotine dependence and psychiatric disorders in the United States: results from the National Epidemiologic Survey on alcohol and related conditions," *Archives of General Psychiatry*, vol. 61, no. 11, pp. 1107–1115, 2004.

[38] J. K. Bobo and C. Husten, "Socio-cultural influences on smoking and drinking," *Alcohol Research & Health*, vol. 24, no. 4, pp. 225–232, 2000.

[39] L. Rew, M. Grady, T. A. Whittaker, and K. Bowman, "Interaction of duration of homelessness and gender on adolescent sexual health indicators," *Journal of Nursing Scholarship*, vol. 40, no. 2, pp. 109–115, 2008.

[40] W. Li and N. Caltabiano, "Prevalence of substance abuse and socio-economic differences in substance abuse in an Australian community-dwelling elderly sample," *Health Psychology Open*, vol. 4, no. 1, pp. 205510291770813–205510291770817, 2017.

[41] T. M. Caldwell, B. Rodgers, A. F. Jorm et al., "Patterns of association between alcohol consumption and symptoms of depression and anxiety in young adults," *Addiction*, vol. 97, no. 5, pp. 583–594, 2002.

[42] K. Graham, A. Massak, A. Demers, and J. Rehm, "Does the association between alcohol consumption and depression depend on how they are measured?," *Alcoholism, Clinical and Experimental Research*, vol. 31, no. 1, pp. 78–88, 2007.

[43] C. F. Helen, L. B. Keri, G. Peihua, and S. Rajita, "Interactive effects of cumulative stress and impulsivity on alcohol consumption," *Alcoholism, Clinical and Experimental Research*, vol. 34, no. 8, pp. 1376–1385, 2010.

Low Utilization of Partograph and Its Associated Factors among Obstetric Care Providers in Governmental Health Facilities at West Shoa Zone, Central Ethiopia

Kefena Etita Bedada,[1] Tufa Kolola Huluka,[2] Gizachew Abdissa Bulto,[3] and Ephrem Yohannes Roga[3]

[1]*Ambo Town Health Office, Ambo, Ethiopia*
[2]*Department of Public Health, College of Medicine and Health Silences, Ambo University, Ambo, Ethiopia*
[3]*Department of Midwifery, College of Medicine and Health Sciences, Ambo University, Ambo, Ethiopia*

Correspondence should be addressed to Gizachew Abdissa Bulto; gizachab@yahoo.com

Academic Editor: Samir Hamamah

Background. Globally, prolonged and obstructed labors were among the common causes of maternal morbidity and mortality in low- and middle-income countries including Ethiopia. The World Health Organization (WHO) recommends the routine use of partograph as a key intervention to avoid prolonged and obstructed labor. Despite the recommendation, studies indicated that the partograph utilization among obstetric care providers (OCPs) is still low. Therefore, this study is aimed at assessing the level of utilization of partograph and associated factors among obstetric care providers working at health facilities in the West Shoa Zone, Central Ethiopia 2019. *Methods.* Facility-based cross-sectional study was conducted from February 1st to 22nd March 2019. A computer-generated simple random sampling technique was used to select 325 study subjects. Data were collected using a self-administered structured questionnaire and using an observational checklist. Additionally, 200 partograph charts were reviewed. Both bivariate and multivariable logistic regression analyses were used to determine the association. *Results.* A total of 322 obstetric care providers were included in the study, giving a response rate of 99.1%. The level of partograph utilization in the study area was revealed to be 31.1% (95% CI: 25.97-36.13). Only 3% of the reviewed partograph was recorded according to the recommended standard. In this study attending training (AOR = 3.94, 95% CI: 1.99-7.78), availability of partograph (AOR = 5.23, 95% CI: 1.69-16.22), perceived as not time-consuming task (AOR = 3.61, 95% CI: 1.19-10.96), adequate number of OCPs available (AOR = 2.92, 95% CI: 1.16-7.33), presence of supervision (AOR = 4.35, 95% CI: 2.11-8.97), having a positive attitude (AOR = 2.48, 95% CI: 1.23-5.02), availability of standard protocol in a health facility (AOR = 4.71, 95% CI: 2.31-9.60), and lack of commitment (AOR = 0.32, 95% CI: 0.16-0.63) were factors significantly associated with partograph utilization. *Conclusion and Recommendation.* Partograph utilization in the study area was found to be low. Almost all reviewed partograph charts were not recorded as to the recommended standard. Attending training, availability of partograph, perceived as it is not time-consuming, the available number of OCPs, presence of supervision, having a positive attitude, available standard protocol, and commitment were factors associated with partograph utilization. Therefore, all concerned stakeholders should emphatically consider those identified factors for intervention.

1. Introduction

Partograph is a simple, low-cost monitoring tool for intrapartum care recommended by the World Health Organization (WHO) which has the potential to identify obstetric complications by graphically representing the vital issues of labor progression [1]. It is the best instrument to help you detect whether labor is progressing normally or abnormally and to warn you as soon as possible if there are signs of fetal distress or if the mother's vital signs deviate from the normal range. It also causes an impact on bettering the quality of intrapartum care, maternal health, and birth outcomes [2–4].

The World Health Organization advocated the general usage of the partograph during labor, and routine use of partograph is helpful to make better decisions for the diagnosis and management of prolonged and obstructed labor [3, 5]. Partograph is one of the most potent and cost-effective tools to prevent unnecessary delays and services as the frontrunner for obstetric care givers [4, 5]. Woman's lifetime risk of dying from preventable or treatable complications of pregnancy and childbirth in sub-Saharan Africa was higher compared to that in developed regions [6–8]. Although prolonged and obstructed labors in the resource-poor settings are among the major causes of deaths, they can be prevented with the proper use of partograph [3, 8–10].

Ground from the developing countries, including Ethiopia, demonstrated that the use of partograph is poor despite preparing the tool that is simple and inexpensive for intrapartum monitoring of labor [11–14]. In Ethiopia, the major sources of maternal and neonatal morbidity and death rate are related to poor labor and delivery care. However, eighty-five percent of deaths can be prevented with cost-effective interventions like using partograph during labor and delivery [12, 15]. Skilled management of labor using a partograph, a simple chart for recording information about the advancement of labor and the status of a woman and her baby during labor, is a key to the appropriate prevention and treatment of prolonged labor and its complications [16].

Globally, about 295,000 women died during and following pregnancy and childbirth in 2017. Majority of these deaths (94%) occurred in low-resource settings, and most could have been prevented [17]. Ethiopian demographic and health survey 2016 showed that the maternal mortality ratio was 471 deaths per 100,000 live births [15]. Moreover, from the study done in Jimma University specialized hospital, the incidence of obstructed labor was 12.2% of which about 45.1% developed uterine rupture and 39.3% had sepsis with other complications [18]. These complications were preventable if correctly followed with partograph [3, 10].

The use of the partograph reduced the incidence of prolonged labor from 6.4% to 3.4%, the proportion of labor requiring augmentation from 9.9% to 8.3%, and intrapartum stillbirth rate from 0.5% to 0.3% [19]. The partograph is a very useful graphical record of the course of labor that yields optimum results when employed in labor management by obstetric care providers. Evidence abounds that the accomplishment of knowledge of its usage and ensuring proper application of that knowledge would culminate in a noteworthy decrease in the incidence and outcomes of prolonged and obstructed labor, which is reported to be associated with 8%–10% of maternal deaths [19–21].

Even though a partograph is an instrument that is helpful to manage obstructed labor and prevent prolonged labor with its ramifications, the level of usage and factors affecting utilization of partograph among obstetric care providers was not yet studied in the study area. Thus, the purpose of this study is to evaluate the extent of usage of the partograph and associated factors that inhibit obstetric care providers from consistent use of partograph in West Shoa Zone public health facilities.

2. Methods

2.1. Study Area and Period. The study was conducted from February 1st to March 22nd, 2019, in West Shoa Zone, Oromia region, Ethiopia. The West Shoa Zone is one of the twenty zones in the Oromia region which contains 22 districts. Ambo is the city of the zone, which is located at 114 km from Addis Ababa. Concerning health facilities, there were 4 primary hospitals, 3 general hospitals, 1 referral hospital, and 92 health centers providing labor and delivery services for over 2.5 million peoples in the West Shoa Zone. According to the data from the West Shoa Zone health office, 1376 obstetric care providers were providing services at those 100 health institutions [22].

2.2. Study Design. The institutional-based cross-sectional study design was conducted to assess the level of partograph utilization and associated factors among obstetric care providers in the governmental health facilities of the West Shoa Zone.

2.3. Source and Study Populations. The source population includes all obstetric care providers (midwives, nurses, Integrated Emergency Surgery Officers, doctors, and health officers) working in all health facilities in the West Shoa Zone. A retrospective document review of all partograph from a recent delivery attended in the last three months at public health facilities from November1st, 2018, to January 30th, 2019. Study populations were all randomly selected obstetric care providers (midwives, nurses, Integrated Emergency Surgery Officers, doctors, and health officers) who have been working in all selected health facilities in West Shoa Zone. Obstetric care providers who were on leave (annual, sick, and maternity leave), who worked less than six-month duration during the data collection period were excluded from the study.

2.4. Sample Size Determination and Sampling Procedure. The sample size was calculated by using single-population proportion formula with the assumptions of proportion (p) of partograph utilization 57.3% taken from a study done in Addis Ababa [23], with 95% confidence level of $ZZ\alpha/2 = 1.96$; 5% of absolute precision gives a large sample size (no. 376) to accommodate all objectives. Since the source population was less than 10,000, the correction factor was used to estimate the final required sample size which is 325 by considering 10% of the nonresponse rate.

By using the simple random sampling method, four hospitals and forty-six health centers were selected. The lists of all obstetric care providers in each health facility were considered a sampling frame. The sample was proportionally allocated to the selected health institutions according to the number of obstetric care providers. A total of 200 client's chart was selected by simple random sampling technique from four hospitals and 46 health centers.

2.5. Operational Definition

2.5.1. Partograph Utilization. Partograph utilization refers to plotting or recording the partograph correctly and interpreting to make appropriate decisions and intervene where necessary. To assess the level of partograph utilization, two steps had been undertaken: the first footprint was asking the participants whether they were using partograph or not (with yes or no doubts). For the second measure, the respondents who replied "yes" in the first step were required to answer "how often" they accept using partograph (occasionally, sometimes, and routinely). Finally, obstetric care providers who were utilizing partograph "routinely" to monitor laboring mothers were considered utilized partograph and those who have been using sometimes and occasionally to monitor labor were considered not utilized [21, 23, 24].

2.5.2. Attitude Scale. There were [10] attitude determining questions used. The responses (5: strongly agree, 4: agree, 3: uncertain, 2: disagree, and 1: strongly disagree) were scored. Providers' attitude towards partograph utilization was assessed by using a 5-point Likert scale as individuals responding strongly agree for positive attitude were given scores of 5 and 1 for those who responded as strongly disagree, while the above scores were turned back for negative attitude questions. In the end, the entire score was dichotomized into favorable and unfavorable attitudes taking the mean score as a cutoff point (mean score or more was considered having favorable attitude and less than the mean score as unfavorable attitude) [25].

2.5.3. Knowledge Scale. There are 15 knowledge-assessing questions used. Correct responses were scored 1 point and incorrect 0. The scores of the items are summed up, and the total was divided by the number of the items, giving a mean score. The obstetric care providers' knowledge was considered good if it is greater than mean score and poor if it is less than mean score [23, 25].

2.6. Data Collection Tools and Procedure. Data were collected using a self-administered structured questionnaire and observational checklist. The questionnaire has different subsections, namely, sociodemographic, training status, knowledge, attitude towards partograph, and utilization of partograph that were used [13, 26]. Five degree holder midwives facilitated the data collection process, and three Integrated Emergency Surgery Officers (IESO) were used as supervisors. Data about the completeness of the WHO partograph was collected by using structured observational checklist by a principal investigator from each selected hospital. The constructed checklists were from the WHO-approved partograph and contain the details of items for administrative data, fetal condition, the progress of labor, drug administration, maternal condition, the time interval of recording the data, time of stopping partograph, and time of delivery.

2.7. Data Quality Control. The training was given for the data collectors and field supervisors for two days before the actual data collection regarding the aim of the study, the data collection tool, and procedures. For data quality assurance, one week before the actual data collection, the questionnaire was pretested on 5% of the total sample size at Holeta town health institutions. The training was focused on the art of interviewing and clarifying questions that would be unclear to answer. They also thoroughly looked into and understood the observation checklists before use. Close supervision was carried out by the investigators day to day during data collection, completeness of data had been checked daily, and corrections were made on the spot. Every day, collected data was reviewed and checked for completeness and consistency of the response.

2.8. Data Processing and Analysis. The collected data were checked visually for completeness, coded and entered into EPI Info version 3.5.1 statistical software, and exported into SPSS version 23 for further analysis. Descriptive summary statistics were done. Both bivariate and multivariable logistic regression analyses were used to determine the association of each independent variable with the dependent variable. Variables with a P value < 0.25 in the bivariate analysis were entered into a multivariable logistic regression model to adjust for the confounders. Odds ratio with 95% confidence intervals was computed to identify the presence of an association, and statistical significance was declared if $P < 0.05$. The findings of the observational assessment were analyzed using descriptive statistics. The outcomes were presented with texts, tables, and summary statistics.

2.9. Ethical Considerations. Ethical clearance was obtained from the Research Review and Ethics Committee of the College of Medicine and Health Sciences, Ambo University. An official letter of cooperation was given to the administrative offices of the selected health facilities. Written informed consent was obtained from each study participant. The purpose of the study was explained, and confidentiality was maintained.

3. Result

3.1. Sociodemographic Characteristics of the Study Participants. A total of 322 obstetric care providers were included in the study making a response rate of 99.1%. About 203 (63%) obstetric care providers were females and 226 (70.2%) of them were working at the health center. The mean age of the respondents was 30.87 years with a standard deviation of 4.92, and the majority of the respondents were in the age range of 25-29 years (147, 45.7%). Regarding their profession, 151 (46.9%) were midwives (diploma and degree) followed by nurse (diploma and degree) 103 (32%). One hundred ninety-six (60.9%) had a degree and above educational levels, and their mean duration of practice was 6.48 years with an SD of 4.78 (Table 1).

3.2. Knowledge and Attitude of Obstetric Care Providers on Partograph Utilization. Most (259, 80.4%) of the respondents defined the partograph correctly. Most of the respondents (267, 82.9%) used partograph before and 208 (64.6%) know the components of partograph. Similarly, 271 (84.2%) respondents knew alert and action lines (Table 2). One hundred eighty-five (57.5%) (95% CI, 52.02-62.9) respondents had good overall knowledge, while 137 (42.5%) of them had poor knowledge of partograph (Figure 1).

More than half of the obstetric care providers (54%) (95% CI 48.6-59.5) generally had a favorable/positive attitude

TABLE 1: Sociodemographic characteristics of obstetric care providers in governmental health facilities in West Shoa Zone, Central Ethiopia, 2019.

Variable ($n = 322$)		Frequency	Percent
Health facility type	Hospital	96	29.8
	Health center	226	70.2
Sex	Male	119	37.0
	Female	203	63.0
Age category in years	20-24	11	3.4
	25-29	147	45.7
	30-34	95	29.5
	35-39	41	12.7
	>40	28	8.7
Professional category	GP & IESO	23	7.1
	HO	45	14.0
	Nurse	103	32.0
	Midwives	151	46.9
Service years	≤3 years	104	32.3
	4-6 years	93	28.9
	7-9 years	53	16.5
	>9 years	72	22.4

TABLE 2: Knowledge of partograph among OCPs in governmental health facilities in West Shoa Zone, Central Ethiopia, 2019.

Variables		Frequency	Percent
Definition of partograph	Correct	259	80.4
	Incorrect	63	19.6
Fetal conditions components	Correct	207	64.3
	Incorrect	115	35.7
Progress of labor components	Correct	216	67.1
	Incorrect	106	32.9
Maternal conditions components	Correct	109	33.9
	Incorrect	213	66.1
Knows alert & action lines	Correct	271	84.2
	Incorrect	51	15.8
The function of alerting at the health center	To give early warning	148	46.0
	It indicates for augmentation	26	8.1
	It does not indicate any	3	.9
The function of alerting at the hospital	As a warning for extra vigilance	67	20.8
	Transfer laboring mothers	17	5.3
	It does not indicate any	9	2.8
The function of the action line at hospital	It indicates the critical point	80	24.8
	Followed for additional 2 hrs	13	4.0
Knows when to start plotting on partograph	Correct	233	72.4
	Incorrect	89	27.6
For whom to use partograph	Correct	284	88.2
	Incorrect	38	11.8
When did you fill partograph	After delivery of the baby	87	27.0
	While the woman is still in labor	235	73.0
Definition of prolonged labor	Correct	149	46.3
	Incorrect	173	53.7
Definition of obstructed labor	Correct	209	64.9
	Incorrect	113	35.1
Overall level of knowledge on partograph	Correct	185	57.5
	Incorrect	137	42.5

toward partograph (Table 3). Medical doctors and IESO (78.3%) and midwives (57.0%) have a more favorable attitude than others (Figure 2).

3.3. Partograph Utilization. Most of the respondents said that they had used partograph (197, 61.2%) to monitor the condition of laboring mothers, most of the respondents (252, 78.3%) reported that the partograph is always available in their health facility, and 297 (92.2%) said that partograph is a mandatory tool to improve the quality of care given to the laboring woman. One hundred sixty-eight (52.2%) have no policy or standard protocol for guidance on the use of partograph. Frequency of partograph utilization by obstetric care providers indicates that 100 (31.1%) of them use it routinely, 106 (32.9%) use partograph sometimes, 73 (22.7%) use partograph occasionally, and 43 (13.4%) do not use partograph. However, less than half (39, 40.6%) of the obstetric care providers from hospitals have used partograph and 61 (27%) respondents were using it in health centers.

Among medical records reviewed, only about 173 (86.5%) records have partograph forms while 7 (3.5%) used plain paper and 20 (10%) used patient history sheets to follow laboring mothers. The pattern of monitoring and recording from components of partograph indicated that only 6 (3%) partograph was recorded as to the WHO's standard (Table 4).

Majority (313, 97.2%) of the respondents said that they learned about partograph during a stay at a university or college. Most of the respondents (197, 61.2%) had never attended training while only 125 (38.8%) had attended a workshop/training on basic or comprehensive emergency obstetric and newborn care. Majority (113, 90.4%) of them have taken the training or orientation a year ago.

3.4. Reasons for Not Using Partograph among Obstetric Care Providers. The reason reported by most of the study participants for not routinely using partograph were partograph chart not available, not trained about partograph, shortage of health care personnel, and the absence of obligation from hospital/health center policy to perform (Table 5). The main reasons mentioned by participants who were aware

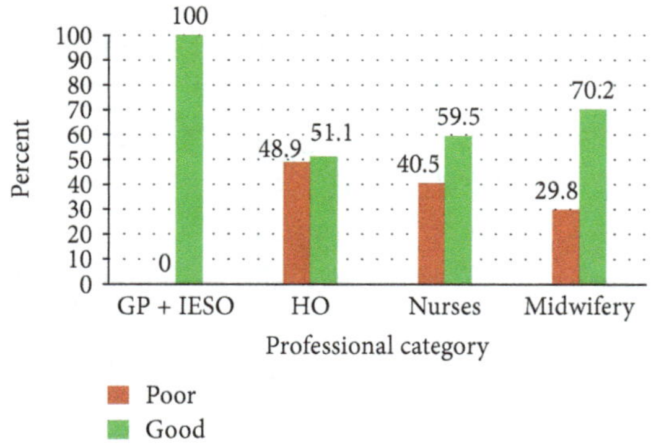

FIGURE 1: Level of knowledge on partograph among OCPs in governmental health facilities in West Shoa Zone, Central Ethiopia, 2019.

of the partograph, but not using the partograph for monitoring women in labor were as follows: lack of orientation/-training on how to use (112, 34.8%), availability of other methods of observation (43, 13.4%), lack of commitment (128, 39.8%), workload (199, 61.8%), and lack of supervision (172, 53.4%).

3.5. Factors Associated with Partograph Utilization among OCPs. In the bivariate analysis, the factors found to be significantly associated with partograph utilization and all candidate variables were analyzed by a multivariable logistic regression model.

Multiple logistic regression analysis indicated that obstetric care providers having a policy or standard protocol for guidance on the use of partograph were almost 5 times more likely to utilize the partograph than those who did not have in their health facility (AOR = 4.71, 95% CI: 2.31, 9.60). Those obstetric care providers who received training on partograph were almost 4 times more likely to use partograph than those who did not (AOR = 3.94, 95% CI: 1.99, 7.78). Those who had a partograph chart always available were 5 times more likely to use partograph than those where partograph is not always available (AOR = 5.23, 95% CI: 1.69, 16.22), and those obstetric care providers who have a favorable attitude toward partograph were two times more likely to utilize partograph than their counterparts (AOR = 2.48, 95% CI: 1.23, 5.02). Furthermore, those respondents that had more health care personnel staff in their health facility were almost three times more likely to utilize partograph than a shortage of health care personnel staff in their health facility (AOR = 2.48, 95% CI: 1.23, 5.02). Likewise, obstetric care providers who reported lack of commitment about the use partograph were 68% less likely to utilize the partograph for monitoring mothers in labor compared to those who were committed to utilizing the partograph (AOR = 0.32, 95% CI: 0.16, 0.63) (Table 6).

4. Discussion

The level of partograph utilization in the study area was revealed to be 31.1% (95% CI: 25.97-36.13). The current finding is in line with the findings from Asella referral and teaching hospitals (26%) [27], the Amhara region (29.3%) [13],

TABLE 3: Attitude towards partograph utilization among OCPs in governmental health facilities in West Shoa Zone, Central Ethiopia, 2019.

Variables	OCPs respondents (n = 322) Unfavorable attitudes N (%)	Favorable attitudes N (%)
Partograph is a tool to monitor labor	90 (28)	232 (72)
Partograph used in all normal labor	105 (32.6)	217 (67.4)
Partograph should be used for high-risk mothers only	131 (40.7)	191 (59.3)
Use of partograph decreases risks of complication on mother and/or newborn	85 (26.4)	237 (73.6)
Partograph helps early identification of cases for transfer, augmentation, and/or surgery	87 (27)	235 (73)
Using partograph increases the quality and regularity of all observations for mother and fetus	80 (24.8)	242 (75.2)
Using partograph is an only time-consuming task without any benefit	178 (55.3)	144 (44.7)
Using partograph is the responsibility of midwife only	79 (24.5)	243 (75.5)
Using partograph is not an appropriate method of monitoring	122 (37.9)	200 (62.1)
Using partograph misleads management as the progress of labor	135 (41.9)	187 (58.1)
Total attitude	Favorable	174 (54)
	Unfavorable	148 (46)

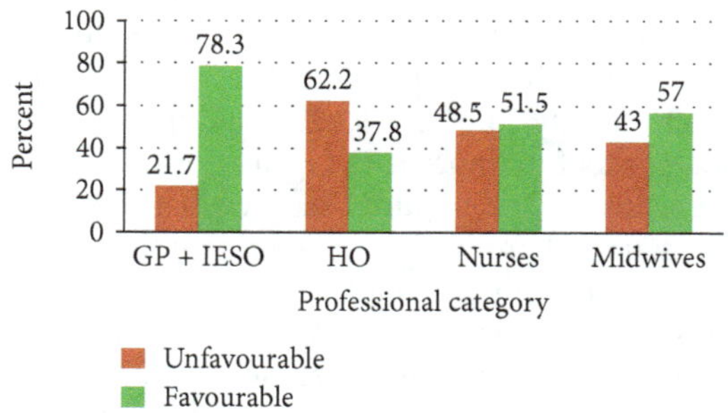

FIGURE 2: Attitude towards partograph utilization among obstetric care providers in governmental health facilities in the West Shoa Zone, Central Ethiopia, 2019.

Uganda (30%) [26], Nigeria (32.4%) [28], and Port Said and Ismailia cities (35.9%) [25].

But the current finding was higher than the findings from Jimma Referral Hospital Ethiopia (6.3%) [29], urban hospitals in Lilongwe-Malawi (3.9%) [30], and Mulanje District Hospital in Malawi (10%) [31]. The higher prevalence rate in this study is attributed to the availability of partograph, having a policy or standard protocol, better supervision, and positive attitudes towards its use.

This finding is lower than that of the studies done in Addis Ababa (57.4%) [23], Western Oromia hospitals (89.1%) [32],

Table 4: Completeness of filled partograph from reviewed records in governmental health facilities of West Shoa Zone, Central Ethiopia, 2019.

Variable	Frequency (N = 200)and percent		
	Recorded as standard	Substandard	Not recorded
FHB	92 (46)	91 (45.5)	17 (8.5)
Membrane & liquor	47 (23.5)	76 (38)	77 (38.5)
Molding of the fetal skull	57 (28.5)	31 (15.5)	112 (56)
Cervical dilatation	130 (65)	44 (22)	26 (13)
Descent of the fetal head	25 (12.5)	83 (41.5)	92 (46)
Uterine contraction	92 (46)	39 (19.5)	69 (34.5)
Additional medication & IV fluids	98 (49)	83 (41.5)	19 (9.5)
Maternal pulse	33 (16.5)	107 (53.5)	60 (30)
Blood pressure	56 (28)	115 (57.5)	29 (14.5)
Temperature	27 (13.5)	8 (4)	165 (82.5)
Protein, acetone & urine volume	14 (7)	59 (29.5)	127 (63.5)
Overall recording status from the reviewed partograph charts	6 (3)	138 (69)	56 (28)

Table 5: Reason mentioned for not using partograph among obstetric care providers in governmental health facilities in West Shoa Zone, Central Ethiopia, 2019.

Variable		Frequency	Percent
Partograph chart was not available	No	277	86.0
	Yes	45	14.0
Not trained about partograph	No	190	59.0
	Yes	132	41.0
Shortage of health care personnel	No	255	79.2
	Yes	67	20.8
Time-consuming task due to the low number of staff	No	263	81.7
	Yes	59	18.3
Its advantage not that much appreciable	No	265	82.3
	Yes	57	17.7
No managerial support and motivation for the use	No	221	68.6
	Yes	101	31.4
Absence of obligation from HFs policy to perform	No	264	82.0

East Gojam Zone (53.85%) [14], Cameroon (58.2%) [33], and the Niger Delta of Nigeria (98.8%) [34]. These differences might be due to the differences in the place of the study that may be explained with different strategies in partograph implementation, selected facility type, data collection methods, sample size, different levels of knowledge, and attitudes of care providers towards partograph utilization.

Attending training or workshop of OCPs was more likely significantly associated with the utilization of the partograph. This finding is consistent with previous studies done in the Amhara region [13], Tanzania [25], and in North Shoa [11] and Eastern Gojam Zone of Ethiopia [14] which is more likely associated with OCPs interviewed that had been previously trained in-service to use the partograph. However, studies done in Western Oromia hospitals indicated less likely utilization than counterparts [32]. This finding points to the need that OCPs should get periodic on-the-job refresher training on the obstetric care that has been overlooked and better make use of the partograph with post-follow-up of training, and this may be possibly explained by the fact that training would improve the status of knowledge about the area of interest.

Those participants who were reporting plotting of the partograph was not an additional time-consuming task were more likely to utilize partograph than those who reported plotting partograph was an additional time-consuming task. This study is not in line with a study done in Nigeria [34] and Addis Ababa [23]. Additionally, studies conducted in Nigeria in the Enugu Metropolis and Southwest Region of Cameroon showed that some midwives often think that completing the partograph is an additional time-consuming task and as such have no understanding of how it can save a woman's life [35, 36]. The probable reason for this discrepancy might be a shortage of staff and consequent workload and may be also ignorance of the importance/benefit of the partograph.

Obstetric care providers having a policy or standard protocol for guidance on the use of partograph in their health facility are more likely to use partograph than counterparts. This implies that it might be that a shortage of health care personnel brings workload which means that where there was a shortage of health care personnel; appropriate actions may vary depending on the setting: augmentation of labor, operative delivery, or just timely referral to a higher level of care. Standard management protocols on the actions to be taken based on partograph that is available for use at first and referral system and should be used to help in decision-making. Obstetric care providers were not likely to use partograph which leads to poor management of laboring women [10, 20, 32].

Those OCPs who were supervised have more likely utilized partograph than the counterpart; for effective utilization of partograph and partograph-based decision-making, OCP's knowledge advancement through refresher training, including practical demonstration, supportive supervision, and on-site partograph audits by trained supervisors, should also be prioritized [26, 36, 37]. The possible reason could be due to the availability of well-designed and coordinated programs like the strength of mentorship and supportive supervision of OCPs. Other reasons might be the competency level and background characteristics of the study participants. Strengthening the integrated supportive supervision with in-services would further enable the workers to implement their decisions in case of an obstetric emergency.

The availability of the partograph was a big hindrance to its utilization. Similarly, a study in Rujumbura Health Sub-district in Southwestern Uganda found that the various health centers had sufficient numbers of the partograph although their utilization was low [26]. However, other sites have documented unavailability as a problem, for example,

TABLE 6: Factors associated with partograph utilization of bivariate and multivariable logistic regression analysis among OCPs in governmental health facilities in West Shoa Zone, Central Ethiopia, 2019.

Variable		Partograph utilization Utilized No. (%)	Nonutilized No. (%)	COR (95% CI)	AOR (95% CI)
Attended training/orientation	Yes	66 (20.5)	59 (18.3)	5.36 (3.21-8.93)*	3.94 (1.99-7.78)*
	No	34 (10.6)	163 (50.6)	1	
Have a policy or standard protocol	Yes	69 (21.4)	85 (26.4)	3.59 (2.17-5.93)*	4.71 (2.31-9.60)*
	No	31 (9.6)	137 (42.6)	1	
Partograph always readily available	Yes	94 (29.2)	158 (49)	6.35 (2.65-15.22)*	5.23 (1.69-16.22)*
	No	6 (1.9)	64 (19.9)	1	
Attitude toward partograph utilization	Favorable.	68 (21.2)	106 (32.9)	2.33 (1.42-3.82)*	2.48 (1.23-5.02)*
	Unfavorable.	32 (9.9)	116 (36)	1	
Plotting partograph is a time-consuming task	No	90 (28)	173 (53.7)	2.55 (1.23-5.27)*	3.61 (1.19-10.96)*
	Yes	10 (3.1)	49 (15.2)	1	
Supervision	Yes	64 (19.9)	86 (26.7)	2.81 (1.72-4.59)*	4.35 (2.11-8.97)*
	No	36 (11.2)	136 (42.2)	1	
Commitment	No	35 (10.9)	159 (49.4)	0.21 (0.13-0.35)*	0.32 (0.16-0.63)*
	Yes	65 (20.2)	63 (19.6)	1	
Adequate manpower	Yes	87 (27)	168 (52.2)	2.15 (1.11-4.16)*	2.92 (1.16-7.33)*
	No	13 (4)	54 (16.8)	1	1

*Statistically significant at P value < 0.05 of adjusted 95% CI; 1 = reference category.

in Central Ethiopia, Nigeria, and South Africa [10, 23, 28, 34]. In our study, the unavailability of partograph may be due to the low preprinted material of partograph by the health institutions and/or the adequacy of the health facility's stationery supply system and other required essential health facility supplies such as blood pressure cuffs and urine test strips that also had gaps not always available.

Having adequate health care personnel staff had three times more likely to utilize partograph than counterparts. The employment of adequate staff was reported by the respondents as a factor that could facilitate their use of the partograph. This is because the increase in the number of workers will bring about a decrease in work overload and thus their provision of quality care. The finding is supported by the studies in Enugu Metropolis and Cambodia which found that more staff on duty was associated with high utilization of the partograph and if there was more partograph completed, there were more staff on duty. This finding is also in line with the finding of Saviola, Arez, Raddi, Sudha, and Metgu in South Asia [38], who inferred that the planned teaching program was effective to improve knowledge and skills on partograph.

The result of this study also revealed the existence of a significant association between participants' attitudes towards the partograph and utilization of it. This is in agreement with the studies done in Nigeria [34] and Ethiopia in Addis Ababa, Oromia, and the Amhara region [11, 13, 23]. This could be because having a good attitude towards partograph utilization might come after having knowledge about partograph that may influence the utilization of partograph.

4.1. Strength and Limitation of the Study. The study was conducted at 50 health facilities found in the West Shoa Zone, which covers half of those health facilities providing the service for over 2.5 million peoples. The limitations of this study could include the fact that there might be social desirability bias which may cause the obstetric care providers who took part in this study to overstate their use of the partograph. However, numerous scientific procedures were employed to minimize the possible effects of social desirability. Since the study design also uses a retrospective review of records for secondary data, some relevant data were missing due to inconsistency and incomplete documentation in the patient files. Progress notes in women's files were used to get the missing data from the partograph.

5. Conclusion

Partograph utilization in the study area was found to be low. Shortage of health care personnel, lack of supervision, partograph chart availability, having a favorable attitude towards partograph, and additional time-consuming tasks for the inadequate staff were factors affecting partograph utilization. Almost all reviewed partograph charts were not recorded as to the recommended standard. Therefore, continuously providing the necessary resources needed for the utilization of the partograph such as partograph charts, observation tools, gloves, blood pressure apparatus, thermometer, and urine analysis kit should have to be maintained. Furthermore, there should be regular supportive supervision by senior care providers, and they should provide on-the-job training on how to use partograph for OCPs and ensure deployment of an adequate number of OCPs based on the available caseloads.

Abbreviations

IESO: Integrated Emergency Surgery Officer
OCP: Obstetric care providers
WHO: World Health Organization.

Authors' Contributions

KEB conceptualized the proposal, participated in data collection, analyzed the data, and drafted the paper. TKH, GAB, and EYR drafted the paper, approved the proposal with some revisions, participated in data collection and analysis, and revised subsequent drafts of the paper. All authors read and approved the final manuscript.

Acknowledgments

We are very grateful to Ambo University for the approval of the ethical clearance and for facilitating the conduct of the study. We extend our appreciation to the West Shoa Zone health office for their support during proposal development and data collection. We would also like to thank all study participants for their time and response.

References

[1] World Health Organization, *The application of the WHO partograph in the management of labo ur*, Report of a WHO multicentre study 1990-91. Maternal Health and Safe motherhood Programme, WHO/FHE/MSN/94.4, Geneva, 1994.

[2] G. J. Hofmeyr, R. A. Haws, S. Bergström et al., "Obstetric care in low-resource settings: what, who, and how to overcome challenges to scale up?," *International Journal of Gynecology & Obstetrics*, vol. 107, Supplement, pp. S21–S45, 2009.

[3] W. P. P. Labour, "A Practical Guide: The Partograph Part I, Principles and Strategy WHO. World Health Organisation. Division of Family Health. Maternal Health and Safe Motherhood Programme. Safe Motherhood Practical Guide: WHO/FHE/MSM/93.8," 1994.

[4] J. Zhang, H. J. Landy, D. W. Branch et al., "Contemporary patterns of spontaneous labor with normal neonatal outcomes," *Obstetrics and gynecology*, vol. 116, no. 6, pp. 1281–1287, 2010.

[5] T. Lavender, A. Hart, and R. M. D. Smyth, "Effect of partogram use on outcomes for women in spontaneous labour at term," *The Cochrane database of systematic reviews*, vol. 8, 2012.

[6] Z. A. Bhutta, M. Chopra, H. Axelson et al., "Countdown to 2015 decade report (2000–10): taking stock of maternal, newborn, and child survival," *The lancet*, vol. 375, no. 9730, pp. 2032–2044, 2010.

[7] M. C. Hogan, K. J. Foreman, M. Naghavi et al., "Maternal mortality for 181 countries, 1980–2008: a systematic analysis of progress towards millennium development goal 5," *The lancet*, vol. 375, no. 9726, pp. 1609–1623, 2010.

[8] N. J. B. R. Kassebaum, Z. A. Bhutta, L. Dandona et al., "Global, regional, and national levels of maternal mortality, 1990-2015: a systematic analysis for the Global Burden of Disease Study 2015," *The Lancet*, vol. 388, no. 10053, pp. 1775–1812, 2016.

[9] A. R. Dalal and A. C. Purandare, "The partograph in childbirth: an absolute essentiality or a mere exercise?," *The Journal of Obstetrics and Gynecology of India*, vol. 68, no. 1, pp. 3–14, 2018.

[10] M. Mathai, "The partograph for the prevention of obstructed labor," *Clinical Obstetrics and Gynecology*, vol. 52, no. 2, pp. 256–269, 2009.

[11] N. Wakgari, A. Amano, M. Berta, and G. A. Tessema, "Partograph utilization and associated factors among obstetric care providers in North Shoa Zone, Central Ethiopia: a cross sectional study," *African health sciences*, vol. 15, no. 2, pp. 552–559, 2015.

[12] E. Yisma, B. Dessalegn, A. Astatkie, and N. Fesseha, "Completion of the modified World Health Organization (WHO) partograph during labour in public health institutions of Addis Ababa, Ethiopia," *Reproductive health*, vol. 10, no. 1, 2013.

[13] F. Abebe, "Assessment of knowledge and utilization of the partograph among health professionals in Amhara region, Ethiopia," *Science journal of clinical medicine*, vol. 2, no. 2, p. 26, 2013.

[14] D. A. Zelellw and T. K. Tegegne, "Level of partograph utilization and its associated factors among obstetric caregivers at public health facilities in East Gojam Zone, Northwest Ethiopia," *PloS one*, J. P. Wouwe, Ed., vol. 13, no. 7, p. e0200479, 2018.

[15] CSACE I, *Ethiopia demographic and health survey 2016*CSA and ICF, Addis Ababa, Ethiopia, and Rockville, Maryland, USA.

[16] F. Care and editor Maternal Health Task Force 2012, *Revitalising the partograph: does the evidence support a global call to action Report of an expert meeting*, New York, 2011.

[17] Organization WH, *Trends in maternal mortality 2000 to 2017: estimates by WHO, UNICEF, UNFPA*, World Bank Group and the United Nations Population Division, World Bank Group and the United Nations Population Division, 2019.

[18] S. Fantu, H. Segni, and F. Alemseged, "Incidence, causes and outcome of obstructed labor in Jimma University specialized hospital," *Ethiopian journal of health sciences*, vol. 20, no. 3, pp. 145–151, 2010.

[19] World Health Organization, *The application of the WHO partograph in the management of labour. Report of a WHO multicentre study 1990-91*, Maternal Health and Safe motherhood Programme, WHO/FHE/MSN/94.4, 1994, Geneva, 1994.

[20] J. E. Lawn, M. Kinney, A. C. C. Lee et al., "Reducing intrapartum-related deaths and disability: can the health system deliver?," *International Journal of Gynecology & Obstetrics*, vol. 107, Supplement, pp. S123–S142, 2009.

[21] B. K. Opoku and S. B. Nguah, "Utilization of the modified WHO partograph in assessing the progress of labour in a metropolitan area in Ghana," *Research Journal of Women's Health*, vol. 2, no. 1, p. 2, 2015.

[22] West Shoa Zone Health Office, "West Shoa Zonal Office:health management information system general report Ethiopia," 2018.

[23] E. Yisma, B. Dessalegn, A. Astatkie, and N. Fesseha, "Knowledge and utilization of partograph among obstetric care givers in public health institutions of Addis Ababa, Ethiopia," *BMC pregnancy and childbirth*, vol. 13, no. 1, 2013.

[24] T. Hailu, K. Nigus, G. Gidey, B. Hailu, and Y. Moges, "Assessment of partograph utilization and associated factors among obstetric care givers at public health institutions in central zone, Tigray, Ethiopia," *BMC research notes*, vol. 11, no. 1, p. 710, 2018.

[25] N. S. Salama, I. M. A. Allah, and M. F. Heeba, "The partograph: knowledge, attitude, and utilization by professional birth

attendances in Port-Said and Ismailia cities," *The Medical Journal of Cairo University*, vol. 78, no. 2, 2010.

[26] S. Ogwang, Z. Karyabakabo, and E. Rutebemberwa, "Assessment of partogram use during labour in rujumbura health Sub district, Rukungiri district, Uganda," *African Health Sciences*, vol. 9, no. 2, 2009.

[27] D. Bekele, K. Beyene, L. Hinkosa, and M. N. Shemsu, *Partograph utilization and associated factors among graduating health professional students in Asella Referal and Teaching Hospital*, Ethiopia, Ethiopia, 2016.

[28] A. Fawole, K. Hunyinbo, and D. Adekanle, "Knowledge and utilization of the partograph among obstetric care givers in South West Nigeria," *African Journal of Reproductive Health*, vol. 12, no. 1, 2017.

[29] S. Kitila, A. Gmariam, A. Molla, and G. Nemera, "Utilization of partograph during labour and birth outcomes at Jimma University," *Journal of Pregnancy and Child Health*, vol. 1, no. 101, p. 10.4172, 2014.

[30] M. Khonje, "Use and documentation of partograph in urban hospitals in Lilongwe-Malawi: health workers' perspective'," *Master of Philosophy Faculty of Medicine, Institute of Health and Society University of Oslo*, 2012, https://www.duo.uio.no/handle/10852/30053.

[31] J. A. Jere, "Use Of Partographs In Women In Labour At Mulanje District Hospital In Malawi (Doctoral dissertation, Faculty of Health Sciences, School of Public Health, University of the Witwatersrand, South Africa)," 2014.

[32] H. Regasa, T. Tilahun, and H. Adem, "Utilization of partograph and associated factors among obstetric care givers in hospitals of Western Oromia, Ethiopia, 2017," *PANACEA JOURNAL OF MEDICAL SCIENCES*, vol. 8, no. 1, pp. 21–24, 2018.

[33] T. Egbe, E. Ncham, W. Takang, E. Egbe et al., "Use of the partogram in the Bamenda health district, north-west region, Cameroon: a cross-sectional study," *Gynecology and Obstetrics Research - Open Journal*, vol. 2, no. 5, pp. 102–111, 2016.

[34] M. M. Opiah, A. B. Ofi, E. J. Essien, and E. Monjok, "Knowledge and utilization of the partograph among midwives in the Niger Delta Region of Nigeria," *African journal of reproductive health*, vol. 16, no. 1, pp. 125–132, 2012.

[35] C.-B. Sama, N. F. Takah, V. K. Danwe, U. F. Melo, T. N. Dingana, and F. F. Angwafo, "Knowledge and utilization of the partograph: a cross-sectional survey among obstetric care providers in urban referral public health institutions in northwest and southwest Cameroon," *PLoS One*, vol. 12, no. 2, article e0172860, 2017.

[36] A. Nwaneri, E. C. Ndie, I. Ehiemere, E. Okafor, P. O. Ezenduka, and A. Emeh, "Evaluation of factors affecting the utilization of partograph by nurses/midwives in primary/secondary health facilities in Enugu Metropolis," *Gynecology & Obstetrics*, vol. 7, no. 8, 2017.

[37] A. N. S. Khan, S. M. Billah, I. Mannan et al., "A cross-sectional study of partograph utilization as a decision making tool for referral of abnormal labour in primary health care facilities of Bangladesh," *PLoS One*, vol. 13, no. 9, article e0203617, 2018.

[38] A. R. Sudha, M. C. Metgud, and A. Saviola, "Effectiveness of a planned teaching program on knowledge and skill in the use of partograph among nurses working in maternity unit," *Journal of South Asian Federation of Obstetrics and Gynaecology*, vol. 1, no. 2, pp. 57–59, 2009.

18

Gonadotropin Stimulation Has Only a Limited Effect on the Concentration of Follicular Fluid Signalling Proteins: An Antibody Array Analysis

Nick A. Bersinger, Markus Eisenhut, Petra Stute, and Michael von Wolff

University Women's Hospital, Division of Gynaecological Endocrinology and Reproductive Medicine, University of Berne, Switzerland

Correspondence should be addressed to Michael von Wolff; michael.vonwolff@insel.ch

Academic Editor: Daniel Vaiman

Objective. The follicular fluid (FF) plays an essential role in the physiology of the follicle and the oocyte. Gonadotropin stimulation affects the FF steroid hormone and anti-Mullerian hormone (AMH) concentrations, which has been suggested to be the reason for lower oocyte competence in conventional gonadotropin stimulated *in vitro* fertilisation (cIVF) compared to natural cycle IVF (NC-IVF). To analyse the effect of gonadotropin stimulation on a broad spectrum of signalling proteins, we ran proteomic antibody arrays on FF of women undergoing both treatments NC-IVF and cIVF. *Method.* Twenty women underwent one NC-IVF and one cIVF treatment cycle. Follicular fluids of the first aspirated follicle were compared between the two groups using a protein microarray which included antibodies against 224 proteins related to cell signalling and reference proteins. Each of the 40 albumin-stripped, matched-pair samples was labelled in the reverse-dye (Cy3/Cy5) procedure before undergoing array hybridisation. Signal analysis was performed using normalisation algorithms in dedicated software. Five proteins yielding a value of $P < 0.05$ in the array experiment (Cystatin A, Caspase-3, GAD65/67, ERK-1, and ERK-2) were then submitted to quantitative determination by ELISA in the same follicular fluids. *Results.* Array analysis yielded only a small number of differentially expressed signalling markers by unadjusted P values. Adjustment as a consequence of multiple determinations resulted in the absence of any significant differential marker expression on the array. Five unadjusted differentially expressed proteins were quantified immunometrically with antibodies from different sources. Follicular fluid concentrations of Cystatin A and MAP kinase ERK-1 concentrations were significantly higher in the cIVF than in the NC-IVF follicles, while GAD-2 (GAD65/67) did not differ. The assays for Caspase-3 and MAP kinase ERK-2 did not have the required sensitivities. *Conclusion.* In contrast to FF steroid hormones and AMH, FF concentrations of signalling proteins are not or only marginally altered by gonadotropin stimulation.

1. Introduction

Follicular fluid (FF) is composed of different elements such as hormones, enzymes, anticoagulants, electrolytes, reactive oxygen species, and antioxidants [1]. It provides the oocyte with nutrients and mediates its communication with the follicle and thereby with the female endocrine system. In conventional in vitro fertilisation (cIVF) therapies, recruitment of the follicles is intensified by high dosages of exogenous gonadotropins, resulting in an unphysiological polyfollicular response. The gonadotropin stimulation has been suggested to be the reason for the lower oocyte competence in cIVF [2].

Indeed, several studies revealed that gonadotropin stimulation alters the concentration of several FF protein components such as cytokines including leukaemia inhibitory factor (LIF) [3–5], steroid hormones [3, 6], and anti-Mullerian hormone (AMH) [6, 7].

AMH is an FF marker for the implantation potential of the oocyte [8–10]. In cIVF follicles, AMH concentrations are reduced.

The cytokine LIF has been suggested to be a FF marker of the oocyte/embryo quality [11, 12]. In cIVF follicles, LIF concentrations are reduced [4].

These findings prompted us not to analyse regulatory proteins which are already well characterised in the context of follicular function but to widen the analysis and to screen the FF for a broad spectrum of signalling proteins using an antibody-based proteomic approach.

Such a protocol, using SDS-PAGE, OFFGEL, and SCX-based separation followed by LC-MS/MS analysis had already been performed by Ambekar et al. [13]. In six women, all undergoing cIVF, 480 proteins had been noted, of which 320 had not been described previously. The identified proteins belonged to diverse functional categories including growth factors and hormones, receptor signaling, enzyme catalysis, defense/immunity, and complement activity.

However, only a small number of women were analysed, and the study was not designed to evaluate the effect of gonadotropins.

To obtain the best possible match between the two treatment groups, we therefore selected a set of women who underwent both NC-IVF and cIVF with the intention to identify differences in a wide spectrum of signalling proteins.

2. Materials and Methods

2.1. Patients. Twenty women undergoing IVF treatment in the University Women's Hospital, Bern, Switzerland, between February 2012 and August 2015 for different infertility causes were enrolled in the study (Table 1). The principal inclusion condition was the availability of follicular fluid from a NC-IVF and from a cIVF treatment cycle for each of them. When several NC-IVF cycles with FF were available for the same patient, they were further matched by selecting the one with the closest patient age and sample storage time to the corresponding cIVF cycle.

2.2. IVF Procedure and Follicular Fluid Collection. In the NC-IVF protocol, cycles were monitored by serum luteinizing hormone (LH) and 17β-estradiol (E_2) levels and by ultrasound. When the diameter of the follicle reached 18 mm or more, serum E_2 concentration was above 800 pmol/L, 5,000 IU of hCG (Predalon®, MSD Merck Sharp & Dohme GmbH, Lucerne, Switzerland) was administered. The aspiration of the follicle and its contents was performed 36 hours later as described [14].

In the cIVF protocol, patients were given 150 to 300 IU of highly purified human menopausal gonadotrophin (Menopur HP®, Ferring AG, Baar, Switzerland) per day starting between days 3 and 5 of the menstrual cycle. The gonadotropin releasing hormone (GnRH) antagonist (Orgalutran®, Ganirelix 0.25 mg, MSD Merck Sharp & Dohme GmbH, Lucerne, Switzerland) was initiated between cycle days 6 and 7 and continued until the induction of ovulation. This was done after adequate follicular growth with 10,000 IU of urinary human chorionic gonadotrophin (hCG) (Pregnyl®, MSD Merck Sharp & Dohme GmbH, Lucerne, Switzerland). Transvaginal oocyte retrieval was performed 36 hours later under ultrasound guidance. The FF aspirated from the first follicle (≥18 mm) was collected separately.

Table 1: Patient's characteristics.

	NC-IVF, $n = 20$	cIVF, $n = 20$
Age (years)	34.6 ± 3.3	34.5 ± 3.1
Follicular diameter (mm)	18.8 ± 2.5	19.8 ± 2.3
Cause of infertility		
Andrological, n	14	
Tubar, n	5	
Others, n	1	

The obtained single-follicle fluids were clarified after the removal of the oocyte and cumulus cells by centrifugation in two steps, first, at 600 x g for 10 min and then at 1300 x g for a further 10 min. The obtained supernatants were stored at -80°C until further processing for antibody arrays and hormone analyses.

Informed written consent was obtained prior to treatment, and the study was approved by the cantonal ethical committee Bern, Switzerland (KEK 2020-01682).

2.3. Antibody Arrays. The Panorama® Antibody Microarray–Cell Signalling Kit (Cat. No. CSAA1) from Sigma-Aldrich (St. Louis, USA) was used. It includes antibodies against 224 proteins related to cell signalling and reference proteins for standardisation in duplicate spots. Several variations of the protocol for different material sources are provided by the manufacturer, as no literature is available for an application to follicular fluids, and also because these fluids contain large amounts of albumin, the serum protocol was followed. As a consequence, the follicular fluids had to be stripped of the bulk protein present in these samples. Proteo-Prep® immunoaffinity columns for albumin and IgG depletion (Cat. No. PROTIA) were obtained from Sigma as recommended, and the provided instructions followed. Briefly, 100 μL of FF containing 55.5 ± 7.9 mg/mL (mean ± SD) total protein (determined by Bradford assay) was loaded onto the column. In the collected effluents of 0.2 to 0.3 mL, the protein concentration was 2.60 ± 0.41 mg/mL. Fulfilling the requirements for running the arrays, the sample volumes were adjusted to 300 μL containing 2.47 ± 0.36 mg/mL total protein (minimum requirement 1 mg/mL) and transferred to the Centre for Functional Genomics and Bio-Chips at the Institute of Biochemistry (Faculty of Medicine), University of Ljubljana, Slovenia, on dry ice. Cy3 and Cy5 dyes were purchased from LKB, Vienna, Austria. Each of the 20 matched-pair samples was labelled once with the Cy3 and once with the Cy5 dye. This reverse-dye approach is a convenient method of normalisation against label-specific interaction differences in array experiments. Each matched pair therefore underwent hybridisation once with the Cy3 label on the NC-IVF and the Cy5 on the cIVF sample and once the other way round, thus yielding a true, normalised duplicate. Labelling and hybridisation procedures were performed according to the manufacturer's protocol and materials (Sigma-Aldrich, CSAA1 Technical Bulletin [15]). The running of the experiment as well as the analysis of the results was performed on the machine at the same institute in Ljubljana using the software dedicated to this approach and also provided by the manufacturer (Sigma). The same method and analysis were applied, and the results described elsewhere in an analogous comparison between two patient groups [16]. The procedure included further normalisation algorithms; in our study, five of the 20 matched pairs were used to establish these algorithms and the results were proper calculated from the remaining 15 pairs. All signals pertaining to protein targets were between those internally provided on the arrays for positive and negative control. Housekeeping proteins included 90 spots (of which 45 proteins of the cytoskeleton), and the smoothing was applied over all spots with protein down weighting.

2.4. Specific Quantitation by ELISA. For the five out of 179 examined FF proteins for which an unadjusted P value of <0.05 was observed in both array duplicates for differential expression between NC-IVF and cIVF (three with NC>c and two with NC<c, see Results), an ELISA assay for their quantification was performed. We used commercial microplate ELISAs manufactured by Cloud-Clone Corporation, Wuhan, China, and available from Brunschwig Chemie, Basel, Switzerland, using antibodies different from those used in the antibody array. For these analyses and in contrast to the protein array experiment, the pairing was not necessary. For this reason, all follicular fluids with a sufficient available volume were included. These numbers varied between 35 and 37. The assay for human Cystatin A (Cat. No. SEA476Hu) had a functional sensitivity of 0.156 ng/mL, and all tested follicular fluids ($N = 37$, three had been used up in the array experiment) yielded a value above this figure. The assay for glutamic acid decarboxylase (GAD-2, Cat. No. SEB258Hu, corresponding to GAD65/67 on the array) came with a sensitivity of 0.1 ng/mL; one of the 37 unknown FF samples yielded a signal below this level. The assay for extracellular signal-regulated kinase-1 (ERK-1) (Cat. No. SEB357Hu) which belongs to the mitogen-activated protein (MAP) kinase family had a detection level of 0.118 ng/mL, but 18 FF samples yielded signal below this limit. The Caspase-3 assay (Cat. No. SEA626Hu) had a functional sensitivity of 0.114 ng/mL, but most FF samples (33 of 37) were found to contain lower amounts of this analyte. Similarly, the assay for the other MAP kinase ERK-2 (Cat. No. SEA930Hu) was not sensitive enough for the analysis of follicular fluids (34/37 below the detection limit of 2 pg/mL). The analysis of the results obtained by ELISA was therefore limited to the three markers Cystatin A, GAD-2, and ERK-1. Intra-assay coefficients of variance for all five assay kits were below 10%. All samples were assayed in one run/one plate according to the manufacturer's instructions. Nontreated FF sample aliquots (i.e., not albumin depleted as done prior to the array hybridisations) were diluted 1 : 3 in the provided diluent. A few samples required a repeat experiment for Cystatin A at a higher dilution (1 : 50). The results were analysed with Graphpad Prism® version 5.

2.5. Statistical Analysis. Statistical analysis was by nonparametric Wilcoxon signed rank test for paired samples. Correlation analysis was done using the paired Wilcoxon test. The association between detectable ERK-1 and the appearance of clusters in the MDS analysis was assessed by Fisher's exact test in a 2 × 2 contingency table.

3. Results

3.1. Patients. Mean patient age was 34.6 ± 3.1 (SD) years, and mean FF storage time was (at -80°C) 22.4 ± 14.9 months. Dependent of the selection process, these values did not statistically differ between the two groups, neither did the diameter of the follicle (the "leading follicle" in the stimulated cycle) at the end of the follicular or stimulation phase, which was 19.3 ± 2.4 mm over all 40 measurements (see Table 1). Serum estradiol levels, influenced by the administration of gonadotrophins, were 845 ± 256 pM in the NC-IVF and 8630 ± 4120 pM in the stimulated (cIVF) group ($P < 0.0001$).

3.2. CSAA1 Arrays. The analysis of the follicular fluid samples, performed over 15 matched NC-IVF/cIVF pairs after extensive internal normalisation using a large number of spotted reference, mostly cytoskeleton proteins, yielded a small number of differentially expressed markers amongst the remaining 179 "unknown" proteins in the array: applying a nonadjusted P value of 0.05, seven showed a higher and eight a lower expression level in the NC-IVF when compared to cIVF treatment cycle in one or both label combination replicates. These are presented in Table 2 as a function of increasing P values. The raw table contained another 482 lines (individual spots of proteins and all types of controls) with unadjusted P values >0.05 (not shown). The full array data table returned with all 179 "unknown" proteins (controls and structural proteins removed) and sorted by name is given in the Supplementary section (Table S1). After the adjustment of P values as a consequence of the multiple determinations, no significant differential expression could be observed for any of the markers available on the array. Table 2 also summarises the array results for the selected markers as a function of the unadjusted P value in either single or crossed-over labelling, including the direction of the differential expression (up or down in NC-IVF versus cIVF). Multidimensional scaling (MDS) analysis as returned by the software consistently yielded a distinct grouping of the samples into two clusters, irrespective of the number of proteins included over the array, ranging from the top 10 to the top 200. The distribution of the samples between the two clusters, however, was not associated with the IVF protocol used (natural or stimulated). An association between the distribution into these two clusters and the detection of MAP kinase ERK-1 above the 0.02 ng/mL detection limit (Figures 1 and 2) was nevertheless observed. Amongst the 16 samples located in cluster A, one had a detectable and 12 a nondetectable ERK-1 level (3 samples were not available for ERK-1 quantitation). Amongst the 13 samples in cluster B, eight had a detectable and three a nondetectable ERK-1 (2 samples

Table 2: Raw data of the first 15 (nonstructural) protein markers as returned by the software and sorted by the unadjusted *P* value as analysed by the CSAA1 Panorama® array. The original raw table included contained another 499 lines (individual spots of proteins and all types of controls) with unadjusted $P > 0.25$ (not shown). The *P* values shown are means between two and four spots.

Rank by *P* (unadjusted)	Protein name	NC-IVF>cIVF		NC-IVF<cIVF		Unadjusted *P* value		Adjusted *P* value	
		Ratio	Log10	Ratio	Log10	Mean	SD	Mean	SD
1	Caspase-3—active			0.977	-0.0103	0.0148	0.0173	0.593	0.151
2	Glutamic acid decarboxylase (GAD65/67)	1.072	0.0301			0.0187	0.0011	0.620	0.002
3	Cystatin A	1.040	0.0172			0.0236	0.0080	0.659	0.058
4	MAP kinase (ERK-1+ERK-2)	1.055	0.0231			0.0321	0.0022	0.700	<0.001
5	JNK (activated)			0.980	-0.0086	0.0467	0.0175	0.751	0.071
6	NF-κB			0.974	-0.0113	0.0515	0.0598	0.731	0.159
7	Nicastrin			0.0983	-0.0074	0.0571	0.0346	0.772	0.101
8	Chk2			0.0983	-0.0074	0.0571	0.0322	0.772	0.101
9	Cdh1	1.017	0.0075			0.0686	0.0747	0.743	0.177
10	Nerve growth factor receptor			0.977	-0.0099	0.0789	0.0565	0.812	0.080
11	FAK (phospho pS772)			0.984	-0.0072	0.0919	0.1055	0.759	0.199
12	Cdk-7/cak			0.986	-0.0061	0.0988	0.0801	0.818	0.089
13	Aop-1	1.023	0.0099			0.1415	0.1954	0.693	0.292
14	DAP kinase	1.015	0.0065			0.1870	0.2442	0.768	0.211
15	Cyclin A	1.032	0.0137			0.2308	0.1754	0.787	0.240

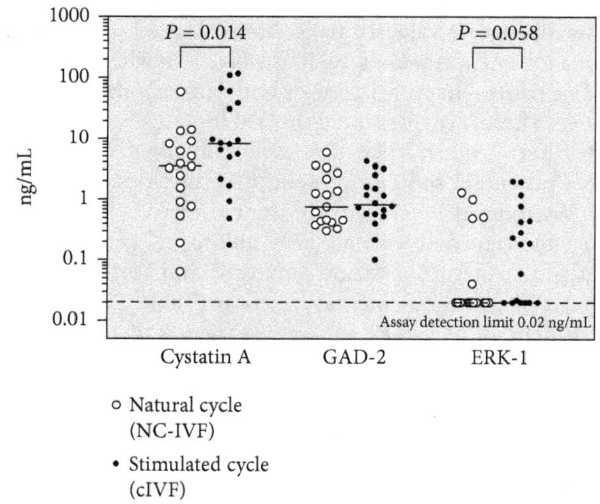

Figure 1: Follicular fluid levels of Cystatin A, GAD-2, and ERK-1 as determined by ELISA. Open circles, NC-IVF. Closed circles, cIVF (conventional stimulation with gonadotrophins). *P* values were obtained by the Wilcoxon signed rank test which takes the efficient pairing into account (the difference in the values between both cycles in the same patient, 15 sample pairs). The graph also includes the results from samples for which the pairing had not been possible due to an insufficient available volume. Please note the logarithmic scale.

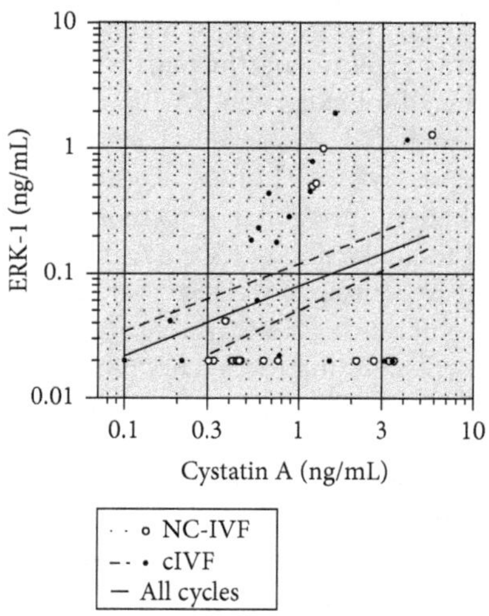

Figure 2: Correlation between the follicular fluid levels of MAP kinase ERK-1 and Cystatin A, as determined by ELISA, in all available samples. Open circles, NC-IVF. Closed circles, cIVF. Please note the double logarithmic scale. Regression lines are shown for the two stimulation protocols as well for the combined group. For *P* values, see text.

not available). This association was statistically significant (Fisher's exact test, $P = 0.002$, quantity control samples excluded). As a consequence of the otherwise poor association between MDS clustering and the IVF stimulation protocol, this analysis was not continued.

3.3. Postarray Quantitation of Selected Marker Proteins by ELISA. A small number of markers, selected as a function of the returned array results but also of the availability of the corresponding immunoassays (specific antibodies), were quantified in the nontreated FF (the fraction obtained from the IVF laboratory after clarification by centrifugation but before protein depletion on the PROTIA columns). As stated in the Materials and Methods, the assays for Caspase-3 and

MAP kinase ERK-2 did not present the required sensitivities. The results for the three other selected markers Cystatin A, GAD-2, and ERK-1 are shown in Figure 1. Cystatin A and MAP kinase ERK-1 levels were found to be significantly higher in the stimulated than in the natural cycles while glutamic acid decarboxylase 2 (GAD-2) did not differ in concentration between the two types of IVF stimulation and treatment (paired nonparametric sign test). Cystatin A and MAP kinase ERK-1 did not reveal a positive correlation between each other, with significance levels of $P = 0.110$ and $P = 0.170$ for the nonstimulated and stimulated cycles, respectively. However, when taken together, irrespective of the type of IVF protocol ($N = 36$), the obtained P value was 0.058, showing a trend towards a positive correlation between each other. These correlations are illustrated in a double logarithmic fashion in Figure 2.

4. Discussion

Our study revealed that the FF concentration of most analysed signalling proteins is not different between women undergoing gonadotropin stimulation and those in natural cycles. Only five proteins such as glutamic acid decarboxylase, Cystatin A, the MAP kinase ERK, Caspase-3, and diphosphorylated JNK yielded a significant difference. However, the antibody array findings did not correspond to the specific additional measurements performed by ELISA. Cystatin A was downregulated in the cIVF group, while in the ELISA, this protein showed higher FF levels in the cIVF than in the NC-IVF group. For GAD-2 (GAD65/67), no difference was observed in the ELISA analysis between the two stimulation groups. The same discrepancy was observed for ERK-1. Caspase-3 and ERK-2 could not be quantified by ELISA.

The reason for the conflicting results might be the use of confirming ELISA antibodies which were different from those supplied by the company which produced the CSAA1 protein array. This might be a weakness which was unexpected at the initiation of the project, but could also be interpreted as a strength of the study. As the differences were only observed in the CSAA1 protein array before P value adjustment and as the differences for the same markers in the ELISA were only marginal (though significant for two of them), the overall significance of the opposite findings can be questioned.

Interestingly, conflicting results were also found in two other antibody-based studies in which the FF cytokine concentrations were analysed. Baskind et al. [4] compared 40 FF and plasma cytokine concentrations in 10 women undergoing NC-IVF and cIVF treatments by fluid-phase multiplex immunoassays. Bersinger et al. [5] performed a similar study in 13 women with 13 mainly different cytokines by Luminex xMAP multiplexing technology. LIF was analysed in both studies. Whereas Baskind et al. [4] described significantly higher LIF concentrations in FF and plasma from NC-IVF compared to cIVF treatments, Bersinger et al. [5] did not find any differences. Conflicting results were also found for interleukin (IL) 6, IL8, IL10, and IL18, analysed by Baskind et al. [4] in plasma and by Bersinger et al. [5] in serum. Baskind et al. [4] did not find any differences whereas Bersinger et al. [5] found significantly higher concentrations in the serum of women undergoing cIVF and in comparison to NC-IVF.

The conflicting results of these and our own studies, all based on protein array technology, could be due to either high variability of specific FF proteins or constituents of FF which affect the accuracy of antibody-based assays.

Fifteen (four in duplicate and 11 in single determinations) FF proteins were found to be differentially expressed between NC-IVF and cIVF by nonadjusted P value; however, this precisely corresponds to the false-positive rate in multiple testing, and for this reason, the adjusted P value had to be applied. According to the adjusted P values, no protein tested on the Panorama array was differentially expressed between the two stimulation protocols.

Even though this seemed to be disappointing as such, it better corresponded to our ELISA results except for Cystatin A and ERK-1. ELISA being a well-controlled quantitative determination method for proteins, we would suggest to investigate these two markers in the follicular fluid of a larger number of samples. We had decided on the perfect match between the two stimulation groups by using one cycle each in the same patient, which strongly reduced the number of available samples (patients) for clinical reasons.

The absence of any significant differential expression by adjusted P value can also be the consequence of the presence of a large number or structural and intracellular proteins on the array. These could be derived from the separation of the cumulus cells in the mature follicle, which has been described [17, 18]. The selected (Panorama) array was developed for the analysis of cell signalling proteins, which we expected to be important players during the hormone-dependent maturation process in the follicle.

The results presented in Figure 1, however, indicate that differences may exist at this level between the two stimulation groups. Moreover, the two mentioned MDS clusters show an association to one or the other stimulation procedure, which is statistically significant ($P = 0.002$ by Fisher's exact test) but not exclusive, i.e., some samples were found in the "wrong" cluster. We were unable to find any clinical feature or irregularity in these particular samples which may explain a hypothetical association with the opposite group. Even with a precise definition of the IVF stimulation groups and subsequent attribution of a cycle into one of these, this illustrates that we are not dealing with a "black and white" situation and that patient-to-patient variations may play an even more important role than anticipated.

Our analysis of the ELISA results revealed a borderline correlation between the concentrations of Cystatin A and MAP kinase ERK-1, the two proteins which were found to show different FF concentrations in NC-IVF and cIVF.

Extracellular signal-regulated kinase-1 (ERK-1), which belongs to the mitogen-activated protein (MAP) kinase family, plays a role in signalling cascades and in transmitting extracellular signals to intracellular targets [19]. The activation of the ERK/MAPK signalling pathway promotes proliferation and has antiapoptotic effects. Activating mutations of this pathway are the most abundant oncogenic factors across all cancer types [20].

Cystatin A, also called acid cysteine proteinase inhibitor (ACPI), is strongly expressed in several different healthy tissues but is also expressed in malignant cells such as neoplastic cells of Hodgkin's disease [21]. Its physiological function is still unknown.

We found a borderline correlation of the concentration of ERK-1 and Cystatin A which might be due to the proliferation activity of growing follicles. However, this is pure speculative. Any specific functions of ERK-1 and Cystatin A in the physiology of the follicle cannot be derived from the literature yet.

5. Conclusion

Overall, our study suggests that concentrations of most FF signalling proteins are not different in follicles following natural or gonadotropin-stimulated cycles. Therefore, it can be assumed that differences in follicular physiology are apparently not substantially based on differences in the concentration of signalling proteins. However, this interpretation needs to be taken with caution as our study also confirmed that protein-based arrays of FF need to be interpreted with great care as they might not have the required sensitivity to pick up subtle differences in concentration.

Authors' Contributions

N.A. Bersinger contributed to the conception and design, acquisition of data, analysis, interpretation, drafting of the article, and final approval. M. Eisenhut contributed to the acquisition of data, analysis, interpretation, drafting of the article, and final approval. P. Stute contributed to the data interpretation, revision of the article, and final approval. M. von Wolff contributed to the conception and design, acquisition of data, interpretation, drafting of the article, and final approval.

Acknowledgments

We thank Anne Vaucher for the collection and processing of the follicular fluid samples as well as for running immunoassays. We also acknowledge IBSA, Institut Biochimique SA, Lugano, Switzerland, for the financial support of this project.

References

[1] L. Basuino and C. F. Silveira, "Human follicular fluid and effects on reproduction," *JBRA Assisted Reproduction*, vol. 20, no. 1, pp. 38–40, 2016.

[2] M. von Wolff, "The role of natural cycle IVF in assisted reproduction," *Best Practice & Research. Clinical Endocrinology & Metabolism*, vol. 33, no. 1, pp. 35–45, 2019.

[3] M. J. de los Santos, V. García-Láez, D. Beltrán-Torregrosa et al., "Hormonal and molecular characterization of follicular fluid, cumulus cells and oocytes from pre-ovulatory follicles in stimulated and unstimulated cycles," *Human Reproduction*, vol. 27, no. 6, pp. 1596–1605, 2012.

[4] N. E. Baskind, N. M. Orsi, and V. Sharma, "Follicular-phase ovarian follicular fluid and plasma cytokine profiling of natural cycle in vitro fertilization patients," *Fertility and Sterility*, vol. 102, no. 2, pp. 410–418, 2014.

[5] N. A. Bersinger, Z. Kollmann, and M. von Wolff, "Serum but not follicular fluid cytokine levels are increased in stimulated versus natural cycle IVF: a multiplexed assay study," *Journal of Reproductive Immunology*, vol. 106, pp. 27–33, 2014.

[6] M. von Wolff, Z. Kollmann, C. E. Flück et al., "Gonadotrophin stimulation for in vitro fertilization significantly alters the hormone milieu in follicular fluid: a comparative study between natural cycle IVF and conventional IVF," *Human Reproduction*, vol. 29, no. 5, pp. 1049–1057, 2014.

[7] N. Jancar, I. Virant-Klun, and E. V. Bokal, "Serum and follicular endocrine profile is different in modified natural cycles than in cycles stimulated with gonadotropin and gonadotropin-releasing hormone antagonist," *Fertility and Sterility*, vol. 92, no. 6, pp. 2069–2071, 2009.

[8] R. Fanchin, D. H. Mendez Lozano, N. Frydman et al., "Anti-Müllerian hormone concentrations in the follicular fluid of the preovulatory follicle are predictive of the implantation potential of the ensuing embryo obtained by in vitro fertilization," *The Journal of Clinical Endocrinology and Metabolism*, vol. 92, no. 5, pp. 1796–1802, 2007.

[9] C. Takahashi, A. Fujito, M. Kazuka, R. Sugiyama, H. Ito, and K. Isaka, "Anti-Müllerian hormone substance from follicular fluid is positively associated with success in oocyte fertilization during in vitro fertilization," *Fertility and Sterility*, vol. 89, no. 3, pp. 586–591, 2008.

[10] R. Pabuccu, C. Kaya, G. S. Cağlar, E. Oztas, and H. Satiroglu, "Follicular-fluid anti-Mullerian hormone concentrations are predictive of assisted reproduction outcome in PCOS patients," *Reproductive Biomedicine Online*, vol. 19, no. 5, pp. 631–637, 2009.

[11] A. Arici, E. Oral, O. Bahtiyar, O. Engin, E. Seli, and E. E. Jones, "Leukaemia inhibitory factor expression in human follicular fluid and ovarian cells," *Human Reproduction*, vol. 12, no. 6, pp. 1233–1239, 1997.

[12] M. Jean, S. Mirallie, P. Barriere et al., "Leukaemia inhibitory factor expression in human follicular fluid," *Human Reproduction*, vol. 14, no. 2, p. 571, 1999.

[13] A. S. Ambekar, R. S. Nirujogi, S. M. Srikanth et al., "Proteomic analysis of human follicular fluid: A new perspective towards understanding folliculogenesis," *Journal of Proteomics*, vol. 87, pp. 68–77, 2013.

[14] M. von Wolff, S. Schneider, Z. Kollmann, B. Weiss, and N. A. Bersinger, "Exogenous gonadotropins do not increase the blood-follicular transportation capacity of extra-ovarian hormones such as prolactin and cortisol," *Reproductive Biology and Endocrinology*, vol. 11, no. 1, p. 87, 2013.

[15] E. Kopf, D. Shnitzer, and D. Zharhary, "Panorama™ Ab microarray cell signaling kit: a unique tool for protein expression analysis," *Proteomics*, vol. 5, no. 9, pp. 2412–2416, 2005.

[16] K. A. Zander, M. T. Saavedra, J. West, V. Scapa, L. Sanders, and T. T. Kingdom, "Protein microarray analysis of nasal polyps from aspirin-sensitive and aspirin-tolerant patients with chronic rhinosinusitis," *American Journal of Rhinology & Allergy*, vol. 23, no. 3, pp. 268–272, 2009.

[17] A. Ai, Z. Tang, Y. Liu et al., "Characterization and identification of human immortalized granulosa cells derived from ovarian follicular fluid," *Experimental and Therapeutic Medicine*, vol. 18, no. 3, pp. 2167–2177, 2019.

[18] H.-M. Chang, J. Qiao, and P. C. K. Leung, "Oocyte–somatic cell interactions in the human ovary—novel role of bone morphogenetic proteins and growth differentiation factors," *Human Reproduction Update*, vol. 23, no. 1, pp. 1–18, 2016.

[19] Y. J. Guo, W. W. Pan, S. B. Liu, Z. F. Shen, Y. Xu, and L. L. Hu, "ERK/MAPK signalling pathway and tumorigenesis," *Experimental and Therapeutic Medicine*, vol. 19, no. 3, pp. 1997–2007, 2020.

[20] Y. B. Khotskaya, V. R. Holla, A. F. Farago, K. R. Mills Shaw, F. Meric-Bernstam, and D. S. Hong, "Targeting TRK family proteins in cancer," *Pharmacology & Therapeutics*, vol. 173, pp. 58–66, 2017.

[21] A. Rinne, "Epidermal SH-protease inhibitor (ACPI, cystatin A) in cancer. A short historical review," *Pathology, Research and Practice*, vol. 206, no. 4, pp. 259–262, 2010.

19

Complementary and Alternative Medicine Use in a Pregnant Population, Northwest Ethiopia

Yohannes Kelifa Emiru,[1] **Betelhem Anteneh Adamu**,[1] **Melak Erara**,[2] **Tigist Chanie**,[3] **and Abyot Endale Gurmu**[1]

[1]*Department of Pharmacognosy, School of Pharmacy, College of Medicine and Health Sciences, University of Gondar, Gondar, Ethiopia*
[2]*Department of Clinical Pharmacy, School of Pharmacy, College of Medicine and Health Sciences, University of Gondar, Gondar, Ethiopia*
[3]*University of Gondar Compressive Specialized Hospital, University of Gondar, Gondar, Ethiopia*

Correspondence should be addressed to Yohannes Kelifa Emiru; johnkelifa@gmail.com and Betelhem Anteneh Adamu; betelhemadamu73@gmail.com

Academic Editor: Robert Gaspar

Background. Complementary and alternative medicine (CAM) appears to be the source of healthcare particularly in the majority of pregnant communities of Africa due to its intrinsic qualities as well as its accessibility and affordability. Despite acknowledged benefits of CAM use in pregnancy, majority of users are unaware of its safety and effects on fetal development. The present study was aimed at examining CAM use among pregnant women in Northwest Ethiopia to provide an opportunity for future investigations on the effectiveness of CAM modalities in the management of pregnancy-related complications across the country. *Methods.* This was an institution-based cross-sectional study which was conducted at Poly Clinic Health Center in the Northwest part of Ethiopia between March and May 2018. Two hundred and eighty two Ethiopian women were conveniently recruited to take part in the study. Structured questioners were used for the survey. Descriptive statistics of sociodemographic and CAM use characteristics were expressed in frequencies and proportions. Chi-square test was performed to determine the difference between CAM user and nonuser. Besides, binary logistic regression analyses were performed to examine predictors of CAM use in the study population. The result was considered statistically significant if P value ≤ 0.05. *Results.* The prevalence rate of CAM use in pregnant women was 89.36% with the commonest practice of spiritual healing (65.2%) and herbal supplement (51.8%) CAM therapies. Use of CAM positively associated with marital status and previous number of children. The odds of using CAM among single/not married women were 3.22 times higher (COR: 3.22, CI: 1.07-9.64) as compared to married women. Pregnant women with no children were 3.30 times more likely (COR: 3.30, CI: 0.92-11.84) to use CAM than those women having ≥3 children. Lower odds of using CAM significantly associated with educational level (COR: 0.20, CI: 0.046-0.93) and antenatal care (COR: 0.45, CI: 0.18-1.13) in a binary logistic regression model. *Conclusions.* A considerable number of pregnant women were utilizing CAM including herbal products as part of their maternity care. This finding provides a reference on the use of CAM for policy-makers, health professionals, and parents. Further studies are needed to investigate the effectiveness and safety of specific CAM modalities with particular focus on herbal medicinal products.

1. Introduction

In resource-constrained health settings, complementary and alternative medicines (CAM) are commonly used because they are often more widely available and more affordable than conventional therapies. The term CAM refers to a wide set of healthcare practices that are not integrated into the current healthcare system and are not part of that country's tradition [1]. It comprises some form of caring approach including acupuncture, especial diets, massage therapy, medicinal plants, biologic feedback, and relaxation techniques [1, 2]. Women have become more informed about their health and use print media, television, radio, and internet to get information on which to base their health decisions. As a result, pregnant women are increasingly recognized CAM and they are leading the utilization trends of CAM for their healthcare and well-being [2, 3]. In the United States of America [4, 5] and Australia [6], for instance, they reported a practice rate of 87% and 91% CAM use during pregnancy, respectively.

Studies revealed the use of CAM throughout the pregnancy period for the treatment of nausea and vomiting, as well as for illnesses due to pregnancy such as fatigue, respiratory, and skin issues and nutritional benefits [7, 8]. Despite known benefits of CAM use in pregnancy, majority of users are unaware of its safety and effects on fetal development and possibility of CAM-drug interaction [1, 7, 9]. Together with this, a substantial proportion of women often fail to disclose their gestational use of CAM to their maternity providers [6, 7]. In Ethiopia, CAM is culturally acceptable and widely utilized, predominantly for the belief that CAM is natural, thus safer than conventional medicine. A previous a study done in Northwest Ethiopia has shown that higher than 48% pregnant women use herbal medicine like ginger (*Zingiber officinale*) and demakese (*Ocimum lamiifolium*) [8]. However, there is paucity of evidence on the prevalence and predictors of other types of CAM modalities such as spiritual healing, biological-based therapies, and manipulative and body-based therapy practices among pregnant women in the nation. Hence, this study was aimed at investigating the prevalence, types, and sociodemographic factors associated with CAM usage among pregnant women in Northwest Ethiopia. The findings of this study will provide supporting evidence that could guide decision making at the system, institutional, and individual level concerning CAM use in pregnancy and provide an opportunity for future investigations on the effectiveness of these modalities in the management of pregnancy-related complications across the country.

2. Methods and Materials

2.1. Study Design and Setting. This was an institution-based cross-sectional study which was carried out at Poly Clinic Health Center (PCHC) from March to May 2018. The source population was pregnant women who attended antenatal care clinics. The study area is found in Gondar Town, North Gondar, which is located 738 km far away from Addis Ababa, capital of Ethiopia. The town is found at 2700 meters above sea level and has a total population of 333,103. PCHC is one of the governmental health centers serving for 101,317 populations.

2.2. Sample Size and Sampling Procedure. A convenience sampling technique was used in this study. Eligible participants had to meet a set of inclusion criteria recruited in the study. These criteria are Ethiopian nationality only (as this study was intended to explore CAM use particularly in Ethiopian population); age ≥ 18 years, willing to participate, and who had provided verbal consent to participate in the study; and completely filled the questionnaire form and answered all questions. Pregnant women who had severe physical and mental illness were excluded.

2.3. Data Collection Tool. The survey questionnaire used in the study was adapted and developed following a detailed review of previous relevant works [1, 8, 10] with some modifications. The questionnaire was constructed in their native language (Amharic) and translated back into English to check its consistency. The content of the questionnaire was piloted among 15 pregnant women visiting Maraki Health Center (one of the public health centers found in Gondar Town) to gather information on its understandability, time consumed by each question, consistency among related variables, and acceptability. Following the results of the pre-test, necessary correctionsand amendments were made on the questionnairebefore the actual data collection was initiated The respondents were interviewed using a structured questionnaire which consists of 4 parts: part I: eleven questions related to sociodemographic characteristic of the respondents; part II: six practice-related questions for CAM users; part III: eleven questions asking the perceived reasons for CAM use; and part IV: four queries demanding types of CAM therapies frequently practiced in the course of pregnancy.

2.4. Ethical Approval. Ethical clearance was obtained from the ethics review committee of School of Pharmacy, College of Medicine and Health Science, University of Gondar. Additionally, the permission to undertake the study was received from the PCHC director. The study subjects were informed about the objective and importance of the study, and oral consent was obtained from each participant. All respondents were assured of the confidentiality regarding the responses obtained from them.

2.5. Statistical Analysis. Statistical analysis was performed using Statistical Package for the Social Sciences (SPSS) version 22.0 for Windows. Descriptive statistics of sociodemographic and CAM use characteristics were expressed in frequencies and proportions. The main outcome variable in the analysis was CAM use. In order to determine the differences in characteristics between pregnant women who have used CAM and those who did not, chi-square test was performed. Moreover, the univariate and multivariate logistic regression analyses were performed to examine predictors of CAM use in the study population. For a variable to be included in the multiple regression model, it had to be significantly associated with the main outcome in the univariate analysis. Odds ratios and their respective 95% confidence intervals were calculated. Statistical significance was set at a P value ≤ 0.05.

3. Results

3.1. Characteristics of CAM and Non-CAM User Pregnant Women. Among the 282 pregnant subjects who had attended the antenatal care, 252 (89.36%) pregnant women reported to be using some form of CAM modalities (Table 1). The vast majority (90.8%) were married, and only 11% had attended

TABLE 1: Sociodemographic characteristics of pregnant women and their association with CAM use in univariate and multiple logistic regression models ($N = 282$).

Characteristics	Overall N (%)	CAM use N (%) Yes	CAM use N (%) No	P value [a]	COR (95% CI)*	P value [a]	AOR (95% CI)*
Age (year)							
<20	17 (6)	15 (6.0)	2 (6.7)		**1 (ref)**		
20-30	176 (62.4)	156 (61.9)	20 (66.7)	0.96	0.96 (0.20-4.52)	—	—
>30	89 (31.6)	81 (32.1)	8 (26.7)	0.71	0.74 (0.14-3.83)	—	—
Religion							
Orthodox	222 (78.7)	200 (79.4)	22 (73.3)	0.123	0.11 (0.007-1.82)	—	—
Muslim	55 (19.5)	48 (19.0)	7 (23.3)	0.99	—	—	—
Protestant	3 (1.1)	3 (1.2)	0 (0.0)	0.19	0.15 (0.008-2.60)	—	—
Catholic	2 (0.7)	1 (0.4)	1 (3.3)		**1 (ref)**		
Marital status							
Married	256 (90.8)	232 (92.1)	24 (80.0)		**1 (ref)**		**1 (ref)**
Single	20 (7.1)	15 (6.0)	5 (16.7)	**0.036**	3.22 (1.07-9.64)	0.18	2.39 (0.663-8.65)
Divorced	4 (1.4)	3 (1.2)	1 (3.3)	0.31	3.22 (0.32-32.19)	0.32	3.50 (0.28-43.20)
Widowed	2(0.7)	2 (0.8)	0 (0.0)	0.99	—	0.99	—
Educational							
Unable to write and read	78 (27.7)	75 (29.8)	3 (10.0)	**0.04**	0.20 (0.046-0.93)	0.14	0.29 (0.05-1.53)
Able to write and read	44 (15.6)	38 (15.1)	6 (20.0)	0.76	0.82 (0.22-2.97)	0.95	1.03 (0.26-4.10)
Primary school	53 (18.8)	50 (19.8)	3 (10.0)	0.13	0.31 (0.069-1.40)	0.30	0.44 (0.09-2.11)
Secondary school	76 (27)	63 (25.0)	13 (43.3)	0.90	1.07 (0.34-3.31)	0.96	1.02 (0.31-3.31)
College/university	31 (11)	26 (10.3)	5 (16.7)		**1 (ref)**		**1 (ref)**
Occupation							
Unemployed/house wife	162 (57.4)	147 (58.3)	15 (50.0)	0.37	0.54 (0.14-2.08)	—	—
Part time	43 (15.2)	40 (15.9)	3 (10.0)	0.29	0.40 (0.07-2.19)	—	—
Full time	58 (20.6)	49 (19.4)	9 (30.0)	0.97	0.98 (0.23-4.06)	—	—
Student	19 (6.7)	16 (6.3)	3 (10.0)		**1 (ref)**		
Monthly income (Ethiopian birr)							
No income	20 (7.1)	20 (7.9)	0 (0.0)	0.99	—	—	—
<500	86 (30.5)	82 (32.5)	4 (13.3)	0.19	0.25 (008-0.79)	—	—
500-999	83 (29.4)	72 (28.6)	11 (36.7)	0.59	0.79 (0.34-1.84)	—	—
>1000	93 (33)	78 (31.0)	15 (50.0)		**1 (ref)**		
Previous number of children							
No	108 (38.3)	92 (36.5)	16 (53.3)	**0.05**	3.30 (0.92-11.84)	0.42	1.82 (0.41-8.05)
1	60 (21.3)	52 (20.6)	8 (26.7)	0.12	2.92 (0.73-11.60)	0.31	2.16 (0.48-9.71)
2	54 (19.1)	51 (20.2)	3 (10.0)	0.89	1.11 (0.21-5.78)	0.73	0.73 (0.12-4.31)
≥3	60 (21.3)	57 (22.6)	3 (10.0)		**1 (ref)**		**1 (ref)**
Pregnancy status							
1st trimester	55 (19.5)	47 (18.7)	8 (26.7)		**1 (ref)**		
2nd trimester	124 (44)	109 (43.3)	15 (50.0)	0.65	0.80 (0.32-2.03)	—	—
3rd trimester	103 (26.5)	96 (38.1)	7 (23.3)	0.12	0.42 (0.14-1.25)	—	—
Antenatal care							
No	47 (16.7)	39 (15.5)	8 (26.7)		**1 (ref)**		**1 (ref)**
Midwife	209 (74.1)	191 (75.8)	18 (60.0)	**0.05**	0.45 (0.18-1.13)	0.62	0.77 (0.27-2.18)
Nurse	10 (3.5)	8 (3.2)	2 (6.7)	0.82	1.21 (0.21-6.84)	0.39	2.30 (0.34-15.59)
Physician	16 (5.7)	14 (5.6)	2 (6.7)	0.67	0.69 (0.13-3.68)	0.93	1.08 (0.18-6.50)

Table 1: Continued.

Characteristics	Overall N (%)	CAM use N (%) Yes	No	P value [a]	COR (95% CI)*	P value [a]	AOR (95% CI)*
Residency							
Urban	241 (85.5)	214 (84.9)	27 (90.0)	0.45	0.62 (0.18-2.16)	—	—
Rural	41 (14.5)	38 (15.1)	3 (10.0)		**1 (ref)**		

CAM: complementary and alternative medicine; [a]P value refers to the significance of the differences between CAM users and non-CAM users using the chi-square test; COR: crude odds ratio; AOR: adjusted odds ratio; CI: confidence interval; *odds ratio and their 95% CI were derived using a binary logistic regression model with CAM use as the dependent variable.

Table 2: The observed responses for the use of CAM in the study participants ($N = 252$).

Queries	Overall n (%)
Responses to quality of life assessment[a]	
Is CAM therapy improving your QOL?	86 (30.5)
My overall health is better	162 (57.4)
I am not depressed all the time	126 (44.7)
I have less fatigue	176 (62.4)
I have more energy	78 (27.7)
I can sleep well	185 (65.6)
I have better memory	162 (57.4)
I do not have frequent nausea/vomiting or other health problem	83 (29.4)
I am not sick all the time	75 (26.6)
Disclosure of CAM use to HCPs	
Yes	95 (33.7)
No	157 (55.7)
Reasons for not reporting to HCPs[a]	
Does not need the HCP's approval	7 (2.5)
The HCPs would be unsupportive and would discourage	52 (18.4)
Insufficient information of CAM	19 (6.7)
The HCPs do not ask about CAM	57 (20.2)
Source of information on CAM use[a]	
Family/friend/relative	140 (49.6)
Media (internet/television/radio/book)	16 (5.7)
Health practitioner	40 (14.2)
Pregnant women who used herbal medicines	12 (4.3)
CAM practitioners	18 (6.4)
Awareness of drug-herb interaction	
Yes	94 (33.3)
No/I do not know	158 (56)
Satisfaction level with CAM use	
Satisfied	59 (20.9)
Average	125 (44.3)
Dissatisfied	68 (24.1)

CAM: complementary and alternative medicine; QOL: quality of life; HCPs: healthcare providers; [a]the values do not sum up to 100% since multiple-choice answers could have been selected.

college/university, whereas 27% had secondary education and 27.7% were unable to write and read. Most of the participants were unemployed (57.4%), and only 33% were earning more than Ethiopian birr (ETB) 1000 per month (≈United States Dollar (USD) 32), while 30.5% and 29.4% had a monthly income of ETB < 500 and 500-99, respectively. In respect of pregnancy status, 44% of women were found in 2nd trimester and majority (74.1%) had visited midwifery for the antenatal care.

In a univariate logistic regression model, those who were single had higher odds of using CAM (COR: 3.22, CI: 1.07-9.64) compared to married or divorced or widowed women. Similarly, no children in previous time showed higher odds of CAM use (COR: 3.30, CI: 0.92-11.84). Pregnant women who were unable to write and read (COR: 0.20, CI: 0.046-0.93) and had visited midwifery for antenatal care (COR: 0.45, CI: 0.18-1.13) reported lower odds of using CAM. However, none of these variables was significantly associated with CAM use in multiple logistic regression analysis as shown in Table 1.

3.2. The Perceived Responses for Questions Linked to CAM Uses and Characterization of Types of CAM Used across Pregnancy Periods. The response in relation to CAM use among study subjects is presented in Table 2. Most of the CAM users were reported having slept well (65.6%) and less fatigue (62.4%) in response to CAM use-related quality of life (QOL) while a small proportion of participants responded having more energy (27.7%) and not sick all the time (26.6%) as CAM use-associated QOL. In the case of level of satisfaction in CAM use, 44.3% respondents had shown an average level of satisfaction for CAM therapies but about 56% of CAM users were not aware of any potential herbal-drug interaction. Majority of the pregnant women (55.7%) informed that they did not disclose CAM use to their HCPs. The reasons for not disclosing CAM use were reported to be 'HCPs do not ask' (20.2%), and 'HCPs may be unsupportive and discourage' (18.4%). Less reported reasons were insufficient information of CAM (6.7%) and CAM use does not need approval of HCPs (2.5%).

Regarding source of information for CAM use, nearly half of the participants relied 'family/friend/relative' (49.6%) while 14.2% answered 'health practitioner'. The utmost strongly agreed reasons for CAM use were accessibility and availability of CAM (28%), family/culture/religious beliefs (22%), more natural (17.4%), and the beneficial effect on quality of life and health of their fetus (15.2%) as described in Table 3.

Table 3: Reasons for using CAM[†] in pregnancy ($N = 252$).

Reasons for using CAM	Responses N (%)		
	Strongly agree	Agree	Disagree
Beneficial effect on quality of life and health[a]	43 (15.2)	99 (35.1)	110 (39.0)
Its more natural	49 (17.4)	151 (53.5)	52 (18.4)
CAM is accessible and available	79 (28.0)	121 (42.9)	52 (18.4)
Improves nutritional status	12 (4.3)	64 (22.7)	176 (62.4)
Less risk for fetus than convectional drugs	20 (7.1)	63 (22.3)	169 (59.9)
Lack of trust on conventional treatments	9 (3.2)	52 (18.4)	191 (67.7)
Dissatisfaction with conventional therapy	6 (2.1)	62 (22.0)	184 (65.2)
Family/culture/religious beliefs	62 (22.0)	127 (45.0)	63 (22.3)
Previous experience of CAM use	21 (7.4)	120 (42.6)	111 (39.4)
Control over situation[b]	13 (4.6)	78 (27.7)	161 (57.1)

CAM: complementary and alternative medicine; [†]the values do not sum up to 100% since data from CAM nonusers have not been selected; [a]beneficial effect on quality of life and physical health of their fetus; [b]CAM therapies gave a sense of control or autonomy over the situation.

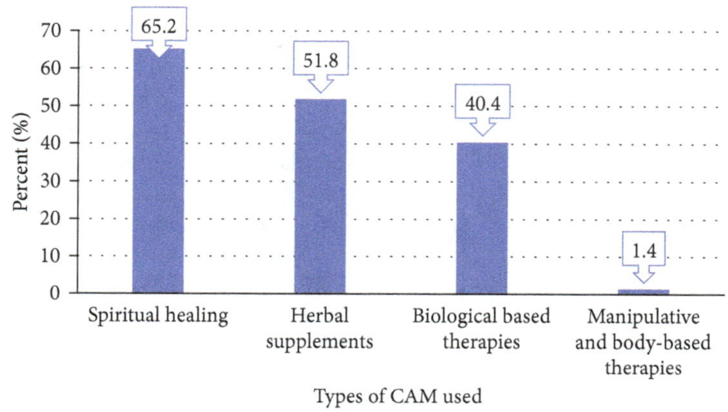

Figure 1: Frequency (%) and types of CAM therapies used during pregnancy.

Spiritual healing (65.2%) and herbal supplements (51.8%) were found to be the commonest types of CAM therapies used throughout pregnancy in the present survey as it is portrayed in Figure 1. The most frequently consumed herbal supplements were ginger (*Zingiber officinale*) (43.6%), garlic (*Allium sativum*) (38.3%), and demakese (*Ocimum lamiifolium*) (36.2%) (Figure 2).

4. Discussion

The present study was aimed at examining the prevalence and types of CAM therapies along with associated factors of CAM use during pregnancy. Despite a scarcity of evidence for efficacy and safety, CAM use is reportedly increasing across the globe [2, 3]. In this study, out of 252 women, 89.36% had reported CAM use at least once during pregnancy for strongly appreciated reasons like accessibility and availability of CAM treatments as well asculture/religion-related beliefs. Similarly, a study in Australia reported CAM use as high as 87% [11]. In contrast, one study done in the United Kingdom evidenced lower (26.7%) prevalence of CAM use in pregnancy. Moreover, three studies [12–14] from the USA reported lesser CAM use among pregnant women. The discrepancy in the prevalence of CAM use may be due to variation in sample size of participants surveyed, knowledge and experience of women, difference in advancement of health system across the countries, and scarcity in availability and access of medical services. In the current work, substantial increment of CAM use was observed in the first and second trimester in line with Mohamed et al.'s [15] study but a study undertaken in Qatar reported the relative decreases in the third trimester.

In this study, the commonest types of CAM modalities used during gestation were spiritual healing and herbal supplements followed by biological-based therapy. In accordance with previous studies conducted in the Northwest part of Ethiopia [8] and Alexandria [16], herbal supplements used by a higher proportion of pregnant women were *Zingiber officinale*, *Allium sativum*, and *Ocimum lamiifolium*. On the other hand, commonly used herbal supplements/preparations in Virginia, Australia, Norway, and Tuscany were reported to be peppermint, raspberry, fennel, and St. John's wort [17–20]. The inconsistency in the pattern of herbal supplement items between the studies might be due to availability, accessibility, affordability, distribution, and traditional claim/belief difference in the use of CAM for pregnancy-related medical conditions. Evidence on efficacy and safety of herbs indicated for pregnant populations is inadequate.

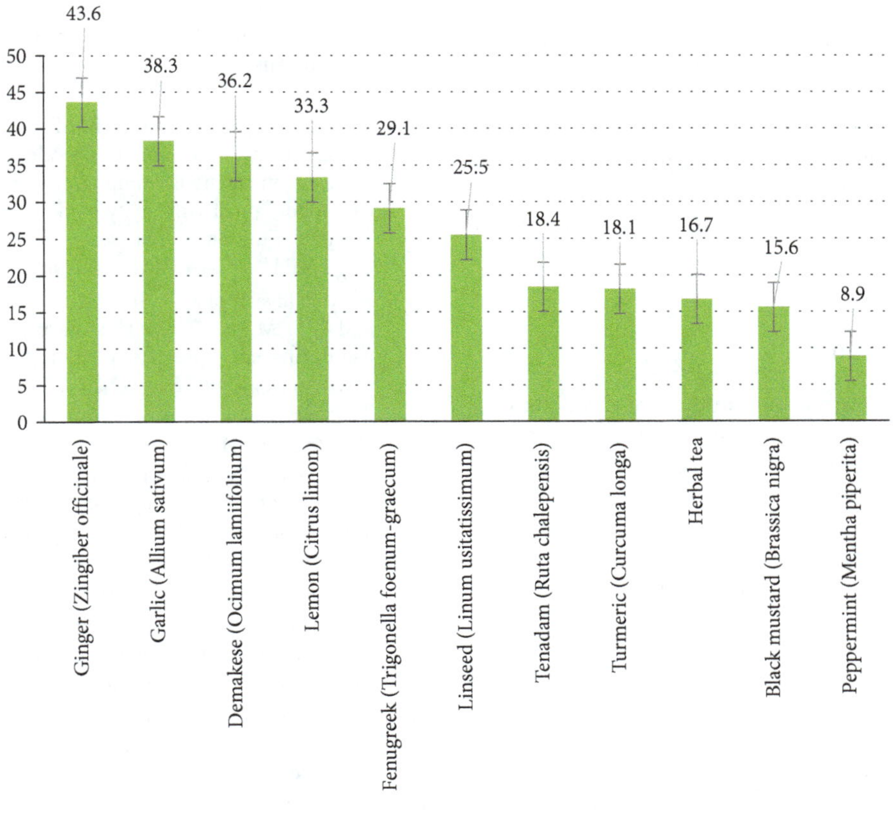

FIGURE 2: Frequency (%) and list of herbal supplements used during pregnancy.

Chamomile and peppermint for morning sickness for instance were shown risky in 6% of studies [21, 22]. *Zingiber officinale* and raspberry leaf were also evidenced as unsafe in 12% and 15% of the studies, respectively [21]. Fenugreek oil also needs to be consumed with caution during pregnancy due to its hypoglycemic effect and its stimulatory effect on oxytocin secretion resulting in uterine contraction [23]. The use of herbal products is not usually tested in clinical trials, and also, they are not included in the FDA pregnancy categories, giving a false impression of safety which could result in immense risk to the mother and fetus and elicit adverse effects including teratogenicity as well [24–26].

Concomitant use of herbs and conventional medications may result to undesired effects [27]. Remarkably, majority of pregnant women in the current study had possessed less awareness to herb-drug interaction while less proportion (33.7%) of women were reported to disclose CAM use to their HCPs. These results agree with the findings of other studies, in which 37.2% of pregnant women informed their HCPs [28]. Although these findings differ from a published study [29], they have reported that 65.8% of pregnant women disclosed uses of some form of CAM therapies to their physicians. Other studies also revealed that the reporting level of pregnant women about CAM uses to their HCPs ranges from 24% to 52% [30, 31]. Most importantly, results of the present study indicated 'HCPs' unsupportiveness and discouragement' and 'omission of HCPs to ask' were the major reasons for nondisclosure of CAM use. Other reasons that were speculated in a previous work [32] included fear and unwillingness to discuss with HCPs.

In this study, family/friends/relatives were found to be the most common sources of information to use CAM in agreement with John and Shantakumari et al.'s findings [33]. However, the findings of the current study do not support the previous researches which showed the health practitioner as a source of information [34–36]. The current study confirmed the association of CAM use with marital status and number of children previously. The odds of using CAM among single/not married pregnant women were 3.22 times higher as compared to married women. Pregnant women with no children were 3.30 times more likely to use CAM than those women having ≥3 children. Contrary to earlier findings [8, 37–40], this study indicated that lower odds of CAM use associated with educational level and antenatal care. Several limitations to this study need to be acknowledged while interpreting the results. First, the study did not identify a causal association related to CAM use and pregnancy. Secondly, a survey data is based on self-report and therefore prone to recall bias.

5. Conclusions

Evidence from this study suggests that a significant proportion of pregnant women were utilizing CAM including herbal products as part of their maternity care. The most obvious finding to emerge from this study is that a considerable number of women failed to disclose the use of CAM modalities for HCPs. These findings provide a reference on the use of CAM in pregnancy for policy-makers, health professionals, and parents. Further studies are warranted to explore the effectiveness and safety of CAM therapies like herbal medicinal products and potential effects of long-term use as well as possible interactions of herbal medicinal products with concomitantly used conventional medicines.

Authors' Contributions

YKE was involved in conception, study tool development, data analysis, final write-up, editing, and approval of the final manuscript. BAA was involved in conception and revising the final manuscript. ME and TC were involved in data collection and write-up of the first draft of the manuscript. AEG was involved in principal supervision and revising the final manuscript. All authors read and approved the final manuscript.

Acknowledgments

The authors would like to appreciate the support of School of Pharmacy, University of Gondar, and PCHC officer in facilitating the data collection process. The authors also would like to thank the study participants.

References

[1] T. Y. Teo, J. Yap, T. Shen, and K. K. Yeo, "Complementary and alternative medicine use amongst patients with cardiovascular disease in Singapore," *BMC Complementary and Alternative Medicine*, vol. 16, no. 1, p. 446, 2016.

[2] S. Warriner, K. Bryan, and A. M. Brown, "Women's attitude towards the use of complementary and alternative medicines (CAM) in pregnancy," *Midwifery*, vol. 30, no. 1, pp. 138–143, 2014.

[3] J. Adams, C. W. Lui, D. Sibbritt et al., "Women's use of complementary and alternative medicine during pregnancy: a critical review of the literature," *Birth*, vol. 36, no. 3, pp. 237–245, 2009.

[4] G. S. Birdee, K. J. Kemper, R. Rothman, and P. Gardiner, "Use of complementary and alternative medicine during pregnancy and the postpartum period: an analysis of the National Health Interview Survey," *Journal of Women's Health*, vol. 23, no. 10, pp. 824–829, 2014.

[5] J. L. Bishopa, K. Northstone, J. R. Green, and E. A. Thompson, "The use of complementary and alternative medicine in pregnancy: data from the Avon Longitudinal Study of Parents and Children (ALSPAC)," *Complementary Therapies in Medicine*, vol. 19, no. 6, pp. 303–310, 2011.

[6] J. Frawley, J. Adams, D. Sibbritt, A. Steel, A. Broom, and C. Gallois, "Prevalence and determinants of complementary and alternative medicine use during pregnancy: results from a nationally representative sample of Australian pregnant women," *Australian and New Zealand Journal of Obstetrics and Gynaecology*, vol. 53, no. 4, pp. 347 352, 2013.

[7] J. Adams, D. Sibbritt, and C. W. Lui, "The use of complementary and alternative medicine during pregnancy: a longitudinal study of Australian women," *Birth*, vol. 38, no. 3, pp. 200–206, 2011.

[8] A. B. Mekuria, D. A. Erku, B. M. Gebresillassie, E. M. Birru, B. Tizazu, and A. Ahmedin, "Prevalence and associated factors of herbal medicine use among pregnant women on antenatal care follow-up at University of Gondar Referral and Teaching Hospital, Ethiopia: a cross-sectional study," *BMC Complementary and Alternative Medicine*, vol. 17, no. 1, p. 86, 2017.

[9] A. R. Pallivalappila, D. Stewart, A. Shetty, B. Pande, R. Singh, and J. S. Mclay, "Complementary and alternative medicine use during early pregnancy," *European Journal of Obstetrics & Gynecology and Reproductive Biology*, vol. 181, pp. 251–255, 2014.

[10] T. Hollyer, H. Boon, A. Georgousis, M. Smith, and A. Einarson, "The use of CAM by women suffering from nausea and vomiting during pregnancy," *BMC Complementary and Alternative Medicine*, vol. 2, p. 1, 2002.

[11] L. Gaffney and C. Smith, "Complementary and alternative medicine in obstetrics," *Birth Issues*, vol. 13, pp. 43–50, 2004.

[12] P. Gibson, R. Powrie, and J. Star, "Herbal and alternative medicine use during pregnancy: a cross-sectional survey," *Obstetrics & Gynecology*, vol. 97, no. 4, pp. S33–S45, 2001.

[13] A. Ranzini, A. Allen, and Y. Lai, "Use of complementary medicines and therapies among obstetric patients," *Obstetrics & Gynecology*, vol. 97, no. 4, article S46, 2001.

[14] J. Headley, K. Northstone, H. Simmons, and J. Golding, "Medication use during pregnancy: data from the Avon Longitudinal Study of Parents and Children," *European Journal of Clinical Pharmacology*, vol. 60, no. 5, pp. 355–361, 2004.

[15] H. Mohamed, J. Abdin, and K. D. Al, "Knowledge, attitude and practice of complementary and alternative medicine (CAM) among pregnant women: a preliminary survey in Qatar," *Middle East Journal of Family Medicine*, vol. 7, no. 10, pp. 5–14, 2010.

[16] I. O. Yasser, F. F. Nadia, and I. A. Mohamed, "Use of herbal medicines among pregnant women attending family health centers in Alexandria," *Middle East Fertility Society Journal*, vol. 19, pp. 42–50, 2014.

[17] D. D. Glover, M. S. Amonkar, B. F. Rybeck, and T. S. Tracy, "Prescription, over-the-counter, and herbal medicine use in a rural, obstetric population," *American Journal of Obstetrics and Gynecology*, vol. 188, no. 4, pp. 1039–1045, 2003.

[18] H. Nordeng and G. C. Havnen, "Use of herbal drugs in pregnancy: a survey among 400 Norwegian women," *Pharmacoepidemiology and Drug Safety*, vol. 13, no. 6, pp. 371–380, 2004.

[19] D. A. Forster, A. Denning, G. Wills, M. Bolger, and E. McCarthy, "Herbal medicine use during pregnancy in a group of Australian women," *BMC Pregnancy and Childbirth*, vol. 6, no. 1, pp. 21–30, 2006.

[20] F. Lapi, A. Vannacci, M. Moschini et al., "Use, Attitudes and Knowledge of Complementary and Alternative Drugs (CADs) among Pregnant Women: A Preliminary Survey in Tuscany," *Evidence-based Complementary and Alternative Medicine*, vol. 7, no. 4, pp. 477–486, 2010.

[21] J. M. Wilkinson, "What do we know about herbal morning sickness treatments? A literature survey," *Midwifery*, vol. 16, no. 3, pp. 224–228, 2000.

[22] T. Fleming, *PDR for herbal medicines*, no. article 121,414, 522, 649, 2009Thomson health care Inc, USA, 4th edition, 2009.

[23] Y. I. Orief, N. F. Farghaly, and M. I. A. Ibrahim, "Use of herbal medicines among pregnant women attending family health centers in Alexandria," *Middle East Fertility Society Journal*, vol. 19, no. 1, pp. 42–50, 2012.

[24] D. Tiran, "The use of herbs by pregnant and childbearing women: a risk-benefit assessment," *Complementary Therapies in Nursing & Midwifery*, vol. 9, no. 4, pp. 176–181, 2003.

[25] D. M. Marcus and W. R. Snodgrass, "Do no harm: avoidance of herbal medicines during pregnancy," *Obstetrics and Gynecology*, vol. 105, 5, Part 1, pp. 1119–1122, 2005.

[26] L. Cuzzolin and G. Benoni, "Safety issues of phytomedicine in pregnancy and pediatrics," in *Herbal Drugs: Ethnomedicine to Modern Medicine*, K. J. Ramawat, Ed., p. 382, Springer-Verlag, Berlin Heidelberg, 2009.

[27] L. Holst, H. Nordeng, and S. Haavik, "Use of herbal drugs during early pregnancy in relation to maternal characteristics and pregnancy outcome," *Pharmacoepidemiology and Drug Safety*, vol. 17, no. 2, pp. 151–159, 2008.

[28] D. H. Adawi, *Prevalence and predictors of herb use during pregnancy (a study at Rafidia Governmental Hospital/ Palestine)*, 2012, August 2018, http://scholar.najah.edu/sites/default/files/all-thesis/deema_adawi.pdf.

[29] F. H. Dabaghian, M. A. Fard, A. Shojaei, S. Kianbakht, N. Zafarghandi, and A. Goushegir, "Use and attitude on herbal medicine in a group of pregnant woman in Tehran," *Journal of Medicinal Plants*, vol. 11, no. 41, pp. 22–33, 2012.

[30] E. Ernst, "Risk associated with complementary therapies," in *Meyler's side effects of drugs*, D. MNG and J. K. Aronson, Eds., p. 1649, Elsevier, Amsterdam, 14th edition, 2000.

[31] G. Pinn and L. Pallett, "Herbal medicine in pregnancy," *Complementary Therapies in Nursing & Midwifery*, vol. 8, no. 2, pp. 77–80, 2002.

[32] Z. Shewamene, T. Dune, and C. A. Smith, "The use of traditional medicine in maternity care among African women in Africa and the diaspora: a systematic review," *BMC Complementary and Alternative Medicine*, vol. 17, no. 1, p. 382, 2017.

[33] L. J. John and N. Shantakumari, "Herbal medicines use during pregnancy: a review from the Middle East," *Oman Medical Journal*, vol. 30, no. 4, pp. 229–236, 2015.

[34] A. T. Elolemy and A. M. Albedah, "Public knowledge, attitude and practice of complementary and alternative medicine in Riyadh region, Saudi Arabia," *Oman Medical Journal*, vol. 27, no. 1, pp. 20–26, 2012.

[35] K. Thomas and P. Coleman, "Use of complementary or alternative medicine in a general population in Great Britain. Results from the National Omnibus survey," *Journal of Public Health (Oxford, England)*, vol. 26, no. 2, pp. 152–157, 2004.

[36] A. Y. Duraz and S. A. Khan, "Knowledge, attitudes and awareness of community pharmacists towards the use of herbal medicines in Muscat region," *Oman Medical Journal*, vol. 26, no. 6, pp. 451–453, 2011.

[37] M. C. Mothupi, "Use of herbal medicine during pregnancy among women with access to public healthcare in Nairobi, Kenya: A cross-sectional survey," *BMC Complementary and Alternative Medicine*, vol. 14, no. 1, p. 432, 2014.

[38] G. Bodeker and F. Kronenberg, "A public health agenda for traditional, complementary and alternative medicine," *American Journal of Public Health*, vol. 92, no. 10, pp. 1582–1591, 2002.

[39] V. N. Addo, "Herbal medicines: socio-demographic characteristics and pattern of use by patients in a tertiary obstetrics and gynaecology unit," *Journal of Science and Technology*, vol. 27, no. 3, pp. 149–160, 2007.

[40] I. Tamuno, A. Omole-Ohonsi, and J. Fadare, "Use of herbal medicine among pregnant women attending a tertiary hospital in Northern Nigeria," *The Internet Journal of Gynecology and Obstetrics*, vol. 15, no. 2, 2011.

20

Early Implanon Discontinuation and Associated Factors among Implanon User Women in Debre Tabor Town, Public Health Facilities, Northwest Ethiopia, 2016

Mengstu Melkamu Asaye, Tewodros Syoum Nigussie, and Worku Mequannt Ambaw

Midwifery Department, College of Medicine and Health Sciences, University of Gondar, P.O. Box 196, Gondar, Ethiopia

Correspondence should be addressed to Mengstu Melkamu Asaye; mengstum@gmail.com

Academic Editor: Robert Gaspar

Background. Implanon discontinuation closely related to higher rates of overall fertility rate, unwanted pregnancies, and induced abortion. This might have social and economic consequences. In Ethiopia the magnitude of early Implanon discontinuation and contributing factors is not well studied. *Objective.* To assess early Implanon discontinuation and associated factors among Implanon user women in Debre Tabor town, 2016. *Methods.* A facility based cross-sectional study was conducted from May 1 to August 2016 through face-to-face interview. A total of 449 Implanon user women were selected by systematic random sampling technique. Epi Info version 7 and SPSS version 20 were used for data entry and analysis, respectively. Factors associated with early Implanon discontinuation were analyzed using binary and multivariable logistic regression model. Variables with p value of <0.05 and 95% confidence interval were considered as statistically significant. *Results.* The overall proportion of early Implanon discontinuation among mothers was 65 % (95%, CI: 60.4%–69.5%). Having no children (AOR = 2.0, 95% CI = [1.3–4.5]), being not counseled for possible side effects (AOR = 1.50, 95% CI = [1.1–3.4]), having no appointment for follow-up (AOR = 2.6, 95% CI = [1.2–4.3]), and having developing side effects (AOR = 1.7, 95% CI = [1.5–4.4]) were found to be statistically significant factors associated with early Implanon discontinuation. *Conclusion and Recommendation.* Early Implanon discontinuation among mothers was found to be high. Hence, counseling about Implanon side effects and appointment for follow-up of Implanon users should be made to increase Implanon retention.

1. Introduction

1.1. Background. Contraceptive discontinuation is a worldwide problem that may be connected with low incentive to avoid pregnancy. Every year, about one-third of the 182 million pregnancies occurring worldwide are unplanned. Contraceptive discontinuation may indicate a missed opportunity to promote and sustain contraceptive use, and therefore it can be used to measure the effectiveness of family planning services [1].

Discontinuation of a contraceptive method often leads to unintended pregnancy, this leads to potentially unsafe induced abortions and unplanned births that expose a risk to the health of the women and ultimately reduced educational attainment [2].

The avoidance of intended pregnancies becomes less dependent on rates of initial adopted contraceptives and more dependent on the ability and willingness of couples to use methods with a maximum effectiveness [3].

In Ethiopia nearly 1 in every 4 married women (37%) of reproductive age group (15–49) does not want any more children. The vast majority of married women want a contraceptive method to either space their next birth or cease childbearing altogether. Among contraceptive users 8% and 11% of married and unmarried sexually active women are using implants [4]. In Amhara region 4% of married women are Implanon user [5] and in Debre Tabor town, the coverage of Implanon utilization is 8.2% [6].

In general, when couples discontinue using a contraceptive method, even for a brief period, the women run the risk of becoming pregnant unintentionally. Those unintended pregnancies often lead to larger than intended family sizes and contribute to higher rates of overall fertility [7].

1.2. Statement of the Problem. Early Implanon discontinuation is defined as discontinuation at less than 2.5 years after insertion of Implanon [8, 9].

In a cross-sectional study in Zaria Nigeria, early Implanon discontinuation was 19% and 69% of removal reason was menstrual disruption [10]. In a community-based cross-sectional study at Ofla Tigray, early Implanon discontinuation was 16% with mean (±SD) of 6.6 ± 2.8 in months [11].

Implanon is an effective form of family planning. Contraceptive discontinuation is a worldwide incident and highly contributes substantially to unplanned pregnancies, unwanted births, and termination of pregnancies [1, 10].

In sub-Saharan Africa including Ethiopia, there are high population and reproductive health challenges, which are indicating higher maternal mortality, higher total fertility rate, and unintended pregnancies [6].

When a woman discontinues the prevailing family planning methods in her body, she may become pregnant unintentionally. This unplanned pregnancy has impacts on larger family size and ultimately contributes to higher overall fertility rates and reflects the effectiveness of family planning program [12], which may have social and economic consequences [3].

When emphasis is given on possible side effect counseling, reassurance, and follow-up, duration of Implanon utilization and women's satisfaction would be increased. Implanon discontinuation rates are poorly documented in Africa [5].

Apart from low utilization, early Implanon discontinuation and its determinants among Implanon user women in Ethiopia are not well studied. The purpose of this study was to assess early Implanon discontinuation and identify its associated factors among Implanon users at Debre Tabor town.

1.3. Literature Review

1.3.1. Proportion of Early Implanon Discontinuation. Contraception and fertility planning should form part of every consultation. Contraception is a means for reducing maternal mortality and morbidity associated with unplanned pregnancy [2] and also prevents pregnancy in women who are medically unfit for pregnancy until their condition has been improved [3].

In a community-based cross-sectional study, United States (US), early Implanon discontinuation was 25.2% with mean duration of utilization 10.4 months and 15% of removal reason was menstrual disruption [14].

In a cohort study conducted in Netherland, discontinuation rate of Implanon after 12 months was 28% but it was 47% at 24 months. History of previously used contraceptive method was associated with highest continuation rates and menstrual disruption was the main reason of early Implanon discontinuation [12].

In a retrospective study at Australia, at 6 months after insertion, 6% of women had removed Implanon. The discontinuation rates showed that 26% removed at one year, 39% discontinued at one and a half years, and 50% removed at two years. Around 40% of women were still using Implanon more than 2.5 years [15].

On the other hand, in a retrospective study in Jordan, many women discontinue contraceptive use within one year of initiating a method. The one-year probability of discontinuing overall contraceptive was 45% [7].

In a retrospective study conducted in low income certain African countries, the discontinuation rates of implants were as follows: Egypt 36%, Yemen 43%, and Cambodia 45% before 2 years after insertion with different reasons [2]. It leads to high prevalence of unintended pregnancy due to its early implant discontinuation.

In a descriptive retrospective study, Ilorin, Nigeria, early Implanon discontinuation rate was 26.5% [16] and on the other hand, in a community-based cross-sectional study at Ofla Tigray, early Implanon discontinuation rates were 16% [11].

1.3.2. Factors Associated with Early Implanon Discontinuation. Discontinuation of contraceptive occurs, when a woman has no need for longer utilization or a woman has not counseled about side effects of the method [2].

In a cross-sectional retrospective study conducted in Port, Nigeria, postinsertion follow-up and counseling of side effects will increase continuation of Implanon utilization and retention [17].

In a retrospective cross-sectional study, Jos, Nigeria, the indication of early Implanon removal was 33.3% due to menstrual disruption. The other indication for early Implanon discontinuation was desire for another pregnancy closely followed by 30% [18], and in another cohort study, unmarried women had 1.62 odds to discontinue compared to married women and younger (14–19 years) and were also associated with early discontinuation [19].

In Columbus, Ohio, discontinuation due to bleeding abnormalities was 77.5% and wanting a baby was the other reason for early Implanon removal. Through counseling of a method prior to placement specially about abnormal bleeding, it increases utilization and retention of Implanon [20].

In a study conducted in Jordan, to increase continuation of a contraceptive method, male involvement counseling was very advantageous. Counseling about possible side effects with counseling material increases 1.6 times of client satisfaction which also increases duration of utilization of a family planning method [21] and in another study on this country, multivariate logistic regression of side effects like menstrual disruption was associated with early removal of implants ($p = 0.002$) and preplacement counseling regarding significant side effects may have an impact on early removal [9].

In a cohort study in Ankara, Turkey, early Implanon discontinuation was 39% due to developing side effects. 18% of the main removal reasons were due to menstrual disruption and 5% due to weight gain [22]. On the other hand, in a cohort study in Philippines, quality of care was correlated for continuation of a contraceptive method. The rate of discontinuation was higher among women who reported that they had not been counseled about side effects of the method [23] and in a study conducted in India, 29% early Implanon discontinuation was due to 30.5% menstrual disruption [24].

In institution based cross-sectional study, in Bangladesh, younger women had higher rate of contraceptive discontinuation of any method, especially those with no children. Women with 1 or 2 living children had 0.49 odds compared to those with no children for contraceptive discontinuation. Women who did not intend to have other children were less likely to discontinue any contraceptive [1].

In a descriptive retrospective study, Ilorin, Nigeria, indications for early discontinuation were as follows: 35% was due to desire of pregnancy followed by 25% being due to menstrual disruption [16].

In Jos Nigeria, mean of 13.4±6.8 months was the duration of Implanon utilization. The suggested removal reasons were 53.1% side effect of the method. From side effects 33.3% was menstrual disruption followed by 13.3% being due to weight gain [18].

In a institution based cross-sectional study in Arsi, Oromia region, 25% of early Implanon discontinuation was mainly due to menstrual disruption whereas 24% was due to plan to conceive in the near future with the mean duration of 19.5 months [13].

On the other hand, in a community base cross-sectional study at Ofla Tigray, the discontinuation rate of Implanon was 16% with different factors. Among the associated factors, women who developed side effects were 2.8 odds, women who were not appointed for follow up and women who were not satisfied by the service given during the insertion of Implanon were more than 3 times more likely to discontinue Implanon as compared to their counterparts [11].

1.4. Conceptual Framework. See Figure 1.

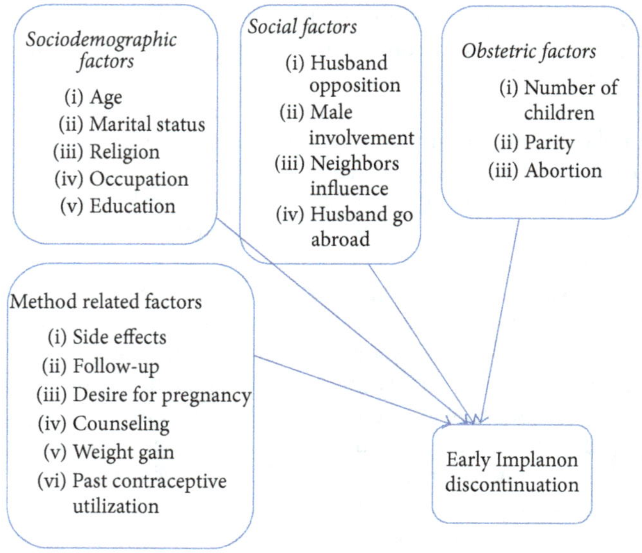

FIGURE 1: Conceptual framework adapted from review of literatures on early Implanon discontinuation and associated factors [11, 13].

1.5. Justification of the Study. Contraceptive implants are the most effective family planning methods available and well-accepted worldwide. Despite its proven long protection, only 8% of married women in Ethiopia use implants and 8.2% of all reproductive age women use Implanon in the study area [4, 6]. Apart from its low utilization, premature removal is common with unknown reasons. Contraceptive discontinuation highly contributes to unplanned pregnancy, abortions, and maternal deaths.

To date there was no study conducted on early Implanon discontinuation and associated factors among Implanon user women in the study area. Therefore, this study aimed to assess early Implanon discontinuation and determinant factors among Implanon user women.

The findings of this study will in general help the health professionals to understand the extent of early Implanon discontinuation. In addition to this, the finding will enhance the capacity of planning and decision making to look for possible solutions to solve the problem in collaboration with concerned stake holders.

Moreover, the findings will help policy makers and planners and other concerning organizations working in the area of family planning and maternal health to plan new strategies based on the identified factors to improve early discontinuation of Implanon in the community.

Finally the findings from this study will help to achieve sustainable development goal 3 (SDGS) of family planning in the country.

2. Objectives

2.1. General Objective

(i) To assess early Implanon discontinuation and associated factors among Implanon user women in Debre Tabor town health institutions, South Gondar Zone, Amhara Region, northwest of Ethiopia, from May 1 to August 30, 2016.

2.2. Specific Objectives

(i) To determine proportion of early Implanon discontinuation among Implanon user women in Debre Tabor town health institutions.

(ii) To identify factors associated with early Implanon discontinuation among Implanon user in Debre Tabor town health institutions.

3. Methods

3.1. Study Design and Period. Facility based cross-sectional study was conducted at Debre Tabor town public health facilities from May 1 to August 30, 2016.

3.2. Study Area. Debre Tabor town is found in South Gondar Zone of Amhara regional state of Ethiopia. It is located 98 kilometer far from Bair Dar, the city of Amhara regional state, and 666 kilometer far from Addis Ababa, the capital city of Ethiopia, to the northwest of the country. The town has four administrative kebeles with a total population of 67,485; among these 13,969 were in the reproductive age group and 96.72% of the population of the town are Orthodox Christians whereas 2.54% is Muslim [25]. There are one general hospital, 4 health centers, and two medium private clinics in the town.

3.3. Source and Study Population

3.3.1. Source Population. The study includes all women of reproductive age group (15–49 years of age) who were using Implanon.

3.3.2. Study Population. The study includes all women who requested removal of Implanon following insertion during the study period at the study areas for any reason.

3.3.3. Inclusion Criteria. The study includes all women who requested removal of Implanon during the study period.

3.4. Sample Size Determination. In this study, sample size was determined using Open Epi version 2 by considering the following statistical assumptions. The odds ratio and counseling status about effectiveness was taken from previous study in Tigray Ethiopia [11].

Assumptions

Two sided significant level (1 − alpha): 95%.

Power (1 − beta, % chance of detecting): 80.

Ratio of sample size: 1.

Percent of not counseled about effectiveness with outcome: 9.6.

Percent of counseled about effectiveness with outcome: 20.

Odds ratio: 2.36.

Continuity correction result = 404 which is the largest sample size from the factors.

Then by adding 10% none response rate

$$n = 404 * \frac{1}{1 - 0.1} = 449. \quad (1)$$

3.5. Sampling Procedure. Public health facilities which gave the service were Debre Tabor Hospital, Debre Tabor-Health Center, Ginbot-20 Health Center, and Hidar 11 Health Center and all were included in the study. The calculated sample size was proportionally allocated to each health facility based on the previous consecutive five month average daily client flow of the units which were obtained by referring client registration log books. The average five-month client flow for Debre Tabor Hospital, Debre Tabor-Health Center, Ginbot-20 Health Center, and Hidar 11 Health Center was 451, 313, 283 and 301, respectively. A total of 1347 women were booked for Implanon removal in five months from review of the previous months' record of each health institutions. The study participants were selected by using systematic random sampling method from Implanon removal women who visited the health institutions during the data collection period. The first client in each health facility was selected by lottery method. We compute *K*th for each health facility and it ranges from 2.66 to 2.78; then every 3rd Implanon user woman in each health facility from their sequence of family planning visit in the study period was selected (Figure 2).

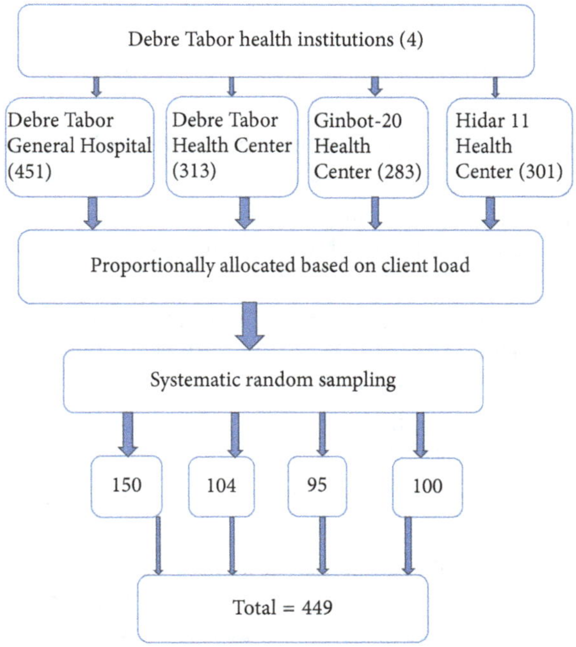

Figure 2: Schematic presentation of sampling procedure for early Implanon discontinuation and associated factors in Debre Tabor town public health facilities, South Gondar Zone, Amhara Region, 2016.

3.6. Study Variables

3.6.1. Dependent Variable

(i) Early Implanon discontinuation

3.6.2. Independent Variables

(i) Sociodemographic character: age, marital status, religion, occupation, and education.

(ii) Obstetric factors: number of children, parity, and abortion.

(iii) Social factors: husband objection, husband involvement, and husband go abroad and neighbors influence.

(iv) Method related factors: side effects, past contraceptive utilization, desire for pregnancy, follow-up, counseling, and weight gain.

3.7. Operational Definitions

(i) Contraceptive: an agent or device intended to prevent conception.

(ii) Counseling: making the women aware of its long protection, side effects, and effectiveness of the method.

(iii) Early Implanon discontinuation: removal of Implanon by health professionals before 2.5 years of utilization.

(iv) Long acting reversible contraceptive: contraceptive methods which serve as 3–10 years but can be removed at any time.

(v) Menstrual disruption: any deviation of a women's regular menstrual cycle.

(vi) Unintended pregnancy: pregnancy without mother's plan.

(vii) Side effect: when the women develop at least one side effect after Implanon insertion like menstrual disruption, insertion arm pain, headache, acne, and others.

3.8. Data Collection Tools. Data were collected using semistructured face-to-face interviewed questionnaire having three parts. The first part contains sociodemographic characteristics of mothers. The second part of the questionnaire was obstetric characteristics of women and the third part was contraceptive related characteristics. One midwife supervisor and four 2nd-year diploma midwifery students were employed for data collection and trained for half of a day about the purpose of the study, timely collection of data, and overall data collection procedure.

3.9. Data Quality Control. To assure the quality of the data the questionnaire was pretested 1 week before the actual data collection time on 23 Implanon discontinuer women at Adiszemen Hospital and appropriate modification was made. The questionnaire was prepared in English and translated into Amharic and retranslated back to English by two language experts. Data collectors and supervisor were trained for half day before one week of the actual data collection time. Interviewers were supervised at each site and regular meetings had been held between the data collectors and the supervisor. The collected data were reviewed and checked for completeness before data entry. Data entry format template was produced and the data were entered into Epi Info version 7 to control data entry errors.

3.10. Data Processing and Analysis. Before analysis data clean-up and cross-checking were done. Data were checked, coded, and entered to Epi Info version 7 then it was exported to SPSS version 20 for analysis. Both descriptive and analytical statistical procedures were utilized. Descriptive statistics like percentage, mean, median, and standard deviation were used for the presentation of sociodemographic data and prevalence of early discontinuation of Implanon. Tables were also used for data presentation. Binary logistic regression was used to identify factors associated with early discontinuation of Implanon. Variables with p value less than 0.2 in bivariate analysis were entered into multivariable logistic regression model. Multiple logistic regression models was fitted to control the possible effect of confounders and finally the variables which had independent association with early discontinuation of Implanon were identified on the basis of OR, with 95% CI and p value less than 0.05. The variables were entered in the multivariate model using the Backward Stepwise regression method. Model fitness was checked using Hosmer and Lemeshow goodness of fit test ($p = 0.65$).

4. Ethical Clearance

Ethical approval and clearance were obtained from Institutional Review Board of University of Gondar. Support letter was obtained from University of Gondar to Amhara Regional Health Bureau and South Gondar Zone Health Office. Letter of cooperation was secured from the administrations of each health institution. Informed verbal consent was obtained from study participants to confirm willingness to participate after explaining the objectives, benefits, and risks of the study. Participation in the study was voluntary and a study participant has the right to accept or refuse participation in the study at any time.

Confidentiality was assured and no personal details were recorded in any documentation related to this study.

5. Result

5.1. Sociodemographic Characteristics. A total of 449 women have responded to the questionnaires making a response rate of 100%. The age of the study participants was between 16 and 45 years with mean (±SD) age 26.7 ± 6.7 years. More than half, 332 (73.5%), of the respondents were married, 394 (87.8%) were Orthodox Christians, 327 (73%) were urban in residence, and all were Amhara in ethnicity.

Among the participants 195 (43.4%) were house wives and 136 (41%) of their husband were employed by occupation and 166 (37%) of the participants and 161 (48.5%) of their husbands had educational status of college and above (Table 1).

5.2. Obstetrics Related Characteristics. Obstetrics history was one of the factors that were assessed in the study. One hundred sixty-nine (37.7%) respondents had given birth one to two times while 154 (34.3%) of the study women were nulliparous. Out of those who had gave birth 95 (21.2%) women had one to two alive children and 47 (10.5%) had more than five alive children.

Among 449 respondents, 101 (22.5%) of them had abortion history and 332 (73.9%) study participants had desire to have more children in the near future. From the participants who desire to have child 154 (46.4%) of them need to have child within two years (Table 2).

5.3. Contraceptive and Counseling Related Characteristics. Majority of the participants 374 (83.3%) used modern contraceptive before the currently discontinued Implanon. Out

TABLE 1: Sociodemographic characteristics of Implanon users in Debre Tabor town public health facilities, northwest Ethiopia, August 2016 ($n = 449$).

Variables	Number	Percentage
Women's age		
16–21	115	25.6
22–27	157	35
28–33	107	23.8
34–39	35	7.8
40–45	35	7.8
Marital status		
Married	332	73.9
Single	71	15.8
Divorced	34	7.6
Widowed	12	2.7
Religion		
Orthodox	394	87.8
Muslim	34	7.6
Others*	21	4.6
Residence		
Urban	327	73
Rural	122	27
Women's education		
Illiterate	93	20.7
Read and write	33	7.3
Primary	81	18
Secondary	76	16.9
College and above	166	37
Husband's education ($n = 332$)		
Illiterate	54	16.26
Read and write	39	11.75
Primary	34	10.24
Secondary	44	13.25
College and above	161	48.49
Women's occupation		
House wife	195	43.4
Employee	120	26.73
Student	87	19.38
Trader	47	10.47
Husband's occupation		
Employee	136	41
Trader	59	18
Student	20	6
Farmer	117	35

* = catholic and protestant.

TABLE 2: Obstetrics characteristics of Implanon user women in Debre Tabor town public health facilities, northwest Ethiopia, August 2016 ($n = 449$).

Variables	Number	Percentage
Parity		
0	154	34.3
1-2	169	37.7
3+	126	28
Living children		
0	156	35
1-2	95	21.2
3-4	91	20.3
5+	47	10.5
History of abortion		
Yes	101	22.5
No	348	77.5
Desire for pregnancy		
Yes	332	73.9
No	117	26.1
When they want become pregnant ($n = 332$)		
Within two years	154	46.4
After two years	178	53.6

of them 221 (59.1%) were using injectable followed by oral contraceptive pills 88 (23.5%).

Two hundred eighty (62.4%) and one hundred three (31.8) of the participants got counseling service about benefit and side effect of Implanon during insertion, respectively. All of study participants got Implanon insertion at government health institutions and 269 (70%) of them choose Implanon by their own.

Two hundred ten (46.8%) of study participants did not have appointment follow-up during their Implanon utilization period.

The suggested reasons for premature removal of Implanon before due date were identified that side effect of Implanon was the major, which accounted for 264 (71%) followed by 61 (16.4%) of plan to conceive in the near future (Table 3).

Among women who developed side effects, menstrual disruption accounted 120 (32.3%) for early Implanon discontinuation followed by 68 (18.3%) insertion arm pain (Figure 3). Proportion of Early Implanon Discontinuation

The main concern of this study was to assess the proportion of early Implanon discontinuation among women who ever used it and request its removal. From 449 study participants who had Implanon removal, 292 (65%, 95% CI, 60.4%–69.5%) were overall early discontinuation. The mean (±SD) overall duration of Implanon utilization in months was 21.5 ± 8.4 (Figure 4).

5.4. Factors Associated with Early Implanon Discontinuation. Finding from bivariate logistic regression analysis revealed that age, residence, parity, number of living children, plan to conceive in the near future, counseling about possible side effects, appointment for follow-up, and developing side effects had associated with early discontinuation of Implanon. However, in multivariable logistic analysis only, women with no living children, being not counseled for possible side effects, having developing side effects, and having no appointment for follow-up given during Implanon insertion

TABLE 3: Contraceptive related characteristics of study participants in Debre Tabor town public health facilities, northwest Ethiopia, August 2016 ($n = 449$).

Variables	Number	Percentage
Ever used contraceptive before Implanon		
Yes	374	83.3
No	75	16.7
Type of contraceptive used before Implanon		
OCP	88	23.5
Injectable	221	59.1
OCP and injectable	60	16
Others*	5	1.4
Place of insertion of Implanon		
Hospital	119	26.5
Health center	271	60.4
Health post	59	13.1
Counseling for benefit of Implanon		
Yes	280	62.4
No	169	37.6
Who choose Implanon		
Own choice	269	59.9
Health professional	130	29
Health extension	27	6
Others**	23	5
Counseling about Implanon side effects		
Yes	143	31.8
No	306	68.2
Follow-up		
Yes	209	46.5
No	240	53.5
Removal due to side effect		
Yes	264	71
No	108	29
Nonside effect removal reasons		
Desire for pregnancy	61	16.4
Husband objection	34	9.2
Divorce	8	2
Husband go abroad	5	1.4

* = IUCD, Jadelle, and Implanon; ** = husband and neighbor.

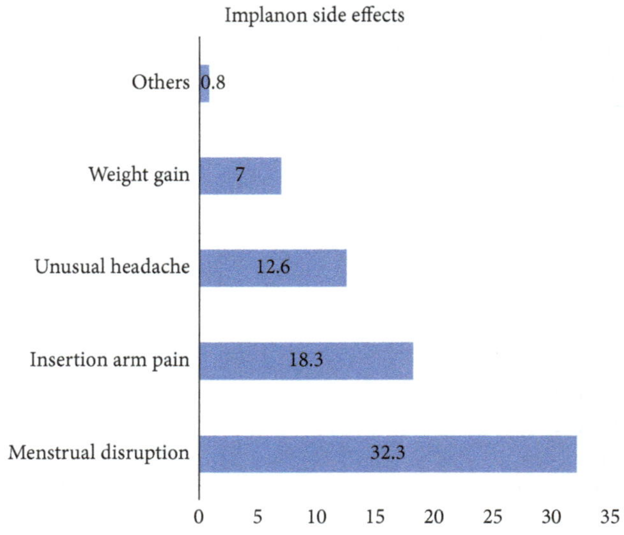

FIGURE 3: The main side effects of Implanon for early discontinuation among Implanon user women in Debre Tabor town public health facilities, South Gondar Zone, Amhara Region, 2016.

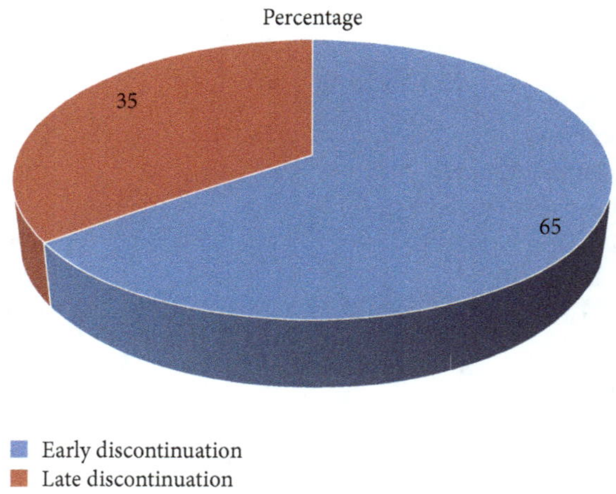

FIGURE 4: Proportion of early Implanon discontinuation among Implanon user women in Debre Tabor town public health facilities, South Gondar Zone, Amhara Region, 2016.

found significant associated factors with early Implanon discontinuation.

According to this study, the odds of discontinue Implanon early among women with no living children were 2 times than those who had living children (AOR = 2.0; 95% CI: 1.3–4.5).

The study suggested that the odds of discontinuing Implanon early among women who did not counsel about possible side effects were 1.5 times than those who got counseling service about Implanon side effects (AOR = 1.5; 95% C.I: 1.1–3.4).

The analysis showed that the odds of discontinue Implanon early among women who did not appointed for follow-up were 2.6 times than those who had appointment follow-up (AOR = 2.6; 95% C.I: 1.2–4.3).

The study also revealed that the odds of discontinue Implanon early among women who develop side effects were 1.7 times than those who had requested premature removal due to none side effects (AOR = 1.7; 95% C.I: 1.5–4.6) (Table 4).

6. Discussion

This study assessed the proportion of early Implanon discontinuation among women who request removal.

The proportion of early Implanon discontinuation among women who ever used Implanon was 65% with mean duration of 21.5 ± 8.4 months. This finding is in agreement with

TABLE 4: Factors associated with early Implanon discontinuation among Implanon user women in Debre Tabor town public health facilities, northwest Ethiopia, 2016.

Variables	Early Implanon discontinuation Yes (%)	No (%)	COR (95% C.I)	AOR (95% C.I)
Age				
16–34	271 (68.8%)	123 (31.2%)	1.6 (1.780–2.727)	--------
≥35	32 (58.2%)	23 (41.8%)	1	
Residence				
Urban	215 (65.5%)	112 (34.3%)	1	
Rural	88 (72.1%)	34 (27.9%)	1.3 (0.854–2.129)	--------
Parity				
≤1	175 (74.5%)	61 (25.8%)	1.9 (1.277–2.843)	--------
≥2	128 (60.1%)	85 (39.9%)	1	
Living children				
No children	116 (74.3%)	40 (25.7%)	2.3 (1.533–2.495)	2.0 (1.29–4.541)**
Have children	145 (62.2%)	88 (37.8%)	1	
Desire of pregnancy				
Yes	230 (69%)	102 (31%)	1.5 (0.831–1.998)	--------
No	70 (60%)	47 (40%)	1	
Side effect counseling				
Yes	80 (60%)	63 (40%)	1	
No	222 (72.5%)	84 (27.5%)	2.1 (1.416–2.561)	1.5 (1.104–3.427)*
Appointment for follow up				
Yes	124 (59.3%)	85 (40.7%)	1	
No	185 (77%)	55 (23)	2.4 (1.897–2.979)	2.6 (1.248–4.305)**
Removal due to side effect				
Yes	200 (75.6%)	64 (24.4%)	2.0 (2.010–3.244)	1.7 (1.452–4.604)*
No	65 (60.2%)	43 (39.8%)	1	

Note. * = statistically significant at $p < 0.05$ and ** = statistically significant at $p < 0.001$.

study conducted at Australia, 60% [15]. However, the current proportion is higher as compared to studies conducted in Netherland, 47% [12], Yemen, 43%, and Cambodia, 45% [2], US, 25.2% [14], India, 37% [24], Zaria, 19% [10], and Ilorin Nigeria, 26.5% [16]. The difference could be attributed to lack of preinsertion counseling particularly about the possible side effects of the method as compared to other studies [7, 20]. In addition to this, it might be due to the educational status of the study participant's as nearly half of the current studies were below primary level as compared to other studies [2, 10, 12, 14, 16, 24]. Moreover, it might be due to lack of efforts made to improve counseling, specially, on those mothers having menstrual disruption problems. This might have an impact on high proportion of early Implanon discontinuation. Lastly, it might be due to sociocultural differences of respondents across the study areas.

Women with no living children, who did not counsel about side effects of Implanon, who had no appointment for follow-up, and those who developed side effects significantly associated with early Implanon discontinuation.

According to this study, the odds of discontinues Implanon early among women with no living children were 2 times than those who had living children. This is in line with study conducted in Bangladesh [1] and Burkina Faso [2]. This is related to the fact that women with no living children might intend to have children and due to the fact that they may have higher discontinuation proportion. In addition to this, 35% of the present study women were between 22 and 27 years of age. Since they were young, they may intend to have more children and discontinue Implanon early [19].

In the present study, the odds of discontinue Implanon early among women who did not counsel about possible side effects were 1.5 times than those who got counseling service of Implanon side effects. This is consistent with study conducted in Tigray [11], Philippine [23], and Jordan [21]. Providing counseling during insertion of Implanon was positively associated with continuation of use [3, 23]. Preplacement counseling about the possible side effects of the method [5] and support by the service providers might be the most important way to help women continue on Implanon contraception. Women and couples who receive better counseling on their method may be more aware of potential side effects and how to cope with them. Preinsertion counseling on Implanon side effects is indispensable to increase the duration of Implanon being used [13]. In addition to this, preplacement counseling regarding significant side effects, including male involvement, may have an impact on early Implanon discontinuation.

The analysis also showed that the odds of discontinue Implanon early among women who did not had appointment for follow-up were 2.6 times than those who had appointment for follow-up. This is in agreement with study conducted in Tigray [11]. This might be because of feeling of confidence due to caring professionals and treating of possible side effects early.

This study also suggested that the odds of discontinue Implanon early among respondents who developed side effects were 1.7 times than those who had requested premature removal due to none side effects. This is consistent with study conducted in turkey [22], Tigray [11], Jos Nigeria [18], and Jordan [9]. It might be because experiencing side effect of the method could contribute for early Implanon discontinuation. In addition to this, respondents who had discontinued Implanon due to side effects might be because of intolerance of the side effects and fear of different complications to occur may lead to discontinuation of the method early. Moreover, this might be because of respondents who might be more concerned about culturally sensitive issues like vaginal bleeding and would want the Implanon to be removed early in order not to interfere with their sexual relationship with their husband.

7. Limitation of the Study

As the study was institutional based and conducted only on Implanon user women who request removal, it might not be generalized to the majority general population including the rural community. Since the study design was cross sectional; therefore, it may be difficult to establish temporal relationship.

8. Conclusion

Proportion of early Implanon discontinuation in this study was found to be high. Factors like women with no living children, mothers who did not receive counseling fort side effects of Implanon, women who had no appointment for follow-up, and those mothers who developed side effects were found statistically associated with early Implanon discontinuation.

9. Recommendation

To South Gondar Health Office and Other Stake Holders. Government health organizations and other stake holders could develop programs to work on health care providers in order to increase retention of Implanon utilization.

To Health Service Providers. Health professionals could be give preinsertion counseling with giving emphasis on possible Implanon side effects.

Follow-up of Implanon users could be made by health professionals to increase retention.

Early side effect management and reassurance is recommended to decrease early discontinuation.

To Researchers. Further comprehensive study including health professionals and a community-based study is recommended.

Abbreviations

AOR: Adjusted Odds Ratio
CSA: Central Statistical Agency
EDHS: Ethiopian Demographic and Health Survey
HEW: Health Extension Worker
IUCD: Intrauterine Contraceptive Device
LARC: Long Acting Reversible Contraceptives
OCPs: Oral contraceptive pills
SDGS: Sustainable Development Goals
SPSS: Statistical Package for Social Science
US: United States
UOG: University of Gondar.

Disclosure

This study is a thesis submitted to the Department of Midwifery, College of Medicine and Health Science, University of Gondar, in partial fulfilment of the requirement for degree of Master of Science in Midwifery.

Acknowledgments

The authors would like to express their gratitude to the University of Gondar for financial support and for conducting this thesis in particular. The authors' gratitude goes to advisors Mr. Tewodros Seyoum and Mr. Worku Mequannt for their invaluable guidance and unreserved comments in the process of thesis development. They would like to forward their deepest and sincere gratitude to South Gondar Zone Health Bureau and Health Facilities for provision of support letter to conduct this thesis. Also they would like to express their heartfelt thanks to their colleagues who helped them by providing useful information about the study area and during this writing. Lastly, they would like to thank all data collectors and study participants.

References

[1] R. A. Mahumud, G. Hossain, A. R. Sarkar et al., "Prevalence and associated factors of contraceptive discontinuation and switching among Bangladeshi married women of reproductive age," *Open Access Journal of Contraception*, vol. 6, no. 7, 2015.

[2] S. Staveteig, L. Mallick, and R. Winter, "Uptake and discontinuation of long-acting reversible contraceptives (Larcs) in low-income countries," *Dhs Analytical Studies*, vol. 54, pp. 17–77, 2015.

[3] WHO, "Research Policy Brief. Contraception: discontinuation and switching in developing countries," in *Reproductive Health Matters*, vol. 12, Department of Reproductive Health and Research, 15 edition, 2012.

[4] S. Gebremedhin, "Trend and socio-demographic differentials of Caesarean section rate in Addis Ababa, Ethiopia: Analysis based on Ethiopia demographic and health surveys data," *Reproductive Health*, vol. 11, no. 1, article no. 14, 2014.

[5] M. Asnake, E. G. Henry, Y. Tilahun, and E. Oliveras, "Addressing unmet need for long-acting family planning in Ethiopia: Uptake

of single-rod progestogen contraceptive implants (Implanon) and characteristics of users," *International Journal of Gynecology and Obstetrics*, vol. 123, no. 1, pp. e29–e32, 2013.

[6] S. A. Yalew, B. M. Zeleke, and A. S. Teferra, "Demand for long acting contraceptive methods and associated factors among family planning service users, Northwest Ethiopia: A health facility based cross sectional study," *BMC Research Notes*, vol. 8, no. 1, article no. 974, 2015.

[7] USAID, "Reducing discontinuation of contraceptive use and unmet need for family planning: policy options," *Jordan Population and Family Health Surveys (JPFHS)*, 2007-2009.

[8] W. J. Van den Bosch, "The progestagen-containing implant (Implanon); who is responsible for what," *Jornal of contraceptive in Netherlands*, vol. 148, no. 36, pp. 1758–1760, 2009.

[9] M. Lori, P. Dickerson, A. Vanessa, M. Diaz, C. Svetlana, and B. Kristin, "Early removal and side effects asssociated with long acting reversible contraception," *Family Medicine*, vol. 45, no. 10, pp. 701–707, 2013.

[10] N. H. Madugu, M. A. Abdul, U. Bawa, and B. Kolawole, "Uptake of hormonal implants contraceptive in Zaria, Northern Nigeria," *Open Journal of Obstetrics and Gynecology*, vol. 5, no. 5, 2015.

[11] K. Birhane, S. Hagos, and M. Fantahun, "Early discontinuation of implanon and its associated factors among women who ever used implanon in Ofla District, Tigray, Northern Ethiopia," *International Journal of Pharma Sciences and Research*, vol. 6, no. 3, 8 pages, 2015.

[12] A. M. Teunissen, B. Grimm, and F. J. M. E. Roumen, "Continuation rates of the subdermal contraceptive Implanon and associated influencing factors," *The European Journal of Contraception & Reproductive Health Care*, vol. 19, no. 1, pp. 15–21, 2014.

[13] A. Burusie, "Reasons for premature removal of implanon among users in arsi zone," *Reproductive System & Sexual Disorders*, vol. 4, no. 1, p. 6, 2015.

[14] P. M. Casey, M. E. Long, M. L. Marnach, and J. E. Bury, "Bleeding related to etonogestrel subdermal implant in a US population," *Contraception*, vol. 83, no. 5, pp. 426–430, 2011.

[15] C. Harvey, C. Seib, and J. Lucke, "Continuation rates and reasons for removal among Implanon® users accessing two family planning clinics in Queensland, Australia," *Contraception*, vol. 80, no. 6, pp. 527–532, 2009.

[16] O. Balogun, N. Olaomo, A. Adeniran, and A. Fawole, "Implanon sub-dermal implant: an emerging method of contraception in Ilorin, Nigeria," *Journal of Medical and Biomedical Science*, vol. 3, no. 1, pp. 1–5, 2014.

[17] J. D. Ojule and E. O. Oranu, "Experience with implanon in Southern Nigeria," *Jornal of Medicine and Medical Science*, vol. 3, no. 11, 5 pages, 2012.

[18] J. T. Mutihir and D. D. Nyango, "Indications for removal of etonogestrel implant within two years of use in Jos, Nigeria," *East African Medical Journal*, vol. 87, no. 11, 4 pages, 2010.

[19] D. Grunloh, T. Casner, G. Secura, J. Peipert, and T. Madden, "Early discontinuation of long-acting reversible contraception," *Contraception*, vol. 88, no. 3, pp. 433–473, 2013.

[20] M. Isley, "Implanon: the subdermal contraceptive implant.," *Journal of Pediatric & Adolescent Gynecology*, vol. 23, no. 6, pp. 364–367, 2010.

[21] S. Kamhawi, C. Underwood, H. Murad, and B. Jabre, "Client-centered counseling improves client satisfaction with family planning visits: evidence from Irbid, Jordan," *Global Health: Science and Practice Journal*, vol. 1, no. 2, pp. 180–192, 2013.

[22] C. I. Duvan, E. Gözdemir, I. Kaygusuz, Z. Kamalak, and N. Ö. Turhan, "Etonogestrel contraceptive implant (implanon): Analysis of patient compliance and adverse effects in the breast-feeding period," *Journal of the Turkish German Gynecology Association*, vol. 11, no. 3, pp. 141–144, 2010.

[23] S. RamaRao, M. Lacuesta, M. Costello, B. Pangolibay, and H. Jones, "The link between quality of care and contraceptive use," *International Family Planning Perspectives*, vol. 29, no. 2, pp. 76–83, 2003.

[24] P. Bhatia, S. Nangia, S. Aggarwal, and C. Tewari, "Implanon: Subdermal single rod contraceptive implant," *The Journal of Obstetrics and Gynecology of India*, vol. 61, no. 4, pp. 422–425, 2011.

[25] Ethiopia. CSA. Housing and Population Census of Ethiopia 2007.

Adherence to Iron and Folic Acid Supplementation and Its Associated Factors among Pregnant Women Attending Antenatal Care at Bwindi Community Hospital, Western Uganda

Christine Nimwesiga,[1] Mereth Murezi,[2] and Ivan Mugisha Taremwa[3]

[1]*Institute of Public Health and Management, Clarke International University, Kampala, Uganda*
[2]*Uganda Nursing School, Bwindi-UCU Affiliate, Uganda*
[3]*Institute of Allied Health Sciences, Clarke International University, Kampala, Uganda*

Correspondence should be addressed to Ivan Mugisha Taremwa; imugisha@ymail.com

Academic Editor: Bryan Larsen

Aims/Objectives. This study assessed the adherence to iron and folic acid supplementation and the associated factors among pregnant women attending antenatal care at Bwindi Community Hospital, in Western Uganda. *Methods.* This was a cross-sectional study that used an interviewer-administered questionnaire and reviewed medical records. Binary and multivariable logistic regression analyses were used to identify factors associated with iron and folic acid supplementation. Adjusted odds ratio (AOR) with 95% confidence interval (CI) and p value < 0.05 were used to assess for statistical significance. *Results.* We enrolled 438 pregnant women aged 16 to 41years. Participants' mean age (±standard deviation (SD)) was 25.9 (±3.17) years. The self-reported adherence to iron and folic acid supplementation (consumed ≥4 tablets a week or 20 tablets in a month daily without missing the prescribed dosage) was 22.37% ($N = 98$). Among the adherent pregnant women, the reported reasons (and their respective proportionality) for adherence were getting advice and counseling from the healthcare worker about the good effects of iron and folic acid supplementation ($N = 34$, 34.69%) and knowledge about the health benefits of iron and folic acid supplementation such as preventing anemia ($N = 16$, 16.33%), among others. On the other hand, the reported reasons (and their respective proportionality) for iron and folic acid nonadherence were forgetfulness ($N = 158$, 46.47%), taking too many pills ($N = 7$, 2.06%), not knowing the usefulness of iron and folic acid supplementation ($N = 29$, 8.53%), fear of the side effects of the medication ($N = 119$, 35.00%), and not getting the supplement from the hospital ($N = 27$, 7.94%). Bivariable and multivariable logistic regression analyses indicated that pregnant women who were primigravida (adjusted odds ratio (AOR) = 4.5), who have parity of 2 or 3 (AOR = 3.4), who perceived importance of iron and folic acid supplementation to prevent anemia (AOR = 2.9), and who considered it important to take iron and folic acid supplementation (AOR = 2.9) showed a statistically significant association with adherence to iron and folic acid supplementation. Moreover, pregnant women who perceived the risk of not taking iron and folic acid supplementation (AOR = 5.2), those who received sufficient health education regarding the goals of iron and folic acid supplementation as well as the dangers of not taking the supplements (AOR = 4.4) and adequate counseling, and those who obtained an explanation of the effects of iron and folic acid (AOR = 4.8) showed a significant association with adherence to iron and folic acid supplementation. *Conclusion.* This study found a low adherence of iron and folic acid supplementation and was associated with obstetric and client- and health system-related characteristics. To this end, there is a need for individualized strategies targeting such factors and intensifying health education, guidance, and counseling to optimize adherence to iron and folic acid supplementation.

1. Background

Iron and folic acid deficiency is a widespread nutritional public health challenge among pregnant women [1, 2]. This is a result of increased body demand and poses severe consequences for both the productive and reproductive roles [2, 3], which may augment severe anemia in pregnancy and life-threatening congenital fetal anomalies such as neural tube defects, hemorrhagic newborn disease, and physical and cognitive dysfunctioning [4]. To avert these effects, iron and folic acid supplementation (IFAS) among pregnant women and optimal adherence have been recommended [1, 2, 5]. Overtime, IFAS has been ensured through varied strategies: firstly, the use of tablets with fixed dose combination, and secondly, the inclusion of iron and folic acid tablets in the list of essential drugs in the national drug formularies [6–8]. Despite these interventions, adherence to IFAS remains unacceptably low in Africa [9–12]. In Uganda, two research studies reported a low IFAS adherence among pregnant women, that is, 11.6% over a 30-day period among pregnant women attending Mulago National Referral Hospital (MNRH) [13] and 13.2% in Kiboga District [14]. The various determinants to the adherence of IFAS among pregnant women included knowledge of the pregnant woman in regard to iron and folic acid supplementation, gravidity, counseling offered especially on the management of its side effects, forgetfulness, travel, age, literacy, socioeconomic status, cost of tablets, perceived side effects, supplement stock-outs, and clarity on importance of iron and folic acid supplementation [5, 11–15]. The reported low level of adherence, coupled with the associated barriers, agitates the need to explore the factors associated with iron and folic acid supplementation adherence to improve the outcome of the current strategy. At Bwindi Community Hospital (BCH), despite the nationwide implementation of providing free iron/folate supplements to all pregnant women, the hospital records for five years (2014-2018) indicated an unacceptably very low iron/folic acid adherence (unpublished hospital report, 2018). At BCH, anecdotal evidence shows that adherence is at 38% and this poses a critical healthcare challenge. Although limited studies have been done to identify factors associated with low adherence, in BCH, there is no single study done to determine factors associated with low adherence to iron and folic acid supplementation, hence the need for this study. The objective of this study was to assess the adherence to iron and folic acid supplementation and the associated factors among pregnant women attending antenatal care at Bwindi Community Hospital, in Western Uganda.

2. Methods

2.1. Operational Definition. Adherence was considered for a pregnant woman who took at least 57% of the expected dose of IFAS in the previous week prior to the study, which is an equivalent of taking a single tablet daily for four days in the week consecutively or 20 tablets in a month without missing the prescribed dosage.

2.2. Study Design and Duration. The study used a cross-sectional study design, between the periods of August 2018 and February 2019.

2.3. Study Setting. The study was conducted at the ANC clinic of Bwindi Community Hospital (BCH). Bwindi Community Hospital is a Private Not for Profit (PNFP) facility founded in 2003 by the U.S. missionaries. It is located in Buhoma village, Mukono Parish, Kayonza Subcounty, Kinkiizi West Constituency, and Kanungu District in Western Uganda. The hospital has a bed capacity of 112 and offers varied healthcare services such as comprehensive emergency obstetric care, curative outpatient and inpatient services, family planning, preventive services, growth monitoring, and antenatal care. It serves as a referral for other health facilities within neighborhood and adjoining districts.

2.4. Study Population, Sample Size Estimation, and Sampling. These comprised pregnant women attending ANC, who were attending for at least the second time and were supplemented with iron and folic acid tablets a month prior to the data collection period. Also, the study focused on the current pregnancy to avoid the recall bias. The sample size was estimated using a single population proportion estimation formula, with the following assumptions: the proportion of iron and folic acid adherence was considered at 11.6% [14], 95% confidence interval, 5% allowable error, and a 10% nonresponse rate. A total of 438 pregnant women were enrolled. The study used a random sampling strategy to include 438 participants. Pregnant women were given information about the study and subsequently asked to participate. These were interviewed consecutively, as they were enrolled. Those who were very sick or had an obstetric emergence were not enrolled.

2.5. Study Variables, Data Collection Tools, and Procedure. The dependent variable was adherence to iron and folic acid, while the independent variables were the sociodemographic and obstetric characteristics and client-related and health facility determinants of iron and folic acid supplementation adherence as given in Figure 1.

Data was collected using a pretested interviewer-administered structured questionnaire and ANC cards. The structured questionnaire was developed in English as guided by previous studies [3, 5, 9–15]. The questionnaire captured the sociodemographic and obstetric characteristics and client-related and health system determinants of iron and folic acid supplementation adherence. This was then translated into the local language (Runyankole-Rukiga) by a translator proficient in the language. The corresponding author crosschecked the translation, and modifications were made accordingly. The pretest of the questionnaire was carried out at Kisugu Health Centre IV on 22 (5.02%) of the pregnant women, and modifications were adopted as required to ensure clarity, wording, and logic flow.

Three members of the research team oversaw the data collection process and were supported by three research assistants who were trained midwives and had had a prior involvement in conducting research among pregnant women. For this study, a two-day training was conducted to enable understanding and practice of the data collection tools. The completed questionnaires were reviewed and crosschecked for completeness, accuracy, and consistency on a daily basis by the corresponding author who ensured data quality and compliance. Additionally, close daily supervision was ensured to monitor the performance of the research team and assistants and to deliver immediate corrective actions on mistakes noted. The completed and reviewed questionnaires were kept in a box file, in a lockable

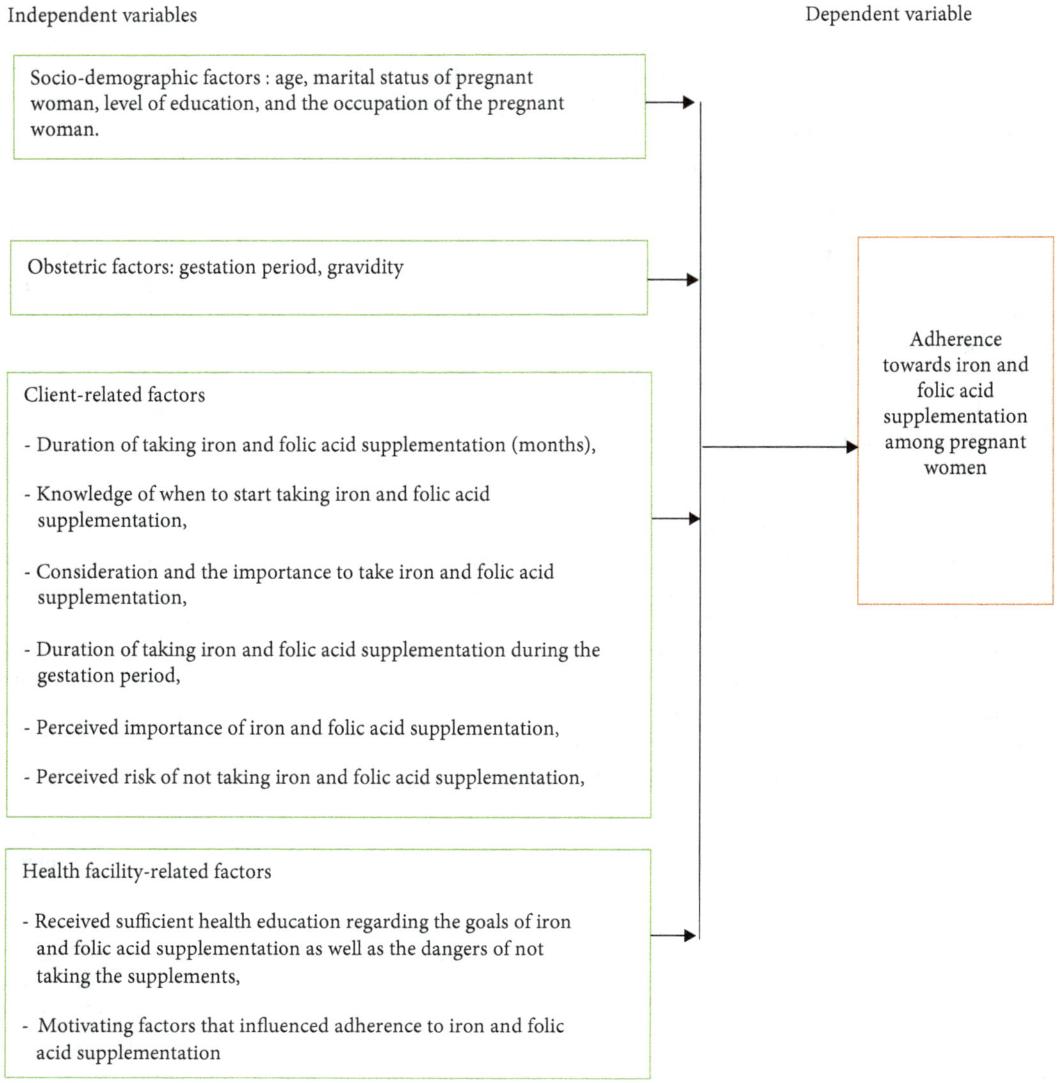

Figure 1: Conceptual framework developed from different literature [3, 9–15].

cupboard, and the key was only accessible to the study team or the corresponding author.

2.6. Data Management and Analysis. Data collected was entered into Epi Info version 7.2 and then exported into the Statistical Package for the Social Sciences (SPSS) version 24.0 for analysis. Descriptive statistics including tables and proportion were used to present the variables. Bivariable and multivariable logistic regression analyses were used to determine the association between dependent and independent variables. Variables with a p value of <0.20 during a bivariable analysis were incorporated into the multivariable logistic regression to control the possible effects of confounders. The analysis used the Hosmer and Lemeshow's goodness-of-fit test with a large p value ($p > 0.05$) to check the good fitness. Also, multicollinearity and confounding effect were checked by using a standard error. The variable without multicollinearity was considered for a multivariable model. The adjusted odds ratio (AOR) with corresponding 95% confidence interval (CI) was computed to see the strength of the association, and a p value of <0.05 was considered statistically significant.

2.7. Ethical Considerations. Ethical approval was obtained from the Research Ethics Committee of Clarke International University, after which administrative permission to carry out the study at Bwindi Community Hospital was obtained from the executive director. The study obtained written informed consent from all the participants who were ≥18years. Participants under 18 years signed a consent form as they are regarded as emancipated minors. The consent process was carried out in privacy, and no incentives were given. The study did not seek consent from a parent or legal guardian on behalf of the participants under the age of 18 years as this was not mandatory as per the guidelines on emancipated minors given in the Uganda National Council for Science and Technology (UNCST). Prior to consent, the study was introduced as part of the directed health talk to the antenatal care attendees. Additionally, anonymity of the participants was ensured at all stages of data analysis by excluding personal identifiers.

3. Results

3.1. Sociodemographic and Obstetric Characteristics of Study Participants. Four hundred and thirty-eight pregnant women aged 16-41years were enrolled. The mean ± standard deviation (SD) age of respondents was 25.9 ± 3.17 years. The majority of the study participants (65.07%, $N = 285$) were in the age group of 20–29 years, 42.24% ($N = 185$) had completed primary level education, and 84% were married. Also, most of the participants (50%) were gravida 2 or 3, and 53.20% ($N = 233$) were in their third trimester of pregnancy, as given in Table 1.

3.2. Adherence to Iron and Folic Acid Supplementation. Of the 438 pregnant women, the self-reported adherence to IFAS (consumed ≥4 tablets a week or 20 tablets in a month daily without missing the prescribed dosage) was 22.37% ($N = 98$). Relatedly, 77.62% ($N = 340$) of the pregnant women had not taken 4 or more tablets of IFAS per week in the past 1 month preceding the study. Among the adherent pregnant women, the reported reasons (and their respective proportionality) for adherence were getting advice and counseling from the healthcare worker about the good effects of iron and folic acid supplementation ($N = 34$, 34.69%) and knowledge about the health benefits of iron and folic acid supplementation such as preventing anemia ($N = 16$, 16.33%) among others. On the other hand, the reported reasons (and their respective proportionality) for iron and folic acid nonadherence were forgetfulness ($N = 158$, 46.47%), taking too many pills ($N = 7$, 2.06%), not knowing the usefulness of IFAS ($N = 29$, 8.53%), fear of the side effects of the medication ($N = 119$, 35.00%), and not getting the supplement from the hospital ($N = 27$, 7.94%).

3.3. Factors Associated with Iron and Folic Acid Supplementation. Bivariable and multivariable logistic regression analyses indicated that pregnant women who were primigravida (adjusted odds ratio (AOR) = 4.5, 95%confidence interval (CI) = 2.21-4.73), those whose parity was 2 or 3 (AOR = 3.4, 95%CI = 2.73-4.02), those who considered it important to take IFAS (AOR = 2.9, 95%CI = 2.39-3.40), those who perceived the importance of iron and folic acid supplementation to prevent anemia (AOR = 2.9, 95%CI = 2.39-3.40), those who perceived it as a risk not to take iron and folic acid supplementation (AOR = 5.2, 95%CI = 4.06 -6.18), those who received sufficient health education regarding the goals of iron and folic acid supplementation as well as the dangers of not taking the supplements (AOR = 4.4, 95%CI = 3.06-5.12) and adequate counseling (AOR = 3.6, 95%CI = 2.16-4.50), and those who obtained an explanation of the effects of IFAS (AOR = 4.8, 95%CI = 3.08-6.42) showed a significant association with adherence to IFAS after adjusting and controlling for all other variables at p value of <0.05.

Table 1: Sociodemographic and obstetric characteristics of participants ($n = 438$).

Variables	Frequency (N)	Percentage (%)
Age (years)		
≤18	16	3.65
19-29	285	65.07
≥30	137	31.28
Marital status		
Married	368	84.02
Single	70	15.98
Level of education		
No formal education	25	5.71
Primary	185	42.24
Secondary	126	28.77
Tertiary	102	23.29
Occupation		
Employed	134	30.59
Unemployed	304	69.41
Gravidity		
Primigravida	131	29.91
2nd-3rd	219	50.00
$\geq 4^{th}$	88	20.09
Parity		
0	34	7.76
1-2	174	39.73
3-4	230	52.51
Gestation period		
1st trimester	115	26.26
2nd trimester	90	20.25
3rd trimester	233	5.20

The analysis indicated that pregnant women who were primigravida were 4.5 times more likely to adhere to IFAS as compared to those who were multigravidae (AOR = 4.5, 95%CI = 2.21-4.73). Also, pregnant women whose parity was 2 or 3 were 3.4 more likely to take four or more iron and folic acid tablets (AOR = 3.4, 95%CI = 2.73-4.02). Moreover, pregnant women who considered it important to take IFAS increased the odds of iron and folic acid adherence (AOR = 2.9, 95%CI = 2.39-3.40). Further, there was a 2.9 times likelihood of adhering to IFAS among those who perceived its importance to prevent anemia (AOR = 2.9, 95% CI = 2.39-3.40). Relatedly, pregnant women who perceived it as a risk not to take IFAS were 5.2 times more likely to adhere (AOR = 5.2, 95%CI = 4.06-6.18). Similarly, pregnant women who received sufficient health education regarding the goals of IFAS as well as the dangers of not taking the supplements were 4.4 times more likely to adhere (AOR = 4.4, 95%CI = 3.06-5.12). Pregnant women who received adequate counseling were 3.6 times more likely to adhere to IFAS (AOR = 3.6, 95%CI = 2.16-4.50), whereas pregnant women who obtained an explanation of the effects of IFAS presented with 4.8 times more likelihood of adhering (AOR = 4.8, 95 %CI = 3.08-6.42), as shown in Table 2.

Table 2: Factors associated with iron and folic acid supplementation among pregnant women.

Variables	Adherence Yes, number (%)	Adherence No, number (%)	Crude odds ratio (95% CI)	Adjusted odds ratio (95% CI)	p value
Sociodemographic characteristics					
Age (years)					
≤18	7 (7.14)	9 (2.65)	1.26 (0.91-2.62)	1.03 (0.77-2.17)	0.215
19-29	59 (60.20)	226 (66.47)	1.13 (0.48-1.86)	1.02 (0.43-1.59)	0.166
≥30	32 (32.65)	105 (30.88)	1	1	
Marital status					
Married	84 (85.71)	284 (83.53)	1.38 (0.94-1.81)	1.17 (0.84-1.49)	0.312
Single	14 (14.29)	56 (16.47)	1	1	
Level of education					
No formal education	11 (11.22)	14 (4.12)	1.20 (0.69-2.16)	1.10 (0.62-2.01)	0.395
Primary	21 (21.43)	164 (48.24)	1.62 (0. 88-2.31)	1.23 (0.76-2.12)	0.098
Secondary	32 (32.65)	94 (27.65)	1.94 (0.96-2.47)	1.66 (0.79-2.21)	0.168
Tertiary	34 (34.69)	68 (20.00)	1	1	
Occupation					
Employed	43 (43.88)	91 (26.76)	1.6 (0.99-2.31)	1.4 (0.72-2.01)	0.114
Unemployed	55 (56.12)	249 (73.24)	1	1	
Obstetric characteristics					
Gravidity					
Primigravida	29 (29.59)	102 (30.00)	4.7 (2.67-5.11)	4.5 (2.21-4.73)	0.002*
2nd-3rd	41 (41.84)	178 (52.35)	1.6 (1.27-2.01)	1.3 (1.19-1.87)	0.712
≥4th	28 (28.57)	60 (17.65)	1		
Parity					
1-2	53 (54.08)	121 (35.59)	3.9 (2.81-4.17)	3.4 (2.73-4.02)	0.003*
3-4	45 (45.92)	219 (64.41)	1	1	
Gestation period					
1st trimester	27 (27.55)	88 (25.88)	1.4 (0.93-1.67)	1.21 (0.74-1.56)	0.716
2nd trimester	44 (44.90)	46 (13.53)	1.7 (0.81-2.2)	1.4 (0.74-2.06)	0.081
3rd trimester	27 (27.55)	206 (60.59)	1	1	
Client-related characteristics					
Duration of taking iron and folic acid supplementation (months)					
1-3	38 (38.78)	211 (62.06)	1.1 (0.43-1.47)	1.08 (0.38-1.38)	0.257
4-6	46 (46.94)	74 (21.76)	1.4 (0.61-1.88)	1.2 (0.54-1.62)	0.377
≥7	14 (14.29)	55 (16.18)	1	1	
Knowledge of when to start taking iron and folic acid supplementation					
Immediately after realising I am pregnant	54 (55.10)	141 (41.47)	1.7 (1.44-2.31)	1.4 (0.96-1.88)	0.094
After 3 months	38 (38.78)	183 (53.82)	1.9 (1.63-2.33)	1.6 (1.42-2.21)	0.791
I do not know	6 (6.12)	16 (4.71)	1	1	
Considered it important to take iron and folic acid supplementation					
Yes	79 (80.61)	284 (83.53)	3.1 (2.49-3.51)	2.9 (2.39-3.40)	0.002*
No	19 (19.39)	56 (16.47)	1	1	

TABLE 2: Continued.

Variables	Adherence Yes, number (%)	No, number (%)	Crude odds ratio (95% CI)	Adjusted odds ratio (95% CI)	*p* value
Duration of taking iron and folic acid supplementation during the gestation period					
Throughout pregnancy	37 (37.76)	34 (10.00)	1.9 (1.71-2.26)	1.6 (1.32-2.13)	0.683
<9 months	59 (60.20)	297 (87.35)	1.3 (1.01-1.83)	1.1 (0.91-1.48)	0.417
I do not know	2 (2.04)	9 (2.65)	1	1	
Perceived importance of iron and folic acid supplementation					
Prevention of anemia	61 (62.24)	113 (33.24)	6.7 (5.80-7.38)	6.2 (5.41-7.17)	0.003*
Good for the baby's growth and health	29 (29.59)	94 (27.65)	1.9 (0.71-2.21)	1.6 (0.62-2.09)	0.455
Prevents complications during delivery	6 (6.12)	46 (13.53)	1.4 (0.98-1.81)	1.1 (0.81-1.57)	0.391
Others	2 (2.04)	87 (25.59)	1	1	
Perceived as a risk not to take iron and folic acid supplementation					
Yes	69 (70.41)	191 (56.18)	5.5 (4.12-6.17)	5.2 (4.06-6.18)	0.002*
No	29 (29.59)	149 (43.82)	1	1	
Days that iron and folic acid supplementation was taken in the previous 1 week					
<4	0 (0.00)	340 (100.00)	1.1 (0.61-1.73)	1.0 (0.55-1.24)	0.741
≥4	98 (100.00)	0 (0.00)	1	1	
Health facility-related characteristics					
Received sufficient health education regarding the goals of iron and folic acid supplementation as well as the dangers of not taking the supplements					
Yes	76 (77.55)	29 (8.53)	4.8 (3.18-5.22)	4.4 (3.06-5.12)	0.001*
No	22 (22.45)	311 (91.47)	1	1	
Motivating factors that influenced adherence to iron and folic acid supplementation					
Availability of iron and folic acid at the hospital	47 (47.96)	27 (7.94)	1.9 (0.19-2.64)	1.4 (0.66-2.14)	0.527
Adequate counseling	29 (29.59)	33 (9.71)	3.9 (2.51-4.71)	3.6 (2.16-4.50)	≤0.001*
Explanation of the effects of iron and folic acid supplementation	13 (13.27)	206 (60.59)	5.1 (3.11-6.98)	4.8 (3.08-6.42)	0.002*
Clear instructions for the use of iron and folic acid supplementation	9 (9.18)	107 (31.47)	1	1	

95% CI denotes 95% confidence interval. * denotes variables with a statistical significance.

4. Discussion

Four hundred and thirty-eight pregnant women aged 16-41 years were enrolled. Of these, the self-reported adherence to IFAS was 22.37%. This value is lower than 55.5% that was reported from Debre Markos Town in Ethiopia [9] and 59.8% obtained from a study conducted in Assela Town, Ethiopia [16]. Additionally, this adherence is lower compared to 64.7% reported from Eritrea [17] and 70.6% from Mizan Aman Town in Ethiopia [15]. The observed low adherence is multifaceted and is in part attributed to the differences in the sociocultural differences and lower literacy rates in the current study setting as up to 47.94% of the studied pregnant women had not attained any formal education at all or had completed up to primary level of education. This is imperative; however, it ought to be recognized that educated women can understand the messages passed from healthcare providers and be put into practicing health messages [18–20]. On the other hand, the obtained adherence was higher than 11.6% reported among pregnant women attending Mulago National Referral Hospital (MNRH) [13], and 13.2% in Kiboga District [14]. The discrepancy in the obtained values is in part attributed to numerous factors related to the study participants and setting.

As it emerged among the adherent pregnant women, the reported reasons for adherence were getting advice and counseling from the healthcare worker about the good effects of IFAS and knowledge about the health benefits of IFAS such as preventing anemia. These reasons had earlier been reported [5, 21–23] and have been described as key determinants to the antenatal care package. On the other hand, the reported reasons for IFAS nonadherence were forgetfulness, taking too many pills, not knowing the usefulness of iron and folic acid supplementation, fear of the side effects of the medication, and not getting the supplement from the hospital [9, 24–26]. Similar to previous reports, forgetfulness of a drug has been a key determinant to bad medication adherence. For example, a study that was done in one of the areas in Uganda indicated that 82% of the pregnant women ever miss to take iron supplements due to forgetting [13]. Relatedly, a study conducted from South Africa indicated that forgetting to take the iron and folic acid supplements was due to busy schedules leading to forgetting [27]. The forgetfulness among the participants could be because being in rural area and with the majority being unemployed, they probably spend most of their time in gardens or become busy with casual labor and forget to carry with them their pills. The practice of too many drugs prescribed at the same time (polypharmacy) has been highlighted as an adherence barrier as supported by the previous research evidence [28, 29]. Polypharmacy was linked to nonadherence because pregnant women experienced medicine fatigue and suffered from frustration of many tablet intakes [30, 31]. Also, not knowing the usefulness of iron and folic acid supplementation was indicated as a hindrance to adherence. Consistent with previous studies, lack of awareness on importance of taking the medication ought to be emphasized among pregnant women [32, 33]. Also, the World Health Organization (2015) emphasizes the need to highlight that all the tablets are necessary to ensure good fetal outcome [4]. These factors negatively affected iron and folic acid supplementation and necessitate a critical consideration to improve the uptake.

The other reason for nonadherence was the fear of the side effects of the iron and folic acid supplementation. As previously explored, fear of having a big baby and related side effects of iron and folic acid supplementation have prevented adherence efforts [4]. Also, a study conducted from South Africa indicated that folic acid and ferrous sulphate made pregnant women feel nauseous, inclined them to vomit, and also caused gastrointestinal upset [27]. This was similar to a study report from the North Western Zone of Tigray, Ethiopia [34]. Besides the listed reasons for nonadherence to iron and folic acid supplementation, not getting the supplement from the hospital was highlighted as a major setback. This collaborates well with previous reports and highlights the negative attributes of drug stock-out in health facilities as some pregnant women may not comply with clinic purchases due to lack of money, as well as exorbitant charges [35–37]. Thus, to improve on the uptake of iron and folic acid supplementation, it is desirable to ensure regular hospital stocks of iron and folic acid tablets and to emphasize their correct use by the pregnant women.

The bivariable and multivariable logistic regression analyses indicated that pregnant women who were primigravida, had parity of 2 or 3, considered it important to take iron and folic acid supplementation, perceived the importance of iron and folic acid supplementation to prevent anemia, and perceived the risk of not taking iron and folic acid supplementation showed a significant association with adherence to iron and folic acid supplementation. In addition, pregnant women who received sufficient health education regarding the goals of iron and folic acid supplementation as well as the dangers of not taking the supplements and adequate counseling and pregnant women who obtained an explanation of the effects of iron and folic acid supplementation showed a significant association with adherence to iron and folic acid supplementation. Primigravida and low parity number (<4) are generally considered factors of adherence to the pregnancy requirements [38]. This is in agreement with previous studies which showed that young parity was associated with compliance [5, 39]; however, it contravenes previous evidence that primigravida and low parity risked missing iron and folic acid supplementation due to lack of knowledge and understanding towards care for their pregnancies [40]. This finding highlights the need to cautiously emphasize the strict need for pregnant women to adhere to iron and folic acid supplementation to ensure the best maternal and fetal outcome [41]. The other factors were the consideration of the importance of IFAS, the perception of the importance of IFAS to prevent anemia during pregnancy, and the perception of risk of not taking IFAS. These factors have been widely studied, and they affirm the importance of pregnant women understanding the positive attributes of IFAS [12, 16, 42]. These factors are as well supported by other research findings [5, 12, 16] and highlight a potential improvement in the uptake of iron and folic acid supplementation in pregnant women to know anemia and its consequences towards the pregnancy outcome. The current study also found that women who received sufficient health education regarding the goals of IFAS and the dangers of not taking the supplements and adequate counseling and pregnant women who obtained an explanation of the effects of IFAS had better adherence than those who did not receive. Similar findings were reported from earlier reports [5, 9, 11, 12]. This suggests that such explanations offer the opportunity to understand the purpose, importance, possible side effects and duration, dosage of the supplement, and tolerance to the associated adverse effects. Also, understanding the dangers of not taking the supplements is critical as pregnant women ensures adherence to subvert the likely consequences. Studies show that lack of health education on IFAS among pregnant women has greatly affected the adherence to IFAS [5, 12, 40, 42], necessitating targeted and focused information, training, and counseling on the importance of IFAS during pregnancy [43]. The understaffing, late coming of mothers, and workload could be contributing to nonhealth education of mothers which are mentioned to contribute to low adherence among participants in this study area. This study finding is similar to previous reports [44, 45] and highlights the need for concerted sensitization for behaviour change. Contrary to previous studies [11, 12], this study did not find a significant statistical association with the sociodemographic variables.

The findings of this study ought to be interpreted in light of the following study limitations: firstly, the 7-day compliance period is short and may not represent compliance throughout the pregnancy period. This period was utilized to minimize recall bias, and this has cross-sectional study design and is guided by previous studies. Also, the estimation of IFAS adherence by the self-report method may underestimate the prevalence of nonadherence when compared with objective measures like pill counts or biological assay medication adherence measures. Secondly, there may have been recall bias and subjectivity because the study heavily relied on verbal reports from the interviewees. Thirdly, the current study was conducted entirely within one center; differences of geographic location were not assessed, and this limits the generalization of study results.

5. Conclusions

This study found a low adherence (22.37%) to iron and folic acid supplementation and was associated with various obstetric and client- and health system-related characteristics. Adherence was linked to advice and counseling to pregnant women and perceived health benefits of iron and folic acid supplementation. On the other hand, numerous reasons for iron and folic acid nonadherence were reported and negatively affected the compliance to antenatal care recommendations. Bivariable and multivariable logistic regression analyses indicated obstetric and client- and health facility-related factors to assess the rate of adherence to IFAS. Based on these, the following recommendations have been proposed: (a) there is a need to increase health education on the goals for IFAS and guidance on how to swallow the drugs as recommended to increase adherence to IFAS, (b) there should be continuous sensitization of the community about the goals and benefits of IFAS, and (c) the community and other local leaders ought to continuously advocate and support early attendance of ANC by pregnant mothers and support mothers on IFAS to enable them finish the required doses.

Abbreviations

AIDS: Acquired immune deficiency syndrome
ANC: Antenatal care
BCH: Bwindi Community Hospital
Hb: Hemoglobin
HIV: Human immunodeficiency virus
HMIS: Health management information system
IFAS: Iron and folic acid supplementation
WHO: World Health Organization.

Acknowledgments

The authors express their utmost gratitude to the participants who voluntarily responded to their questionnaire and the research assistants for the field support.

References

[1] WHO, "Guideline: daily iron and folic acid supplementation in pregnant women," 2012, https://apps.who.int/iris/bitstream/handle/10665/77770/9789241501996_eng.pdf.

[2] WHO, "Daily iron and folic acid supplementation during pregnancy," 2019, https://www.who.int/elena/titles/daily_iron_pregnancy/.

[3] A. Mousa, A. Naqash, and S. Lim, "Macronutrient and micronutrient intake during pregnancy: an overview of recent evidence," *Nutrients*, vol. 11, no. 2, p. 443, 2019.

[4] WHO, "Recommendations on antenatal care for a positive pregnancy experience," 2016, https://apps.who.int/iris/bitstream/handle/10665/250796/9789241549912eng.pdf?sequence=1.

[5] M. W. Kamau, W. Mirie, and S. Kimani, "Compliance with iron and folic acid supplementation (IFAS) and associated factors among pregnant women: results from a cross-sectional study in Kiambu County, Kenya," *BMC Public Health*, vol. 18, no. 1, p. 580, 2018.

[6] WHO, "Periconceptional daily folic acid (400 μg) supplementation for prevention of neural tube defects," https://www.who.int/selection_medicines/committees/expert/20/applications/Folic_acid.pdf.

[7] WHO, "National medicines list/formulary/standard treatment guidelines," 2014, http://www.who.int/selection_medicines/country_lists/en/.

[8] Medecins Sans Frontiers (MSF), "Folic acid 400 μg tablet," https://www.who.int/selection_medicines/committees/expert/20/applications/MSF-comment-folic-acid-tablet_Mar-15.pdf?ua=1.

[9] M. Desta, B. Kassie, H. Chanie et al., "Adherence of iron and folic acid supplementation and determinants among pregnant women in Ethiopia: a systematic review and meta-analysis," *Reproductive Health*, vol. 16, no. 1, p. 182, 2019.

[10] Z. Y. Kassa, T. Awraris, A. K. Daba, and Z. Tenaw, "Compliance with iron folic acid and associated factors among pregnant women through pill count in Hawassa City, South Ethiopia: a community based cross-sectional study," *Reproductive Health*, vol. 16, no. 1, p. 14, 2019.

[11] A. S. Abinet, A. G. Lakew, and A. H. Mamusha, *Compliance with Iron-Folate Supplement and Associated Factors among Antenatal Care Attendant Mothers in Misha District*, Community Based Cross-Sectional Study. Journal of Environmental and Public Health, South Ethiopia, 2015, Available from: https://www.hindawi.com/journals/jeph/2015/781973/.

[12] B. B. Nasir, A. M. Fentie, and M. K. Adisu, "Adherence to iron and folic acid supplementation and prevalence of anemia among pregnant women attending antenatal care clinic at Tikur Anbessa Specialized Hospital, Ethiopia," *PLoS One*, vol. 15, no. 5, article e0232625, 2020.

[13] T. S. Kiwanuka, S. Ononge, P. Kiondo, and F. Namusoke, "Adherence to iron supplements among women receiving antenatal care at Mulago National Referral Hospital, Uganda-cross-sectional study," *BMC Research Notes*, vol. 10, no. 1, p. 510, 2017.

[14] M. A. Mbule, Y. B. Byaruhanga, M. Kabahenda, and A. Lubowa, "Determinants of anaemia among pregnant women in rural Uganda," *Rural and Remote Health*, vol. 13, no. 2, p. 2259, 2013.

[15] S. Shewasinad and S. Negash, "Adherence and associated factors of prenatal iron folic acid supplementation among pregnant women who attend ante natal care in health facility at Mizan-Aman Town, Bench Maji Zone, Ethiopia," *Journal of Pregnancy and Child Health*, vol. 4, p. 335, 2015.

[16] H. Assefa, S. M. Abebe, and M. Sisay, "Magnitude and factors associated with adherence to Iron and folic acid supplementation among pregnant women in Aykel Town, Northwest Ethiopia," *BMC Pregnancy and Childbirth*, vol. 19, no. 1, p. 296, 2019.

[17] M. Getachew, M. Abay, H. Zelalem, T. Gebremedhin, T. Grum, and A. Bayray, "Magnitude and factors associated with adherence to iron-folic acid supplementation among pregnant women in Eritrean refugee camps, northern Ethiopia," *BMC Pregnancy and Childbirth*, vol. 18, no. 1, p. 83, 2018.

[18] P. Rasheed and L. S. Al-Sowielem, "Health education needs for pregnancy: a study among women attending primary health centers," *Journal of Family and Community Medicine*, vol. 10, no. 1, pp. 31–38, 2003.

[19] M. A. Al-Ateeq and A. A. Al-Rusaiess, "Health education during antenatal care: the need for more," *International Journal of Women's Health*, vol. 7, pp. 239–242, 2015.

[20] K. D. Konlan, J. A. Saah, R. M. Amoah et al., "Factors influencing the utilization of focused antenatal care services during pregnancy, a study among postnatal women in a tertiary healthcare facility, Ghana," *Nursing Open*, vol. 7, no. 6, pp. 1822–1832, 2020.

[21] M. Kamau, S. Kimani, and W. Mirie, "Counselling and knowledge on iron and folic acid supplementation (IFAS) among pregnant women in Kiambu County, Kenya: a cross-sectional study," *AAS Open Research*, vol. 1, p. 21, 2018.

[22] M. W. Kamau, S. T. Kimani, W. Mirie, and I. K. Mugoya, "Effect of a community-based approach of iron and folic acid supplementation on compliance by pregnant women in Kiambu County, Kenya: a quasi-experimental study," *PLoS ONE*, vol. 15, no. 1, p. e0227351, 2020.

[23] A. D. Gebremariam, S. A. Tiruneh, B. A. Abate, M. T. Engidaw, and D. T. Asnakew, "Adherence to iron with folic acid supplementation and its associated factors among pregnant women attending antenatal care follow up at Debre Tabor General Hospital, Ethiopia, 2017," *PLoS One*, vol. 14, no. 1, 2019.

[24] T. G. Gebremichael and T. G. Welesamuel, "Adherence to iron-folic acid supplement and associated factors among antenatal care attending pregnant mothers in governmental health institutions of Adwa Town, Tigray, Ethiopia: cross-sectional study," *PLoS One*, vol. 15, no. 1, p. e0227090, 2020.

[25] T. G. Gebremichael, H. Haftu, and T. A. Gereziher, "Time to start and adherence to iron-folate supplement for pregnant women in antenatal care follow up; northern Ethiopia," *Patient Preference and Adherence*, vol. 13, pp. 1057–1063, 2019.

[26] M. Nechitilo, P. Nguyen, A. Webb-Girard et al., "A qualitative study of factors influencing initiation and adherence to micronutrient supplementation among women of reproductive age in Vietnam," *Food and Nutrition Bulletin*, vol. 37, no. 4, pp. 461–474, 2016.

[27] Z. Kalipa, D. T. Goon, E. M. Yako, and A. Okeyo, "Factors influencing adherence to folic acid and ferrous sulphate nutritional intake among pregnant teenagers in Buffalo City Municipality, South Africa," *Pakistan Journal of Nutrition*, vol. 16, no. 7, pp. 531–537, 2017.

[28] Z. A. Marcum and W. F. Gellad, "Medication adherence to multidrug regimens," *Clinics in Geriatric Medicine*, vol. 28, no. 2, pp. 287–300, 2012.

[29] D. E. Patton, C. A. Cadogan, C. Ryan et al., "Improving adherence to multiple medications in older people in primary care: selecting intervention components to address patient-reported barriers and facilitators," *Health Expectations*, vol. 21, no. 1, pp. 138–148, 2018.

[30] S. A. Iacob, D. G. Iacob, and G. Jugulete, "Improving the adherence to antiretroviral therapy, a difficult but essential task for a successful HIV treatment-clinical points of view and practical considerations," *Frontiers in Pharmacology*, vol. 8, p. 831, 2017.

[31] R. W. Grant, N. G. Devita, D. E. Singer, and J. B. Meigs, "Polypharmacy and medication adherence in patients with type 2 diabetes," *Diabetes Care*, vol. 26, no. 5, pp. 1408–1412, 2003.

[32] R. Devkota, G. M. Khan, K. Alam, B. Sapkota, and D. Devkota, "Impacts of counseling on knowledge, attitude and practice of medication use during pregnancy," *BMC Pregnancy and Childbirth*, vol. 17, no. 1, p. 131, 2017.

[33] K. J. Marwa, A. Njalika, D. Ruganuza, D. Katabalo, and E. Kamugisha, "Self-medication among pregnant women attending antenatal clinic at Makongoro Health Centre in Mwanza, Tanzania: a challenge to health systems," *BMC Pregnancy and Childbirth*, vol. 18, no. 1, p. 16, 2018.

[34] A. Demis, B. Geda, T. Alemayehu, and H. Abebe, "Iron and folic acid supplementation adherence among pregnant women attending antenatal care in North Wollo Zone, northern Ethiopia: institution based cross-sectional study," *BMC Research Notes*, vol. 12, no. 1, p. 107, 2019.

[35] R. Stone, "Pregnant women and substance use: fear, stigma, and barriers to care," *Health Justice.*, vol. 3, no. 1, p. 2, 2015.

[36] B. H. Wagenaar, S. Gimbel, R. Hoek et al., "Stock-outs of essential health products in Mozambique - longitudinal analyses from 2011 to 2013," *Tropical Medicine & International Health*, vol. 19, no. 7, pp. 791–801, 2014.

[37] N.-H. Z. Leung, A. Chen, P. Yadav, and J. Gallien, "The impact of inventory management on stock-outs of essential drugs in sub-Saharan Africa: secondary analysis of a field experiment in Zambia," *PLoS One*, vol. 11, no. 5, article e0156026, 2016.

[38] M. Amoakoh-Coleman, K. Klipstein-Grobusch, I. A. Agyepong, G. A. Kayode, D. E. Grobbee, and E. K. Ansah, "Provider adherence to first antenatal care guidelines and risk of pregnancy complications in public sector facilities: a Ghanaian cohort study," *BMC Pregnancy and Childbirth*, vol. 16, no. 1, p. 369, 2016.

[39] A. Titilayo, M. E. Palamuleni, and O. Omisakin, "Sociodemographic factors influencing adherence to antenatal iron supplementation recommendations among pregnant women in Malawi: analysis of data from the 2010 Malawi Demographic and Health Survey," *Malawi Medical Journal*, vol. 28, no. 1, pp. 1–5, 2016.

[40] O. Ogundipe, C. Hoyo, T. Østbye et al., "Factors associated with prenatal folic acid and iron supplementation among 21,889 pregnant women in northern Tanzania: a cross-sectional hospital-based study," *BMC Public Health*, vol. 12, no. 1, p. 481, 2012.

[41] P. P. Pal, S. Sharma, T. K. Sarkar, and P. Mitra, "Iron and folic acid consumption by the ante-natal mothers in a rural area of India in 2010," *International Journal of Preventive Medicine*, vol. 4, no. 10, pp. 1213–1216, 2013.

[42] W. B. Lyoba, J. D. Mwakatoga, C. Festo, J. Mrema, and E. Elisaria, "Adherence to iron-folic acid supplementation and associated factors among pregnant women in Kasulu communities in north-western Tanzania," *International Journal of Reproductive Medicine*, vol. 2020, Article ID 3127245, 11 pages, 2020.

[43] L. Maina-Gathigi, J. Omolo, P. Wanzala, C. Lindan, and A. Makokha, "Utilization of folic acid and iron supplementa-

tion services by pregnant women attending an antenatal clinic at a regional referral hospital in Kenya," *Maternal and Child Health Journal*, vol. 17, no. 7, pp. 1236–1242, 2013.

[44] D. Warri, "Perceptions of pregnant women of reasons for late initiation of antenatal care: a qualitative interview study," *BMC Pregnancy and Childbirth*, vol. 20, no. 1, p. 70, 2020.

[45] I. Kisuule, D. K. Kaye, F. Najjuka et al., "Timing and reasons for coming late for the first antenatal care visit by pregnant women at Mulago hospital, Kampala Uganda," *BMC Pregnancy and Childbirth*, vol. 13, no. 1, p. 121, 2013.

22

A Comparative Study to Assess the Efficacy of Two Different Estradiol Formulations during In Vitro Fertilization

Manish Banker,[1] **Parul Arora**,[1] **Jwal Banker**,[2] **and Sandeep Shah**[1]

[1]*Nova IVF Fertility, Ahmedabad, India*
[2]*IVI RMA, Madrid, Spain*

Correspondence should be addressed to Parul Arora; drparul20arora@gmail.com

Academic Editor: Vikas Roy

Improvements in stimulation protocols, introduction of vitrification, and changes in clinical practices have contributed to improved efficacy and safety of assisted reproductive technology (ART) procedures. This has also led to a concomitant increase in number of cycles requiring hormone replacement therapy (HRT) protocol for performing an embryo transfer. Successful implantation is dependent on endometrial thickness which in turn is regulated by temporal regulation of hormones. Careful control of estrogen levels determines uterine receptivity. One of the most used drugs for achieving appropriate endometrial lining of >7 mm in HRT is estradiol valerate. Although different estrogen formulations with varying physicochemical properties exist, there is not enough literature to support if the differences translate into a discernible clinical outcome in an in vitro fertilization (IVF) setting. *Objective and Method.* In this study, retrospective in nature, we compare the efficacy of oral estradiol hemihydrate with estradiol valerate in HRT cycles in 2,529 Indian women, undergoing treatment at a center in India between Jan 2017 and May 2019. *Results.* Our results primarily indicate that between the estradiol valerate and estradiol hemihydrate treatment groups, the implantation rate (IR) was 47.42% and 49.07%, respectively (P value 0.284), and the endometrial thickness (mean ± SEM in mm) that was achieved was 9.25 ± 0.038 mm and 9.57 ± 0.058 mm (P value < 0.001), respectively. There were no significant differences observed in the secondary outcome measures including clinical pregnancy rate, abortion rate, ectopic pregnancy, and live birth rate. *Conclusions.* Hence, this study concludes that oral estradiol hemihydrate and estradiol valerate are therapeutically equivalent and provide similar clinical outcomes in an IVF setting.

1. Introduction

Ever since the first child born in 1978, assisted reproductive technology (ART) has emerged as one of the most significant and successful medical interventions contributing to approximately 0.1% of the global citizens [1]. Faddy et al. in his mathematical modelling projected that there would be approximately 157 million to 357 million people borne through ART by the turn of 21st century [1]. The European IVF-monitoring consortium for the European Society of Human Reproduction and Embryology (ESHRE) report using real-world data from 38 different countries reported that there was a 9.4% increase in the number of ART treatments that accounted for an increase in 7% of child births in 2015 compared to 2014 [2].

The successful cryopreservation of human embryos was first reported in 1983 using slow-cooling technique leading to the first live birth in 1984 [3]. These significant developments changed the course of in vitro fertilization (IVF) treatment and heralded further developments to follow in ART. Eventually, the method of rapid cooling and thawing known as vitrification was introduced which bypassed the difficulties and drawbacks associated with slow cooling. A comprehensive world report on ART for 2004 by the International Committee for Monitoring Assisted Reproductive Technologies (ICMART), noted that the change in clinical practice with reduced number of embryos transferred per attempt yielded favorable outcomes with a considerable decrease in the incidence of multiple births [4]. According to the ICMART 2011 report, the percentage of hormone replacement therapy (HRT) cycles, representing the fraction of frozen-thawed embryo transfer (FET) and oocyte donation cycles to the total embryo transfers, is about 55% [5]. Frozen embryo transfer and blastocyst transfer have been performed more often and have been shown to improve the cumulative pregnancy rates for each patient while eliminating multiple pregnancies [5]. Performance of fresh embryo transfer was seen to decline from 85.5% in 2010 to 79.8% in 2011 with a simultaneous increase in FET from 29.7% in 2010 to 31.3% in 2011 [5]. Frozen embryo transfer has improved neonatal outcomes and seemed to be associated with reduced ectopic pregnancy risk [6]. Earlier studies have illustrated either improvements or no change in ART outcomes following FET [7–12]. Moreover, with the advancements in vitrification techniques, FET provides temporal flexibility and allows the deferred use of all viable embryos obtained from a single egg collection. This has led to the suggestion of a "freeze all" strategy that might facilitate reintroducing the frozen-thawed embryos to a more "physiological" milieu, in harmony with the natural cycle, improving the outcomes [7, 13]. These advancements are quite valuable to those at risk of ovarian hyperstimulation syndrome (OHSS) and those requiring genetic testing to detect chromosomal abnormalities. As a result of such increasing trends due to a change in clinical practice, the percentage of cycles requiring HRT is expected to be higher.

Successful implantation is influenced by the intricate and synchronized crosstalk between good-quality embryos and a receptive endometrium. This initial process is modulated by the spatial-temporal regulation of different hormones at the uterine and ovarian level [14], specifically by estrogen and progesterone. Using a mouse model, a study by Ma et al. [15] has demonstrated that a very narrow range of estrogen levels determines the "window" of uterine receptivity, suggesting the careful regulation of estrogen levels as one of the major factors influencing the outcome in IVF and embryo transfer (IVF-ET) programs.

The regulation of estrogen levels is essential to control uterine receptivity for implantation [15, 16]. Endometrial thickness increases throughout the follicular phase under the influence of estrogen [17]. Following adequate estrogen priming of the endometrium, progesterone prepares the endometrium for implantation [18]. Estrogen enables contraction of spiral arteries resulting in hypoxia in the functional layers and promotes endometrial proliferation. [19]. Since exogenous administration of estrogen is required to increase the serum estrogen within a required range, it is important to be selective and understand the nature of such estrogen interventions. The pharmacological and clinical similarities or dissimilarities need good quality clinical validations.

The common forms in current use are estradiol valerate and micronized estrogens. One of them, estradiol valerate, has been regularly employed in IVF [20, 21]. There is not enough literature to ascertain whether the different esters and salts of estradiol act differently and if any such differences translate into valid clinical significance. Monitoring endometrial thickness in cycles using a HRT protocol provides the best model to study and compare the different estrogen compounds because the endometrium in these cycles is completely under the control of exogenously administered drugs [22, 23]. The aim of our study is to analyzeretrospectively if oral estradiol hemihydrate and estradiol valerate are equally efficacious or dissimilar when used in a HRT protocol. Since we are comparing two different estrogen products, the strongest predictors of estrogenic activity, viz., endometrial thickness and implantation rate (IR), are analyzed as primary outcomes. Secondary outcome measures included in the study are clinical pregnancy rate, abortion rate, live birth rate, and ectopic pregnancy. This study compares the clinical efficacy of two estrogen products in IVF treatment.

2. Materials and Methods

This is a retrospective study examining the treatment outcomes of HRT cycles in women during the period from January 2017 to December 2017 (estradiol valerate group) and from October 2018 to May 2019 (estradiol hemihydrate group), at Nova IVF Fertility, Ahmedabad, India. All women ($n = 2529$) who underwent an embryo transfer using the HRT protocol with the transfer of a single/double blastocyst were included in the study. These embryos were either frozen-thawed embryos using self or donor oocytes (OD), or donor embryos (ED), or fresh transfers with embryos using donor oocytes or donor embryos (OD/ED). These samples will be accordingly referred to as thaw self or thaw OD/ED or fresh OD/ED, respectively. Since the study was retrospective in nature, prior ethics approval was not sought. All the participants had consented (written informed) to sharing of their treatment records and outcome before initiating treatment at the clinic, and patient data to produce this paper was used only after their consent for use of their data for research purposes was provided.

2.1. Exclusion Criteria. Women suspected or diagnosed to have an endometrial pathology (suspected adhesions, polyps, fibroids, or poor endometrium during HRT) during endometrial preparation or history of poor endometrium were excluded from the study. Women who did not have viable fresh or frozen blastocyst/s for transfer on the embryo transfer day were also excluded.

2.2. Study Protocol. The HRT regimen commenced from day 2 of the menstrual period and used estradiol valerate tablets or estradiol hemihydrate 2 mg orally twice daily for 4 days and then 4 mg twice daily for 10 days. Measurement of endometrial thickness was done between the two echogenic borders of endometrium at the midsagittal plane. During the study period Jan 1st–Dec 31st, 2017, all the recruited women were administered estradiol valerate for endometrial preparation. During the study period from 1st October 2018 to 31st May 2019, all women were administered estradiol hemihydrate for endometrial preparation during HRT cycle. Women in either group were assessed on day 10/11 of the menstrual cycle after the initiation of HRT. A transvaginal scan was performed for assessment of endometrial thickness. Adequate endometrial preparation was defined as an endometrial thickness of at least 7 mm with trilaminar appearance [22]. In case the endometrium was not adequate, the estradiol preparation was added vaginally (2 mg twice daily) and the sonography repeated after 4–5 days. Once the endometrium was adequately prepared, serum progesterone levels were measured after the endometrial assessment. Progesterone supplementation was initiated if the serum progesterone values were <0.5 ng/mL. Progesterone was administered orally (dydrogesterone 10 mg twice daily along with micronized progesterone vaginal suppositories 400 mg twice daily). A maximum of two blastocysts were transferred after 5 days of progesterone supplementation. Serum beta human chorionic gonadotropin (B-hCG) levels were measured 14 days after embryo transfer to confirm pregnancy.

2.3. Outcome Measures. Outcomes were measured and compared across all HRT cycles using thaw self or thaw OD/ED or fresh OD/ED between the two treatment groups receiving either estradiol valerate or estradiol hemihydrate. Since the objective of the study is to see if there were differences between the two estradiol products, (1) endometrial thickness and (2) IR in HRT cycles were chosen as primary outcome measures. These two measures are directly linked to estrogen activity. Clinical pregnancy rate, abortion rate, ectopic pregnancy rate, and live birth rate were considered as secondary outcome measures.

2.4. Statistical Analysis. Statistical analyses of the data were performed using GraphPad Prism 8 software and Microsoft Excel. For the descriptive analyses, results were expressed for numerical data as means ± standard deviations, for categorical variables as number and percentage. The minimum and maximum values are also provided in some cases. The null hypothesis assumed was that the average effect of the two treatments with estradiol valerate or with estradiol hemihydrate is not different. The statistical analysis comparing the data pertaining to primary outcome measures was performed using Welch's t-test, and $P < 0.05$ was considered significant. For the secondary outcome measures, statistical analysis using t-test for difference in proportions was used and $P < 0.05$ was significant.

3. Results and Discussion

3.1. Demographic Characteristics. The demographic descriptions of treatment groups are given Tables 1 and 2. There were no significant differences between the two treatment groups. Table 2 lists the individual demographic variables for the groups classified based on the embryo transfer cycle. There was no significant difference in the variables among these groups.

A total of 3,552 embryo transfers using the HRT protocol, corresponding to 2,476 patients, during the study period were analyzed. The embryo transfer cycle was categorized into three: (a) frozen-thawed transfer using self-oocytes (thaw self), (b) frozen-thawed embryo transfer from OD/ED (thaw OD/ED), or (c) fresh OD/ED transfer cycles (fresh OD/ED). Estrogenic preparation of the endometrium was achieved in all the three embryo transfer cycle categories with forms of estradiol formulations (Table 1). This is a retrospective study, and the two-sample population were assessed for variability. Demographic variables including age, partner age, body mass index (BMI), and years of infertility were comparable between the two treatment groups receiving either estradiol valerate or estradiol hemihydrate (Tables 1 and 2).

3.2. Primary Outcome Measures

3.2.1. Endometrial Thickness as a Direct Measure of the Treatment Outcome. The HRT treatment regimen was initiated on day 2 of the menstrual cycle by administering oral estrogen in the form of either estrogen valerate or hemihydrate. In all the treatment groups after estrogen administration, there was an increase in the endometrial thickness (Table 3). Irrespective of the different embryo transfer cycles, the two treatment groups receiving either estradiol hemihydrate or estradiol valerate displayed an adequate endometrial line thickness (Table 3). The endometrial assessment was first performed after 10 days of estrogen initiation. The endometrial line thickness was assessed by transvaginal scan, and it was 9.251 ± 0.038 mm and 9.566 ± 0.0579 mm in the estradiol valerate and hemihydrate groups, respectively (Tables 3 and 4).

3.2.2. Comparison of Implantation Rate. Implantation rate (IR), calculated as the proportion of gestational sacs observed on ultrasonography to the number of transferred embryos, for the two treatment groups is presented in Table 5. IR, expressed as percentage (%), is comparable between the two treatment groups. IR for estradiol valerate versus estradiol hemihydrate in the thaw-self category was 46.52% vs. 47.89%; in the fresh OD/ED category, it was 57.3% vs. 56.7%; and in the thaw OD/ED embryo transfer cycle group, it was 40.98% vs. 44.77%, respectively (Table 5). The statistical analysis of the test of proportions did not indicate any significant difference between the two treatment groups.

3.3. Secondary Outcome Measures. The pregnancy outcome was not statistically different between the two groups. Clinical pregnancy rate was comparable between the two groups (58.61% in the estradiol valerate group and 59.57% in the estradiol hemihydrate group). Clinical abortion rate was about 17.86–26.85% in the estradiol valerate-treated group and was about 17.04–22.97% in the estradiol hemihydrate group. Occurrence of ectopic pregnancy events was negligible with only three in the estradiol valerate-treated frozen-thawed embryo transfer cycle and only one observed in the estradiol hemihydrate frozen-thawed using self-oocyte cycle. The occurrence of ectopic pregnancy is nil in the fresh OD/ED or thaw OD/ED groups irrespective of estradiol valerate or estradiol hemihydrate treatment groups. The live birth rate (LBR) was similar between the two groups (Table 6). There was no significant difference in the LBR between estradiol valerate and estradiol hemihydrate treatment groups (45.63% and 47.93%, respectively; relative risk, 0.95; P value = 0.532). Comparing the LBR in the two treatment groups, individually for the thaw self or fresh OD/ED or thaw OD/ED categories, it also did not show any

TABLE 1: Demographic details of the two treatment groups.

	Estradiol valerate	Estradiol hemihydrate	P value
N	1556	920	
Age (mean ± SD)	33.84 ± 5.44	33.78 ± 5.24	0.6566 (NS)
BMI (mean ± SD)	26.891 ± 5.12	26.63 ± 5.17	0.261 (NS)
Partner age (mean ± SD)	36.56 ± 6.22	36.56 ± 6.40	0.8549 (NS)

NS: not statistically significant; SD: standard deviation; BMI: body mass index.

TABLE 2: Description of patient population in the two treatment groups.

Variable	Estradiol valerate			Estradiol hemihydrate		
	Thaw self	Fresh OD/ED	Thaw OD/ED	Thaw self	Fresh OD/ED	Fresh OD/ED
N	734	415	407	453	202	265
Age (years)						
Mean	30.62	36.59	36.82	31.13	36.50	36.27
SD	3.52	5.254	5.27	3.48	4.98	4.646
Min	20	20	23	21	24	23
Max	43	52	50	51	48	49
20–29	265	33	33	162	17	31
30–39	467	260	247	287	125	157
≥40	2	113	130	6	60	78
BMI (kg/m^2)						
Mean	26.76	27.05	27.01	26.73	26.51	26.54
SD	5.05	5.03	5.34	5.42	4.63	5.14
Partner age (years)						
Mean	33.67	38.88	39.12	34.39	39.09	38.94
SD	4.12	6.45	7.6	4.36	6.48	6.34
Min	23	22	24	23	25	22
Max	67	60	60	52	63	63
20–29	104	14	16	59	8	11
30–39	573	225	195	319	103	135
≥40	56	176	192	53	89	118
Years of infertility (years)						
Mean	4.24	7.53	8.041	4.26	7.045	7.135
SD	3.075	6.503	6.654	3.33	6.079	5.729
Min	0	0	0	0	0	0
Max	18	32	30	17	25	25

OD/ED: donor oocyte/donor embryo; SD: standard deviation; Min: minimum; Max: maximum.

TABLE 3: Endometrial line thickness corresponding to different treatment groups.

	Thaw self		Fresh OD/ED		Thaw OD/ED	
	Estradiol valerate	Estradiol hemihydrate	Estradiol valerate	Estradiol hemihydrate	Estradiol valerate	Estradiol hemihydrate
N	734	453	415	202	407	265
Mean thickness (mm)	9.25	9.63	9.324	9.69	9.17	9.37
SEM	0.0592	0.089	0.065	0.114	0.073	0.099
P value	0.00047**		0.0056*		0.054	

OD/ED: donor oocyte/donor embryo; SEM: standard error mean. $^*P < 0.01$; $^{**}P < 0.001$.

Table 4: Endometrial line thickness corresponding to the two treatment groups.

	Endometrial line thickness	
	Estradiol valerate	Estradiol hemihydrate
N	1555	920
Mean days	9.251 mm	9.566 mm
SEM	0.038	0.0579
P value	$P < 0.0001^{***}$	

SEM: standard error mean; ***statistical significance of $P < 0.0001$.

Table 5: Implantation rates of the two treatments.

	Total number of embryos transferred	Implantation rate (IR) (%) (ratio)
Thaw self		
Estradiol valerate	1285	46.69% (600/1285)
Estradiol hemihydrate	765	47.89% (365/765)
P value	0.646	
Fresh OD/ED		
Estradiol valerate	728	57.3% (402/728)
Estradiol hemihydrate	342	56.7% (197/342)
P value	0.4611	
Thaw OD/ED		
Estradiol valerate	718	40.98% (293/718)
Estradiol hemihydrate	452	44.77% (203/452)
P value	0.167	
Total		
Estradiol valerate	2731	47.42% (1295/2731)
Estradiol hemihydrate	1559	49.07% (765/1559)
P value	0.284	

OD/ED: donor oocyte/donor embryo.

significant variation. The rates of biochemical pregnancy (PR), clinical pregnancy (CPR), and clinical abortion (CAB) also did not differ significantly between the two groups (Table 6). Overall, the statistical analysis for difference in proportions did not indicate any difference between the two treatment groups irrespective of the embryo transfer protocols.

4. Discussion

The advent of technological advancement, especially vitrification and changes implemented in the practice of ART, has seen significant trend towards increasing number of cycles having an embryo transfer using HRT. This also facilitates genetic testing of embryos, assists those at risk of OHSS, and has a role in fertility preservation [13].

Estrogen supplementation is a crucial and integral part of all HRT protocols. The three common forms of estrogen are estrone (E1), estradiol (E2), and estriol (E3) [15, 24–27]. Estradiol, also referred to as estradiol-17β, is the most common and potent form of estrogen [28]. Estrogen could be administered as natural estrogens, conjugated equine estrogen (CEE), or synthetic estrogens. However, estradiol in the natural form has a disadvantage of poor bioavailability [28].

Oral estrogen medications owing to their ease of administration and rapid reversibility are usually preferred in HRT. However, estrogen administered by oral route succumbs to increased rate of metabolism in the gut and liver resulting in higher estrone/estradiol ratio. With a prospect of improving the bioavailability and further enhance the clinical outcomes, alterations of physicochemical characteristics of estradiol have led to the development of varying esters or forms of estradiol. Therefore, esters of estradiol or other synthetic estrogens with chemical variations having potential to offer pharmacological advantages have been regularly employed for the IVF process. Microcrystalline estradiol offers increased surface area and therefore expected to offer greater bioavailability: the smaller the crystal, the better the absorption. Crystals of estradiol hemihydrate contain minimum water and is a repeated stacked arrangement of two molecules of estradiol associated with one molecule of water. Following dissolution, the water molecule does not have a pharmacological role. Estradiol and its hemihydrate form are identical in terms of bioequivalence and activity, with only 3% difference in potency by weight (attributed due to presence of water molecules in hemihydrate form). Estradiol hemihydrate is more hydrated than anhydrous estradiol and is more insoluble in water in comparison, which may result in slower absorption rates with specific formulations of the drug such as vaginal tablets. Administration of 1 mg of oral micronized estradiol resulted in an E2 C_{max} of 40–50 pg/mL and an E1 C_{max} of 200 pg/mL. Pharmacokinetic parameters with oral administration of 2 mg of micronized estradiol had a T_{max} of 8.2 hours and a terminal half-life of 13.5 hours for estradiol. For estrone, T_{max} was 6.3 hours and terminal half-life was estimated to be 11.2 hours [29, 30]. Estradiol valerate is an ester of the C17-hydroxy group of estradiol with valeric acid. This formulation prevents the usual metabolism of estradiol to estrone until hydrolysis has taken place. Upon hydrolysis in the intestines to estradiol and valeric acid, the resulting estradiol is rapidly absorbed. During oral treatment, the peak levels of estradiol obtained with either 2 mg estradiol hemihydrate or estradiol valerate were 40 pg/mL on day 1 and 80 pg/mL on day 21 [28, 31]. In terms of indication, AUC (area under the curve), dosing behavior, and adverse effects, there is no difference between both the molecules [32]. Therefore, after oral administration, the pharmacokinetics of estradiol valerate or micronized estradiol remain comparable and the bioavailability is about 5% [30, 33]. Accordingly, estradiol hemihydrate and the valerate are dose equivalent [33]. Although there are clear differences in the physicochemical properties of these

TABLE 6: Measures of secondary outcome of the two treatments.

	Enrolled number of patients N	Pregnancy rate (PR) N_{PR} (%)	Clinical pregnancy rate (CPR) N_{CPR}/N (%)	Clinical abortion (CAB) N_{CAB}/N_{CPR} (%)	Ectopic (EC) N_{EC}/N_{CPR} (%)	Live birth rate (LBR) N_{LBR}/N (%)
Thaw self						
Estradiol valerate	734	457 (62.26%)	416/734 (56.68%)	91/416 (21.88%)	3/416 (0.72%)	322/734 (43.87%)
Estradiol hemihydrate	453	288 (63.58%)	265/453 (58.50%)	49/265 (18.49%)	1/265 (0.38%)	215/453 (47.46%)
P value		0.648	0.535	0.286	—	0.227
Fresh OD/ED						
Estradiol valerate	415	308 (74.21%)	280/415 (67.47%)	50/280 (17.86%)	0	230/415 (55.42%)
Estradiol hemihydrate	202	150 (74.25%)	135/202 (66.83%)	23/135 (17.04%)	0	112/202 (55.45%)
P value		0.9912	0.874	0.837	—	0.382
Thaw OD/ED						
Estradiol valerate	407	252 (61.92%)	216/407 (53.07%)	58/216 (26.85%)	0	158/407 (38.82%)
Estradiol hemihydrate	265	167 (63.02%)	148/265 (55.85%)	34/148 (22.97%)	0	114/265 (43.02%)
P value		0.773	0.48	0.403	—	0.631
Total						
Estradiol valerate	1556	1017 (65.36%)	912/1556 (58.61%)	199/912 (21.82%)	3/912 (0.33%	710/1556 (45.63%)
Estradiol hemihydrate	920	605 (65.76%)	548/920 (59.57%)	106/548 (19.34%)	1/548 (0.18%)	441/920 (47.93%)
P value		0.84	0.625	0.259	—	0.532

PR: pregnancy rate; CPR: clinical pregnancy rate; CAB: clinical abortion; EC: ectopic pregnancy; LBR: live birth rate; OD/ED: donor oocyte/donor embryo; NPR, NCR, NEC, and NLBR: number of instances of pregnancy, clinical pregnancy, ectopic pregnancy, and live birth rate, respectively.

formulations of estradiol, whether these translate into a clinically discernible difference is debatable. A recent study comparing the estradiol levels according to dose and formulation in postmenopausal women using hormonal replacement therapy found similar serum estradiol levels with estradiol valerate and hemihydrate [34].

Our study, for the first time, compares two oral formulations of estradiol with varying physicochemical characteristics from the standpoint of clinical outcomes up to live birth rates. Specifically, we analyzed the clinical outcomes in an IVF setting upon exogenous introduction of estrogen in the form of either oral estradiol valerate or estradiol hemihydrate, administered at 2 mg twice daily and then 4 mg. In this study, we have considered only those cycles with the HRT protocol. Our results indicate that treatments with either estradiol valerate or estradiol hemihydrate improved the endometrial receptivity, indicated by increase in endometrial thickness (Tables 3 and 4). The endometrial thickness achieved by both compounds is adequate though there is a significant increase (of 0.351 mm; $P < 0.0001$) in thickness in the hemihydrate group. The cut-off for a thin endometrium has remained variable across different studies, and the clinical outcomes are affected for every millimeter variation in endometrial thickness only below 8 mm for fresh embryo transfer and 7 mm for FET cycles [35]. Although statistically significant, the difference in endometrial thickness between the two treatment groups is minimal (0.351 mm), both above 9 mm, and hence should not translate into any clinically significant difference. The implantation rate measured as the proportion of gestational sacs observed on sonography to the number of embryos transferred did not significantly differ between the two treatment groups (Table 5). These primary results suggest that estradiol hemihydrate is not inferior to estradiol valerate in terms of efficacy. Recent studies by Vartanyan et al. also report increased thickness with estradiol hemihydrate as compared to valerate though it was administered transdermally. They also reported higher implantation rates in the transdermal hemihydrate group [36]. Further, there was no significant difference between the secondary outcomes including clinical pregnancy rate, abortion rate, and ectopic pregnancy. Ultimately, the desired clinical outcome for the success of the treatment is the LBR. There was no difference observed in the LBR outcome of the treatments using these two compounds in all the three subgroups studied. We have not observed any adverse symptoms attributable to overdose of estradiol in any of our study subjects.

5. Conclusions

Although it is a retrospective real-life data analysis of the two different preparations of estradiol, this is the first study where the two oral estradiol compounds have been compared for their clinical effects across various treatments in ART involving HRT cycles. The results of this large study ($n = 2476$) show that there is no significant difference between these two different forms of estradiol in terms of efficacy in endometrial preparation (measured as endometrial thickness) and the clinical outcomes (measured as implantation rates, clinical pregnancy rates, abortion rates, and live birth rates) [28, 37].

Additional Points

What is Known. There has been gradual and sustained increase in assisted reproductive technology (ART) cycles requiring hormone replacement therapy (HRT) due to improvements in stimulation protocols, introduction of vitrification, and changes in clinical practice. Estrogens have been used for successful endometrial preparations in HRT. Due to the major concern with lower bioavailability, several formulations of estrogens have been developed. *What is New.* While there are esters and salt formulations of estrogen with varying physicochemical properties, this large-scale retrospective analysis reviews for the first time to our knowledge any potential clinical advantages of one over the other. Specifically, we have compared for the first time oral estrogen valerate and estrogen hemihydrate in the context of endometrial preparation for various HRT treatment groups in in vitro fertilization (IVF) treatment. We report that these two estradiol preparations are similar in our study.

Authors' Contributions

All the four authors contributed to the concept and design of the study, interpretation of the data, critical revision of the manuscript, and approval of the manuscript. Dr. Manish Banker and Dr. Parul Arora were involved in the data acquisition. Dr. Manish Banker, Dr. Parul Arora, and Dr. Jwal Banker were involved in the statistical analysis and drafting the manuscript.

Acknowledgments

The authors thank Medlish Communications for providing medical writing services.

References

[1] M. J. Faddy, M. D. Gosden, and R. G. Gosden, "A demographic projection of the contribution of assisted reproductive technologies to world population growth," *Reproductive Biomedicine Online*, vol. 36, no. 4, pp. 455–458, 2018.

[2] C. de Geyter, C. Calhaz-Jorge, M. S. Kupka et al., "ART in Europe, 2015: results generated from European registries by ESHRE," *Human Reproduction Open*, vol. 2020, no. 1, 2020.

[3] G. H. Zeilmaker, A. T. Alberda, I. van Gent, C. M. Rijkmans, and A. C. Drogendijk, "Two pregnancies following transfer of intact frozen-thawed embryos," *Fertility and Sterility*, vol. 42, no. 2, pp. 293–296, 1984.

[4] E. A. Sullivan, F. Zegers-Hochschild, R. Mansour et al., "International Committee for Monitoring Assisted Reproductive Technologies (ICMART) world report: assisted reproductive technology 2004," *Human Reproduction*, vol. 28, no. 5, pp. 1375–1390, 2013.

[5] G. D. Adamson, J. de Mouzon, G. M. Chambers et al., "International Committee for Monitoring Assisted Reproductive Technology: world report on assisted reproductive technology,

2011," *Fertility and Sterility*, vol. 110, no. 6, pp. 1067–1080, 2018.

[6] O. Ishihara, R. Araki, A. Kuwahara, A. Itakura, H. Saito, and G. D. Adamson, "Impact of frozen-thawed single-blastocyst transfer on maternal and neonatal outcome: an analysis of 277,042 single-embryo transfer cycles from 2008 to 2010 in Japan," *Fertility and Sterility*, vol. 101, no. 1, pp. 128–133, 2014.

[7] M. Roque, M. Valle, A. Kostolias, M. Sampaio, and S. Geber, "Freeze-all cycle in reproductive medicine: current perspectives," *JBRA Assisted Reproduction*, vol. 21, no. 1, pp. 49–53, 2017.

[8] M. Noble and T. Child, "The role of frozen–thawed embryo replacement cycles in assisted conception," *Obstetrics and Gynecology*, vol. 22, no. 1, pp. 57–68, 2020.

[9] K. M. Wong, M. van Wely, F. Mol, S. Repping, and S. Mastenbroek, "Fresh versus frozen embryo transfers in assisted reproduction," *Cochrane Database of Systematic Reviews*, vol. 3, no. 3, 2017.

[10] A. Maheshwari, S. Pandey, E. Amalraj Raja, A. Shetty, M. Hamilton, and S. Bhattacharya, "Is frozen embryo transfer better for mothers and babies? Can cumulative meta-analysis provide a definitive answer?," *Human Reproduction Update*, vol. 24, no. 1, pp. 35–58, 2018.

[11] C. Blockeel, P. Drakopoulos, S. Santos-Ribeiro, N. P. Polyzos, and H. Tournaye, "A fresh look at the freeze-all protocol: a SWOT analysis," *Human Reproduction*, vol. 31, no. 3, pp. 491–497, 2016.

[12] Y. Zheng, Z. Li, M. Xiong et al., "Hormonal replacement treatment improves clinical pregnancy in frozen-thawed embryos transfer cycles: a retrospective cohort study," *American Journal of Translational Research*, vol. 6, no. 1, pp. 85–90, 2013.

[13] K. A. Rodriguez-Wallberg, M. Waterstone, and A. Anastácio, "Ice age: Cryopreservation in assisted reproduction - An update," *Reproductive Biology*, vol. 19, no. 2, pp. 119–126, 2019.

[14] H. Matsumoto, "Molecular and cellular events during blastocyst implantation in the receptive uterus: clues from mouse models," *The Journal of Reproduction and Development*, vol. 63, no. 5, pp. 445–454, 2017.

[15] W. G. Ma, H. Song, S. K. Das, B. C. Paria, and S. K. Dey, "Estrogen is a critical determinant that specifies the duration of the window of uterine receptivity for implantation," *Proceedings of the National Academy of Sciences of the United States of America*, vol. 100, no. 5, pp. 2963–2968, 2003.

[16] C. Simón, J. J. Garcia Velasco, D. Valbuena et al., "Increasing uterine receptivity by decreasing estradiol levels during the preimplantation period in high responders with the use of a follicle- stimulating hormone step-down regimen," *Fertility and Sterility*, vol. 70, no. 2, pp. 234–239, 1998.

[17] S. Gupta, A. Tempe, and L. Sahu, "Supplementation with estradiol valerate and gonadotropins in clomiphene citrate stimulated IUI cycles," *International Journal of Biomedical and Advance Research*, vol. 5, no. 4, p. 211, 2014.

[18] N. Ranisavljevic, J. Raad, T. Anahory, M. Grynberg, and C. Sonigo, "Embryo transfer strategy and therapeutic options in infertile patients with thin endometrium: a systematic review," *Journal of Assisted Reproduction and Genetics*, vol. 36, no. 11, pp. 2217–2231, 2019.

[19] Y. Mouhayar and F. I. Sharara, "Modern management of thin lining," *Middle East Fertility Society Journal*, vol. 22, no. 1, pp. 1–12, 2017.

[20] Z. Kalem, M. Namli Kalem, and T. Gurgan, "Methods for endometrial preparation in frozen-thawed embryo transfer cycles," *Journal of the Turkish German Gynecological Association*, vol. 17, no. 3, pp. 168–172, 2016.

[21] P. Devroey and G. Pados, "Preparation of endometrium for egg donation," *Human Reproduction Update*, vol. 4, no. 6, pp. 856–861, 1998.

[22] J. Zhao, Q. Zhang, and Y. Li, "The effect of endometrial thickness and pattern measured by ultrasonography on pregnancy outcomes during IVF-ET cycles," *Reproductive Biology and Endocrinology*, vol. 10, no. 1, 2012.

[23] R. F. Casper and E. H. Yanushpolsky, "Optimal endometrial preparation for frozen embryo transfer cycles: window of implantation and progesterone support," *Fertility and Sterility*, vol. 105, no. 4, pp. 867–872, 2016.

[24] M. P. Thomas and B. V. Potter, "The structural biology of oestrogen metabolism," *The Journal of Steroid Biochemistry and Molecular Biology*, vol. 137, pp. 27–49, 2013.

[25] G. J. Pepe and E. D. Albrecht, "Actions of placental and fetal adrenal steroid hormones in primate pregnancy," *Endocrine Reviews*, vol. 16, no. 5, pp. 608–648, 1995.

[26] R. M. Kamel, "The onset of human parturition," *Archives of Gynecology and Obstetrics*, vol. 281, no. 6, pp. 975–982, 2010.

[27] S. D. Silberstein and G. R. Merriam, "Physiology of the menstrual cycle," *Cephalalgia*, vol. 20, no. 3, pp. 148–154, 2000.

[28] H. Kuhl, "Pharmacology of estrogens and progestogens: influence of different routes of administration," *Climacteric*, vol. 8, supplement 1, pp. 3–63, 2005.

[29] M. B. O'connell, "Pharmacokinetic and pharmacologic variation between different estrogen products," *Journal of Clinical Pharmacology*, vol. 35, no. 9S, pp. 18S–24S, 1995.

[30] W. Kuhnz, C. Gansau, and M. Mahler, "Pharmacokinetics of estradiol, free and total estrone, in young women following single intravenous and oral administration of 17 beta-estradiol," *Arzneimittel-Forschung*, vol. 43, no. 9, pp. 966–973, 1993.

[31] T. Price, K. Blauer, M. Hansen, F. Stanczyk, R. Lobo, and G. Bates, "Single-dose pharmacokinetics of sublingual versus oral administration of micronized 17 β -estradiol," *Obstetrics and Gynecology*, vol. 89, no. 3, pp. 340–345, 1997.

[32] C. J. Timmer and T. B. Geurts, "Bioequivalence assessment of three different estradiol formulations in postmenopausal women in an open, randomized, single-dose, 3-way crossover study," *European Journal of Drug Metabolism and Pharmacokinetics*, vol. 24, no. 1, pp. 47–53, 1999.

[33] B. Düsterberg and Y. Nishino, "Pharmacokinetic and pharmacological features of oestradiol valerate," *Maturitas*, vol. 4, no. 4, pp. 315–324, 1982.

[34] S. M. Kim, S. E. Kim, D. Y. Lee, and D. S. Choi, "Serum estradiol level according to dose and formulation of oral estrogens in postmenopausal women," *Scientific Reports*, vol. 11, no. 1, 2021.

[35] K. E. Liu, M. Hartman, A. Hartman, Z. C. Luo, and N. Mahutte, "The impact of a thin endometrial lining on fresh and frozen–thaw IVF outcomes: an analysis of over 40 000 embryo transfers," *Human Reproduction*, vol. 33, no. 10, pp. 1883–1888, 2018.

[36] E. Vartanyan, K. Tsaturova, and E. Devyatova, "Thin endometrium problem in IVF programs," *Gynecological Endocrinology*, vol. 36, supplement 1, pp. 24–27, 2020.

23

Biochemical Assessment of Renal and Liver Function among Preeclamptics in Lagos Metropolis

Oloruntoba Ayodele Ekun,[1] **Oluwatumininu Mary Olawumi**,[1] **Christian Chigozie Makwe**,[2] **and Nkeiruka Ogochukwu Ogidi**[1]

[1]*Department of Medical Laboratory Science, College of Medicine, University of Lagos, Nigeria*
[2]*Department of Obstetrics and Gynaecology, College of Medicine, University of Lagos, Nigeria*

Correspondence should be addressed to Oloruntoba Ayodele Ekun; ayodele1619.oe@gmail.com

Academic Editor: Daniel Vaiman

Objectives. Preeclampsia is a pregnancy specific syndrome. Studies have shown that preeclampsia has multiorgan dysfunction effects. This study evaluated biomarkers of renal and liver function among preeclamptic Nigerian women. *Study Design.* This was a cross-sectional study conducted among 49 preeclamptic women and 50 normotensive healthy pregnant women. *Method.* The baseline data comprising age, gestational age, and blood pressure were obtained. Venous blood and spot urine samples were collected from each participant. Plasma obtained from blood samples taken into lithium heparinized vacutainer bottles was assayed for electrolytes, urea, creatinine, total protein, albumin, and uric acid, while sera samples from blood samples taken into serum separation tube- (SST-) gel vacutainer were assayed for aspartate transaminase and alanine transaminase using ion selective electrode technique and Cobas autoanalyzer. Spot urine samples were assayed for protein and creatinine using Pyrogallol's reagent and Jaffe's methods, respectively. Microalbuminuria (protein/creatinine ratio) was generated from spot urine protein and creatinine data. *Result.* The plasma sodium, total protein, and albumin in preeclamptic group were significantly decreased ($p<0.05$) when compared with control. There was statistically significant increase ($p<0.05$) in microalbuminuria, plasma potassium, urea, creatinine, uric acid levels, serum AST, and ALT activities in preeclamptic group. A positive association ($p<0.05$) between alanine aminotransferase and biomarkers of renal function was observed. *Conclusion.* Preeclampsia has deleterious effects on renal and liver function as shown by alteration of these parameters.

1. Introduction

Preeclampsia has been described as a systemic syndrome of pregnancy, which is characterized by a new onset high blood pressure (systolic ≥140 mmHg or diastolic ≥90 mmHg) and proteinuria of ≥ 0.3 grams per 24 hours that occurs after 20 weeks of gestation in a woman that was previously normotensive [1]. It has been suggested to be a disease of the placenta, which possibly resulted from impaired trophoblast differentiation and invasion during early pregnancy. This impairment possibly stimulates sustained oxidative stress and a systemic inflammatory response in the affected women [2]. As recommended by the International Society for the Study of Hypertension in Pregnancy, the diagnosis of preeclampsia should requires blood pressures of 140/90 mmHg or higher on two occasions combined with either urinary protein excretion of ≥300mg/day or new onset of maternal organ dysfunction (creatinine ≥ 90μmol/l), liver involvement (elevated transaminases), haematological complication (thrombocytopenia platelet <150,000/cmm), neurological complications, and fetal growth restriction [3]. Laboratory tests, such as liver function tests, quantification of urinary protein, or serum creatinine, may be helpful in characterizing the degree of end-organ damage, but none is specific for preeclampsia. It has been observed that preeclampsia has deleterious effects on maternal and perinatal health, particularly in the developing nations of the world [2]. It is a major complication of pregnancy [1]. It has been suggested that pregnant women with preeclampsia or eclampsia are likely to be at higher risk of end stage kidney disease and high blood pressure later in life [4, 5]. While most studies have been undertaken in high-income settings, some inconsistencies exist especially in developing settings where preeclampsia risk factors have been less explored [6].

A previous study suggested that women with severe preeclampsia possibly exhibits more prominent signs and symptoms of end-organ damage that may result in life-threatening disease [7]. Multiple organ systems may be affected in severe preeclampsia including dysfunction of the central nervous system (could lead to blurred vision, altered mental status, severe headache, and cerebrovascular accident), liver (which results in elevated serum transaminases), [3, 7] cardiovascular system (systolic blood pressure ≥160 mm Hg or diastolic ≥110 mm Hg), lungs (pulmonary edema, cyanosis), and/or kidneys [7]. Twenty-four hour urinary protein level is twice the normal limit in nonpregnant women [8].

Preeclampsia is more common in women with an underlying kidney disease. On the other hand, it has been suggested that preeclampsia itself increases the risk of kidney disease later in life [9]. It is a disease with worldwide significance to mothers and infants; it may have health hazards that increase maternal, fetal, and infant morbidity and mortality [8, 9]. It has been shown that preeclampsia has greatest impact in developing countries, where it accounts for 20-80% of strikingly increased maternal mortality, while in developed countries, preeclampsia has a major effect on fetuses and neonates [7–9].

2. Materials and Methods

2.1. Participants Selection and Study Design. A cross-sectional study was conducted on female preeclamptic patients attending Lagos University Teaching Hospital (LUTH), Ifako General Hospital, Isolo General Hospital, Lagos Island Maternity Hospital, and Amuwo Odofin Mother and Child Centre. A total of ninety-nine participants were recruited into this study, comprising 50 apparently healthy normotensive pregnant participants without urinary protein and 49 preeclamptic participants. This study was conducted between July and November 2017. Blood and spot urine samples were collected in the morning from all consenting participants, since proteinuria is known to exhibit circadian rhythm [10, 11]. The blood samples were collected into lithium heparinized and serum separation tube- (SST-) gel vacutainer bottles; the samples were centrifuged at 3,000 revolution per minute (rpm) for five minutes. Plasma and serum were extracted from lithium heparinized and SST-gel vacutainer, respectively. The samples were kept frozen at -20°C pending analysis.

2.2. Ethical Consideration. Approval was obtained from the Research and Ethics Committee of College of Medicine of University of Lagos (CMUL) and Lagos State Health Service Commission (HSC) prior to the commencement of the study. Informed consent was sought and obtained from each participant prior to the commencement of this study.

2.3. Inclusion Criteria. The inclusion criteria for this study include the following:

Apparently healthy pregnant volunteers with gestational age greater than 20 weeks, preeclamptic women with no previous history of hypertension and proteinuria before gestational age of 20 weeks and above.

2.4. Exclusion Criteria. The exclusion criteria for this study include the following:

pregnant women with other medical conditions such as viral hepatitis, diabetes mellitus renal failure, autoimmune diseases, anaemia, tuberculosis, chronic hypertension, and myeloproliferative disorders.

2.5. Methodology. Electrolytes were analyzed with SFRI 4000 ion selective electrode (ISE), while plasma urea, creatinine, uric acid, total protein, albumin, serum aspartate amino transferase, and alanine amino transferase were analyzed using Cobas C111 autoanalyzer by Roche. Spot urine creatinine and protein were determined using Biosystem BTS 350 semi-autoanalyzer by Biosystems SFA Pro.

2.6. Data Analysis. The data from the study was analyzed using SPSS version 21.0. Quantitative data were expressed as mean, standard deviation, and standard error of mean. Independent t-test was used to compare the groups. Pearson correlation coefficient was used to evaluate the degree of association. The level of significance for all the inferential statistics was set at $p<0.05$

3. Results

Table 1 presents the mean age, the gestational age, systolic pressure, and diastolic pressure of the participants in this study. There was a significant ($p<0.05$) increase in both the systolic and diastolic blood pressure among preeclamptic group. The comparative statistical analysis of plasma electrolytes, urea, creatinine, albumin, total protein, and uric acid among participants was presented in Table 2. There was a significant decrease ($p<0.05$) in the mean plasma sodium, total protein, and albumin among preeclamptic volunteers when compared with control group. A significant increase ($p<0.05$) in the mean plasma value of potassium, urea, creatinine, and uric acid as well as spot urine protein (albumin) creatinine ratio (microalbuminuria) among preeclamptic patients when compared with normotensive control (Table 2) was observed. There was a significant elevation ($p<0.05$) of transaminases in preeclamptic patients when compared with control (Table 3). A significantly higher plasma total protein and albumin ($p<0.05$) were observed among normotensive control group. The level of association of the parameters among preeclamptic group studied was evaluated (Table 4). There was a significant and positive association between the systolic and diastolic pressure ($p<0.05$) among preeclamptic women. Gestational age was observed to correlate positively with systolic and diastolic blood pressure ($p<0.001$, $p = 0.01$). A negative association was observed between plasma sodium and urea, sodium and creatinine ($p=0.01$, $p< 0.001$). There was a positive association between plasma potassium ($p< 0.001$) and creatinine, potassium and uric acid ($p = 0.01$), urea and uric acid as well as creatinine and urea ($p<0.001$).

TABLE 1: Baseline characteristics of the studied participants.

Variable	Preeclampsia mean ±SD (n=49)	Control mean ±SD (n=50)	t value	p value
Age (year)	33.18 ± 4.55	32.44 ± 4.99	-0.77	0.44
Gestational Age (weeks)	29.45 ± 3.03	29.80 ± 4.02	0.49	0.63
Systolic BP (mmHg)	172.55 ± 24.16	113.02 ± 9.95	-16.09	<0.0001*
Diastolic BP (mmHg)	112.47 ± 17.73	70.20 ± 9.09	-14.97	<0.0001*

*Significant probability (probability <0.05), BP: blood pressure.

TABLE 2: Comparative analysis of renal function parameters in preeclamptic and normotensive participants.

Variable	Preeclampsia mean ±SD (n=49)	Control mean ±SD (n=50)	t value	p value
Sodium (mmol/L)	130.39 ± 6.30	133.16 ± 6.75	2.11	0.04*
Chloride (mmol/L)	104.89 ± 6.75	105.62 ± 3.58	0.69	0.50
Potassium (mmol/L)	4.83 ± 1.08	4.14 ± 0.52	-4.05	<0.0001*
Bicarbonate (mmol/L)	15.73 ± 3.73	17.10 ± 3.41	1.90	0.06
Plasma Urea (mmol/L)	3.80 ± 2.09	1.26 ± 0.66	-8.21	< 0.0001*
Plasma Creatinine (μmol/L)	93.82 ± 38.39	45.57 ± 11.20	-8.53	<0.0001*
Uric Acid (μmol/L)	398.24 ± 160.36	213.66 ± 50.00	-7.76	<0.0001*
Spot urine Creat (mg/L)	316.19 ± 205.24	222.06 ± 130.69	-2.73	0.01*
Spot urine Prot (mg/L)	1666.24 ± 1188.26	512.12 ± 343.13	-6.59	<0.0001*
Albumin/creatinine (μg/mg)	632.38 ± 527.09	246.25 ± 82.26	-5.12	<0.0001*

* Significant probability (probability <0.05).

TABLE 3: Comparison of liver function parameters in preeclampsia and control.

Analytes	Preeclampsia (n=49) mean ± SEM	Control (n=50) mean ± SEM	t-value	p-value
Plasma T. Prot (g/L)	49.55 ± 7.82	57.80 ± 7.28	5.44	<0.0001*
Albumin (g/L)	23.10 ± 3.76	32.42 ± 5.22	10.18	<0.0001*
AST (U/L)	112 ± 18.61	16.83 ± 2.58	-5.14	<0.0001*
ALT (U/L)	31.75 ± 4.63	4.78 ± 0.42	-5.86	<0.0001*

* Significant probability (probability <0.05).

TABLE 4: Degree of association between parameters studied among preeclamptic group.

Variable	Correlation coefficient "r"	p value
Gestational age vs systolic BP	0.42	<0.001 *
Gestational age vs Diastolic BP	0.35	0.010*
Potassium vs Creatinine	0.43	<0.001*
Potassium vs Uric acid	0.39	0.010*
Sodium vs Urea	-0.35	0.01*
Sodium vs Creatinine	-0.58	< 0.001*
Urea vs Creatinine	0.46	<0.001*
Urea vs Albumin	-0.41	<0.001*
Urea vs Uric Acid	0.71	<0.001*
Uric Acid vs Creatinine	0.53	<0.001*
Uric Acid vs Albumin	-0.29	0.040*
ALT vs Uric Acid	0.500	<0.001*
ALT vs Urea	0.455	0.001*
ALT vs Creatinine	0.589	<0.001*

4. Discussion

Preeclampsia has been a dreaded disease affecting women and their pregnancy for a long time. The disorder could be accompanied by possible numerous complications both to the woman and the unborn child. This has triggered phobia in some pregnant women and aroused the interest of obstetricians everywhere. It has been shown that development of preeclampsia involves a multifactorial process and multiorgan dysfunction with no individual factor strictly essential or sufficient for causing it [12].

In this study, there was no difference ($p>0.05$) in the mean age and gestational age of the preeclamptic test group when compared with the normotensive control. As observed in this study, there was a significant decrease ($p<0.05$) in the mean plasma sodium value among preeclamptic test group when compared with the control. This observation suggests that preeclampsia could be associated with hyponatremia. Our observation is corroborated by the previous study of Indumati et al. [13] who demonstrated a linear decrease in the mean sodium value among preeclamptic volunteers when compared with the normal pregnancy. Available data suggests that preeclamptic women with hyponatremia may present with severe symptoms [14]. Thus hyponatremia in patients with preeclampsia may be associated with increased risk of maternal seizures [15]. Razavi et al. [16] showed that hyponatremia tends to occur more frequently among preeclamptic women with severe disease. Our finding regarding plasma sodium agreed with the previous studies of Razavi et al. [16] and Dwivedi et al. [17]. While the mechanism of hyponatremia in preeclampsia is unclear, it has been suggested, however, that syndrome of inappropriate antidiuretic hormone secretion (SIADH) and low effective plasma volume which possibly leads to a nonosmotic release of ADH may be involved in the development of hyponatremia in preeclamptic patients [18].

Furthermore, there was a significant increase in the mean plasma potassium level of the preeclamptic volunteers in this study when compared with the normotensive pregnant control. Our observation with regard to potassium is in consonance with the previous study of Dwivedi et al. [16]. In preeclampsia, it has been reported that a decrease glomerular filtration rate (GFR) and renal plasma flow (RPF) possibly decreases sodium delivery to the distal nephron as well as causing decreased potassium secretion [19]; thus suggesting the possibility of inhibition of urinary potassium excretion prior to administration of magnesium in some preeclamptic women [19]. An increase in the mean plasma potassium as observed in preeclamptic patients may also possibly be secondary to the effect of magnesium sulphate infusion therapy as Hudali and Takkar [20] as well as Iglesias et al. [21] reported hypocalcaemia and hyperkalemia during magnesium infusion therapy in preeclamptic patients. It is thought that administration of magnesium in the treatment of preeclampsia possibly reduces the activity of plasma renin and angiotensin converting enzymes resulting in low levels of renin, angiotensinogen, angiotensin II, and aldosterone [19, 22, 23]. Thus magnesium infusion possibly increases sodium and chloride excretion but suppresses potassium excretion by the kidney [24, 25]. An increase in potassium value as observed in our study was similar to the previous finding by Handwerker et al. [26] where a significant increase in ionized magnesium and potassium was observed among preeclamptic women. On the other hand, Adewolu [27] showed no significant difference between the mean plasma potassium values in preeclampsia and normal pregnancy.

Also, our study showed that the mean plasma urea, creatinine, and uric acid levels were significantly raised ($p<0.05$) among preeclamptic population when compared with normotensive control pregnant women. Our observation was similar to the previous study by Vyakaranm et al. [28] that reported an increase in the mean uric acid and creatinine values among preeclamptic patients. Previous study has shown that blood urea nitrogen (BUN) and creatinine levels among preeclamptic women are similar to the levels seen in nonpregnant women because of reduced glomerular filtration rate (GFR) and reduced renal plasma flow (RPF) [11] as against normal pregnancy that is characterized by increase in GFR [29, 30] as well as RPF. Thus elevated levels of creatinine may be due to decrease urinary clearance secondary to reduced GFR and increased reabsorption [31]. A significant increase in the mean uric acid level as seen among preeclamptic volunteers in this study is in consonance with previous studies by Salako. et al. [32] and Mert et al. [33] that indicated a significant elevation in serum uric acid in preeclampsia test group when compared with normotensive control.

Also, it has been shown that uric acid concentration falls initially by 25% to 35% in normal pregnancy partly due to estrogen, expanded blood volume, and increased glomerular filtration rate [34]. However, it later rises to a nonpregnant women level at term. However, in preeclamptic patients, uric acid tends to increase much earlier than the onset of hypertension and proteinuria [35] and fall in GFR [36]. Thus elevated uric acid as observed in this study may suggest an antioxidant effect in response to oxidative stress [37]; this may be protective on one hand; however it has been shown that hyperuricemia elicits proinflammatory effect which may lead to endothelia dysfunction [38] possibly causing vascular damage and hypertension [39, 40], thus worsening the outcome. Recent studies have suggested an association between serum uric acid in preeclampsia and the severity of the disease [41, 42]. Thus increased renal function biomarkers parameters as observed among preeclamptic group in this study are in consonance with previous study by Manjareeka and Nanda [43] whereas Salako et al. [32] reported no significant difference in creatinine level of preeclampsia and normotensive pregnant women.

Moreover, the mean plasma total protein and albumin as observed in this study were significantly ($p<0.05$) lower among preeclamptic group when compared with normotensive control group. This could possibly be a consequence of urinary loss of protein as observed in this study with spot urine protein which was significantly higher ($p<0.05$) among preeclamptic test group when compared with the normotensive control. It has been shown that proteinuria as seen in preeclampsia might be the consequence of a loss of both size and charge selectivity of the glomerulus [44]. Hence Muller-Deile and Schiffer [11] reported that a common reason for proteinuria in pregnancy is preeclampsia. In this study, there were significantly raised ($p<0.05$) spot urinary protein (albumin) and urine protein creatinine ratio (UPC) among preeclamptic patients when compared with the normotensive control volunteers. Previous study has shown that accuracy of UPC ratio in predicting 300mg protein in 24-h urine collection in pregnant patients with suspected preeclampsia had a sensitivity of 90%–99% and specificity of 33%–65% [11, 45]. In addition, Durnward et al. [46] suggested that UPC ratio can predict severe preeclampsia and can be used for rapid diagnosis of severe preeclampsia as the correlation of UPC ratio and 24-hr proteinuria increases with the amount of proteinuria. It appears that a significant increase in albumin-creatinine ratio (microalbuminuria) among preeclamptic group could possibly be an indication of renal pathology, an observation which may support the multiorgan dysfunction effect of preeclampsia as a disease.

Furthermore, we observed that transaminases (ALT and AST) were significantly elevated among preeclamptic women ($p<0.05$). Our observation is similar to the previous studies by Hazari et al. [47] and Dacaj et al. [48]. It is thought that elevated transaminases among preeclamptic women are possibly due to hypoxic effect of preeclampsia on their livers, since hypoxia results in necrosis with a resultant degeneration of hepatocytes [48].

An assessment of the degree of association among the parameters studied in preeclampsia shows that gestational ageing is positively ($p<0.05$) associated with increase in both systolic and diastolic blood pressures. There were positive correlations ($p<0.05$) between urea and creatinine, total protein and albumin, and potassium and creatinine. Positive associations ($p<0.05$) were also observed between uric acid and urea, as well as between alanine aminotransferase and biomarkers of renal function (uric acid, urea, and creatinine). On the other hand, negative association existed between uric acid and albumin, as well as between albumin and urea. The positive association between alanine aminotransferase and markers of renal function suggests that preeclampsia is possibly associated with increased risk of hepatic and renal pathology.

5. Conclusion

Our study shows that preeclampsia has deleterious effects on renal and liver functions as shown by deraignment in biomarkers of renal and liver function with respect to normotensive pregnancies. Preeclampsia results in significant electrolyte imbalance. Thus there is a need for close monitoring of women with preeclampsia.

Acknowledgments

The authors are grateful to the doctors and nurses in various centers used for this study.

References

[1] J. M. Roberts and C. A. Hubel, "Oxidative stress in preeclampsia," *American Journal of Obstetrics & Gynecology*, vol. 190, no. 5, pp. 1177-1178, 2004.

[2] R. Pijnenborg, L. Vercruysse, and M. Hanssens, "The uterine spiral arteries in human pregnancy: facts and controversies," *Placenta*, vol. 27, no. 9-10, pp. 939–958, 2006.

[3] ISSHP, A. L. Tranquilli, G. Dekker et al., "The classification, diagnosis and management of the hypertensive disorders of pregnancy: a revised statement from the ISSHP," *Pregnancy Hypertension: An International Journal of Women's Cardiovascular Health*, vol. 4, no. 2, pp. 97–104, 2014.

[4] A. G. Kattah, D. C. Scantlebury, S. Agarwal et al., "Preeclampsia and ESRD: The Role of Shared Risk Factors," *American Journal of Kidney Diseases*, vol. 69, no. 4, pp. 498–505, 2017.

[5] A. M. Hildebrand, M. A. Hladunewich, and A. X. Garg, "Preeclampsia and the Long-term Risk of Kidney Failure," *American Journal of Kidney Diseases*, vol. 69, no. 4, pp. 487-488, 2017.

[6] A. B. Alper, Y. Yi, and L. S. Webber, "Estimation of glomerular filtration rate in preeclamptic patients," *American Journal of Perinatology*, vol. 24, pp. 569–574, 2007.

[7] M. D. Lindheimer, S. J. Taler, and F. G. Cunningham, "Hypertension in pregnancy," *Journal of the American Society of Hypertension*, vol. 4, no. 2, pp. 68–78, 2010.

[8] B. J. Wilson, M. S. Watson, G. J. Prescott et al., "Hypertensive diseases of pregnancy and risk of hypertension and stroke in later life: Results from cohort study," *British Medical Journal*, vol. 326, no. 7394, pp. 845–849, 2003.

[9] D. Ayansina, C. Black, S. J. Hall et al., "Long term effects of gestational hypertension and pre-eclampsia on kidney function: Record linkage study," *Pregnancy Hypertension: An International Journal of Women's Cardiovascular Health*, vol. 6, no. 4, pp. 344–349, 2016.

[10] M. G. Koopman, R. T. Krediet, G. C. M. Koomen, J. Strackee, and L. Arisz, "Circadian rhythm of proteinuria: Consequences of the use of urinary protein:Creatinine ratios," *Nephrology Dialysis Transplantation* , vol. 4, no. 1, pp. 9–14, 1989.

[11] J. Müller-Deile and M. Schiffer, "Preeclampsia from a renal point of view: Insides into disease models, biomarkers and therapy," *World Journal of Nephrology*, vol. 3, no. 4, pp. 169–181, 2014.

[12] T. Sunitha, K. Sameera, and G. Umaramani, "Study of Biochemical changes in Preeclamptic women," *International Journal of Biological & Medical Research*, vol. 3, no. 3, pp. 2025–2028, 2012.

[13] V. Indumati, M. V. Kodliwadmath, and M. K. Sheela, "The role of serum electrolytes in pregnancy induced hypertension," *Journal of Clinical and Diagnostic Research*, vol. 5, no. 1, pp. 66–69, 2011.

[14] G. Sandhu, S. Ramaiyah, G. Chan, and I. Meisels, "Pathophysiology and Management of Preeclampsia-Associated Severe Hyponatremia," *American Journal of Kidney Diseases*, vol. 55, no. 3, pp. 599–603, 2010.

[15] JP. Hayslett, DL. Katz, and JM. Knuson, "Dilutional hyponatraemia in preeclampsia," *American Journal of Obstetrics and Gynecology*, vol. 179, pp. 1312–1316, 1998.

[16] A. Razavi, S. Chasen, R. Gyawali, and R. Kalish, "289: Preeclampsia associated hyponatremia," *American Journal of Obstetrics & Gynecology*, vol. 212, no. 1, p. S156, 2015.

[17] S. Dwivedi, US. Berman, and D. Sharma, "Mineral levels in Women with Pre-Eclampsia in Third Trimester of pregnancy," *Journal of Clinical and Biomedical Sciences*, vol. 6, no. 1, pp. 28–32, 2016.

[18] H. J. Wilson and L. E. Shutt, "Syndrome of inappropriate ADH secretion in a woman with preeclampsia," *International Journal of Obstetric Anesthesia*, vol. 16, no. 4, pp. 360–362, 2007.

[19] Y. Chen, S. Lin, H. Chen, F. Sun, and C. Wu, "Hyperkalemia associated with prolonged magnesium sulfate administration in preeclampsia," *Acta Nephrologica*, vol. 24, no. 1, pp. 8–15, 2010.

[20] T. Hudali and C. Takkar, "Hypocalcemia and hyperkalemia during magnesium infusion therapy in a pre-eclamptic patient," *Clinical Case Reports*, vol. 3, no. 10, pp. 827–831, 2015.

[21] M.-H. Iglesias, E. M. Giesbrecht, P. Von Dadelszen, and L. A. Magee, "Postpartum hyperkalemia associated with magnesium sulfate," *Hypertension in Pregnancy*, vol. 30, no. 4, pp. 481–484, 2011.

[22] P. August, T. Lenz, K. L. Ales et al., "Longitudinal study of the renin-angiotensin-aldosterone system in hypertensive pregnant women: deviations related to the development of superimposed preeclampsia," *American Journal of Obstetrics & Gynecology*, vol. 163, no. 5, pp. 1612–1621, 1990.

[23] D. M. Shah, "Preeclampsia: new insights," *Current Opinion in Nephrology and Hypertension*, vol. 16, no. 3, pp. 213–220, 2007.

[24] B. I. Heller, J. F. Hammarsten, and F. L. Stutzman, "Concerning the effects of magnesium sulfate on renal function, electrolyte excretion, and clearance of magnesium 1," *The Journal of Clinical Investigation*, vol. 32, no. 9, pp. 858–861, 1953.

[25] L. C. Chesley and I. Tepper, "Some effects of magnesium loading upon renal excretion of magnesium and certain other electrolytes," *The Journal of Clinical Investigation*, vol. 37, no. 10, pp. 1362–1372, 1958.

[26] S. M. Handwerker, B. T. Altura, and B. M. Altura, "Ionized serum magnesium and potassium levels in pregnant women with preeclampsia and eclampsia," *Obstetrics, Gynaecology and Reproductive Medicine*, vol. 40, no. 3, pp. 201–208, 1995.

[27] O. Adewolu, "Serum sodium, potassium, calcium and magnesium in women with pregnancy induced hypertension and preeclampsia in Oredo local Government, Benin Metropolis: A pilot study," *African Journal of Medical and Health Sciences*, vol. 12, no. 1, pp. 1–5, 2013.

[28] S. Vyakaranam, A. Bhongir, D. Patlolla, and R. Chintapally, "Study of serum uric acid and creatinine in hypertensive disorders of pregnancy," *International Journal of Medical Science and Public Health*, vol. 4, no. 10, pp. 1424–1428, 2015.

[29] J. M. Davison and W. Dunlop, "Renal hemodynamics and tubular function in normal human pregnancy," *Kidney International*, vol. 18, no. 2, pp. 152–161, 1980.

[30] E. A. Sims and K. E. Krantz, "Serial studies of renal function during pregnancy and the puerperium in normal women," *The Journal of Clinical Investigation*, vol. 37, no. 12, pp. 1764–1774, 1958.

[31] A. Jeyabalan and K. P. Conrad, "Renal function during normal pregnancy and preeclampsia," *Frontiers in Bioscience*, vol. 12, no. 7, pp. 2425–2437, 2007.

[32] B. L. Salako, O. Olayemi, A.-T. A. Odukogbe et al., "Microalbuminuria in pregnancy as a predictor of preeclampsia and eclampsia," *West African Journal of Medicine*, vol. 22, no. 4, pp. 295–300, 2003.

[33] I. Mert, A. S. Oruc, S. Yuksel et al., "Role of oxidative stress in preeclampsia and intrauterine growth restriction," *Journal of Obstetrics and Gynaecology Research*, vol. 38, no. 4, pp. 658–664, 2012.

[34] J. Carter and A. Child, "Serum Uric Acid Levels in Normal Pregnancy," *Australian and New Zealand Journal of Obstetrics and Gynaecology*, vol. 29, no. 3, pp. 313-314, 1989.

[35] R. W. Powers, L. M. Bodnar, R. B. Ness et al., "Uric acid concentrations in early pregnancy among preeclamptic women with gestational hyperuricemia at delivery," *American Journal of Obstetrics & Gynecology*, vol. 194, no. 1, pp. 160–e8, 2006.

[36] E. D. M. Gallery, S. N. Hunyor, and A. Z. Győry, "Plasma volume contraction: A significant factor in both pregnancy-associated hypertension (preeclampsia) and chronic hypertension in pregnancy," *QJM: An International Journal of Medicine*, vol. 48, no. 4, pp. 593–602, 1979.

[37] A. Many, C. A. Hubel, S. J. Fisher, J. M. Roberts, and Y. Zhou, "Invasive cytotrophoblasts manifest evidence of oxidative stress in preeclampsia," *The American Journal of Pathology*, vol. 156, no. 1, Article ID 64733, pp. 321–331, 2000.

[38] C. Lam, K.-H. Lim, D.-H. Kang, and S. A. Karumanchi, "Uric acid and preeclampsia," *Seminars in Nephrology*, vol. 25, no. 1, pp. 56–60, 2005.

[39] S. Watanabe, D.-H. Kang, L. Feng et al., "Uric acid, hominoid evolution, and the pathogenesis of salt-sensitivity," *Hypertension*, vol. 40, no. 3, pp. 355–360, 2002.

[40] D.-H. Kang, J. Finch, T. Nakagawa et al., "Uric acid, endothelial dysfunction and pre-eclampsia: searching for a pathogenetic link," *Journal of Hypertension*, vol. 22, no. 2, pp. 229–235, 2004.

[41] L. S. Voto, R. Illia, H. A. Darbon-Grosso, I. Francisco Uranga, and M. Margulies, "Uric acid levels: A useful index of the severity of preeclampsia and perinatal prognosis," *Journal of Perinatal Medicine*, vol. 16, no. 2, pp. 123–126, 1988.

[42] S. A. Bainbridge and J. M. Roberts, "Uric acid as a pathogenic factor in Preeclampsia," *Placenta*, vol. 29, pp. 67–72, 2008.

[43] M. Manjareeka and S. Nanda, "Elevated levels of serum uric acid, creatinine or urea in preeclamptic women," *International Journal of Medical Science and Public Health*, vol. 2, no. 1, pp. 43–47, 2013.

[44] P. Moran, P. H. Baylis, M. D. Lindheimer, and J. M. Davison, "Glomerular ultrafiltration in normal and preeclamptic pregnancy," *Journal of the American Society of Nephrology*, vol. 14, no. 3, pp. 648–652, 2003.

[45] R. Papanna, L. K. Mann, R. W. Kouides, and J. C. Glantz, "Protein/creatinine ratio in preeclampsia: A systematic review," *Obstetrics & Gynecology*, vol. 112, no. 1, pp. 135–144, 2008.

[46] C. Durnwald and B. Mercer, "A prospective comparison of total protein/creatinine ratio versus 24-hour urine protein in women with suspected preeclampsia," *American Journal of Obstetrics & Gynecology*, vol. 189, no. 3, pp. 848–852, 2003.

[47] N. R. Hazari, V. S. Hatolkar, and S. M. Munde, "Study of Serum Hepatic Enzymes in Preeclampsia," *International Journal of Current Medical and Applied Sciences*, vol. 2, no. 1, pp. 1–8, 2014.

[48] R. Dacaj, S. Izetbegovic, G. Stojkanovic, and S. Dresha, "Elevated Liver Enzymes in Cases of Preeclampsia and Intrauterine Growth Restriction," *Medical Archives*, vol. 70, no. 1, pp. 44–47, 2016.

24

Determinants of Home Delivery among Mothers in Abobo District, Gambella Region, Ethiopia

Asmelash Abera Mitiku,[1] Abraham Lomboro Dimore,[2] and Solomon Berhanu Mogas[2]

[1]*Gambella Regional Health Bureau, Gambella Region, Ethiopia*
[2]*Department of Epidemiology, Jimma University, Jimma, Oromia, Ethiopia*

Correspondence should be addressed to Asmelash Abera Mitiku; asme26abera@gmail.com

Academic Editor: Robert Gaspar

Introduction. Home delivery is one of the major reasons for high maternal mortality ratio in sub-Saharan Africa. Sub-Saharan Africa and South Asia together contribute over 85% of maternal deaths, of which, only half of deliveries are institutional. However, data are scarce on the availability of information with regard to the determinant factors for this high prevalence of home delivery in the study area. *Objective.* This study is aimed at determining factors associated with home delivery, among mothers in Abobo Woreda, Gambella region, Southwest Ethiopia, 2019. *Methods.* A case control study conducted from 12 March 2019 up to 2 April 2019 on 88 cases and 176 controls. Cases include mothers who gave birth at home and those mothers who gave birth at health facility in the last one year preceding the study included as controls. Data entry was made using Epi-Data version 3.1, and analysis was made using SPSS version 20. A binary logistic regression analysis was conducted to assess candidate variables and subsequently a multivariable regression to determine the statistical associations. Adjusted odds ratio (AOR) with 95% confidence interval (CI) was calculated to determine strength of association, and p value <0.05 was used to establish significant associations. *Results.* No formal education (AOR: 5.07; 95% CI: 2.18-11.50), poor knowledge on obstetric complications (AOR: 3.83; 95% CI: 1.98-7.40), negative attitude towards delivery service (AOR: 3.25; 95% CI: 1.70-6.19), poor household wealth index (AOR: 4.55; 95% CI: 2.01-10.31), and no antenatal care visit (AOR: 3.29; 95% CI: 1.63-6.63) were found to be significantly associated with home delivery. *Conclusions.* The findings do support that no formal education, poor knowledge on obstetric complications, negative attitude towards delivery service, poor household wealth index, and no antenatal care visit showed a significant association with home delivery.

1. Introduction

Even though, most pregnancies and births are uneventful, too many women still suffer and die from serious health issues during pregnancy and childbirths [1]. Maternal mortality (MM) is not merely due to particular pathologies but has strong association with women's social determinants of health [2]. The target of Sustainable Development Goal (SDG 3.1) is to reduce global maternal mortality ratio (MMR) to less than 70 deaths per 100,000 live births with annual rate of 7.3% reduction and with a maximum target of no more than 140 deaths per 100,000 live births for any country [1].

Globally, due to pregnancy related causes, an estimated 303,000 maternal deaths occurred every year. From the total deaths, 99% were from developing countries and 66% in sub-Saharan Africa alone [3, 4]. According to the Ethiopian Demographic and Health Survey (EDHS) 2016 report, the MMR in Ethiopia was 412/100,000 live births [5].

It has become increasingly clear that MMR in sub-Saharan Africa is highly attributed to home delivery, and most births take place at home [2]. Globally, about two-thirds of births take place in the HF [6]. However, in developing countries, home delivery is widely practiced. Mothers deliver in unhygienic environment, without skilled birth attendant and lifesaving medications [7]. Sub-Saharan Africa and South Asia together contribute over 85% of maternal deaths, and of which only half of deliveries are institutional [6]. Previous studies across the sub-Saharan Africa report a significant proportion of mothers still deliver at home [8–10]. Furthermore, a cross-sectional study conducted in Abobo District showed that significant number of women (91.5%) had given birth at home [11]. There is enthusiasm by the government to reduce the high prevalence of home delivery in Ethiopia. However, data are scarce on the availability of information with regard to the determinant factors for this high prevalence of home delivery. Therefore, given the scarcity of studies conducted to examine predictors as to why women give birth at home, the current study adds potential determinant factors (enabling, predisposing, and need based) for home delivery in rural settings to current literatures. In addition to this, the finding from the current study provides evidence for decision makers, stakeholders, and health professionals aimed to reduce MMR by decreasing home delivery specifically in the study area and generally to areas with similar rural settings. Therefore, the study is aimed at identifying determinants of home delivery in the study area.

2. Materials and Methods

2.1. Study Setting, Design, and Population. The study was conducted at Abobo District, Anguwa Zone, Gambella region state, Southwest Ethiopia. The district has 19 kebeles (the smallest administrative unit in Ethiopia) with a total population of 31,209 (15,292 males and 15,917 females). Among the total population, 8,146 women were in the reproductive age group. There are four health centers found in the district and providing child delivery services for the population.

A community-based case control study was conducted. The study population includes mothers who gave birth in the last one year preceding the current study. Cases were permanent resident mothers who gave birth in the last one year outside of health institutions irrespective of the delivery attendant. Controls were mothers who gave birth in the last one year in health institutions (health center in this case) irrespective of the delivery attendant. The current study was conducted from March 12 to April 2, 2019.

2.2. Sampling. Sample size was calculated using the Epi Info version 7 software program by considering 80% power, 95% confidence level, 10% nonresponse rate, a1 : 2 case to control ratio, and taking exposure factors from different studies [12–14]. The sample size was 264 (88 cases and 176 controls).

Stratified random sampling technique was used to select the study participants. All the 19 kebeles (two urban and 17 rural) found in Abobo Woreda were taken. Then, sampling frame was prepared for cases and controls separately for each kebele with their corresponding household identification numbers by making house-to-house survey. Sample size was allocated by proportional to the size allocation (PPS) of each kebele. Finally, 88 cases and 176 controls were selected by simple random sampling technique within each strata using computer-generated random number by Excel sheet.

2.3. Data Collection. Face to face interview technique was used to collect data by making house to house visit. The questionnaire was adapted from different literatures and Ethiopian Demographic and Health Survey (EDHS) [5, 12, 14]. Data were collected by using seven trained diploma nurses.

2.4. Measurement. Knowledge on danger signs of pregnancy: those who mentioned at least four danger signs of pregnancy were classified as having good knowledge.

Knowledge on obstetric complications of labor or delivery: those who mentioned at least three obstetric complications were classified as having good knowledge.

Attitude towards delivery services: those who scored greater than or equal to the mean were labeled as having positive attitude [14].

2.5. Operational Definitions. Predisposing factors: this implies the proclivity to utilize health care services. An individual is more or less likely to use health services based on demographics, position within the social structures, and beliefs of health services benefits.

Enabling factors: this implies resources found within the family and the community.

Need-based factors: this includes the perception of need for health services, whether individual, social, or clinically evaluated perceptions of need.

Household wealth index: this includes household ownership of selected assets, such as televisions, bicycles, housing constructions, type of water access, and sanitation facilities.

2.6. Quality Control. Survey was conducted to prepare sampling frame for cases and controls. Diploma nurses who have been working in the study area were recruited to collect data. To increase the quality of data, training was given to data collectors on the objective and data collection tools of the study.

2.7. Data Analysis. Data cleaning, coding, and entry were made using the Epi-Data version 3.1 software. Analysis was conducted using Statistical Package for Social Science (SPSS) version 20. To determine associations between dependent and independent variables, logistic regression analysis was used. Bivariate analysis was performed to select variables for multivariable analysis; p value <0.25 was used as a cutoff point. Multivariable logistic regression was used to determine significant association between the outcome and independent variable. Multicollinearity diagnostic was done by checking variance inflation factor (VIF), and no problems were identified. Backward stepwise logistic regression was used to determine independent predictors with p value <0.05 with their respective AOR and 95% CI. The model fitness was checked by Hosmer-Lemeshow goodness of fit test, and the model was declared as fit model since p value was greater than 0.05.

2.8. Ethical Clearance. Ethical clearance was obtained from Jimma University Institute of Health Ethical Review Committee. Permission letters were also obtained from regional health bureau and Abobo District health office. Confidentiality was assured by excluding their name during the period of data collection. The study purpose, procedure, duration, possible risks, and benefits of the study were clearly explained for the study participants. Before any kinds of data collection, informed verbal consent was obtained from each study participant.

Table 1: Sociodemographic characteristics of cases and controls in Abobo District, Gambella region, Southwest Ethiopia, 2019.

Variables	Category	Cases (88) No. %	Controls (176) No. %
Age of mothers	15-24	19 (21.6)	47 (26.7)
	25-29	22 (25.0)	71 (40.3)
	≥30	47 (53.4)	58 (33.0)
Residence	Rural	60 (68.2)	121 (68.8)
	Urban	28 (31.8)	55 (31.3)
Educational status of mothers	No formal education	42 (47.7)	29 (16.5)
	Primary (1–8)	24 (27.3)	72 (40.9)
	Secondary and above	22 (25.0)	75 (42.6)
Educational status of husbands	No formal education	17 (19.3)	35 (19.9)
	Primary (1–8)	34 (38.6)	59 (33.5)
	Secondary and above	37 (42.0)	82 (46.6)
Occupational status of mothers	Housewives/farmer	65 (73.9)	126 (71.6)
	Students	9 (10.2)	22 (12.5)
	Merchants	5 (5.7)	13 (7.4)
	Government employee	9 (10.2)	15 (8.5)
Occupational status of husbands	Farmer	55 (62.5)	91 (51.7)
	Students	10 (11.4)	13 (7.4)
	Daily laborer	6 (6.8)	14 (8.0)
	Merchants	3 (3.4)	17 (9.7)
	Government employee	14 (15.9)	41 (23.3)
Family size	<5	36 (40.9)	79 (44.9)
	≥5	52 (59.1)	97 (55.1)
Parity	One birth	22 (25.0)	35 (19.9)
	Two birth	17 (19.3)	44 (25.0)
	Three birth	14 (15.9)	35 (19.9)
	Four birth	19 (21.6)	30 (17.0)
	Fifth and above birth	16 (18.2)	32 (18.2)

3. Results

3.1. Sociodemographic Characteristics of Cases and Controls. In this study, a total of 88 cases and 176 controls were included with a response rate of 100% in both groups. Of total respondents, 47 (53.4%) cases and 58 (33.0%) controls were above age of 30 years. The median ± IQR (interquartile range) age of cases and controls were 30.00 ± 10 and 28.00 ± 6 years, respectively. About 60 (68.2%) cases and 121 (68.8%) controls were rural residents. Concerning educational status, 22 (25.0%) cases and 75 (42.6%) controls had secondary and above educational status. Regarding ethnicity, majority of the study participant 55 (62.5%) cases and 102 (58.0%) controls were Anyuak (Table 1).

3.2. Knowledge, Attitude, and Decision on the Place of Delivery. Thirty-four (38.6%) cases and ninety-eight (55.7%) controls had good knowledge about danger signs of pregnancy. Regarding knowledge about obstetric complications, 26 (29.5%) cases and 118 (67.0%) controls had good knowledge.

Regarding about attitude towards delivery services, six questions related to benefits of giving birth at HF, health professionals' skill, health services staffing, and availability of supplies were asked. Accordingly, 30 (34.1%) cases and 125 (71.0%) controls had positive attitude towards delivery services (Table 2).

4. Socioeconomic and Health Service-Related Factors

Concerning the household wealth index, 20 (22.7%) cases and 70 (39.8%) controls were in the rich wealth tertile (category).

Regarding to health service-related characteristics, majority of cases 87 (98.9%) and controls 173 (98.3%) mentioned that there was health facility in their residence (Table 3).

5. Need-Based Factors for Cases and Controls

Of total respondents, 40 (45.5%) cases and 142 (80.7%) controls had history of ANC visit for her last pregnancy. From those who had ANC visit, 14 (35.0%) cases and 103 (72.5%) controls had four and above number of visit. Regarding to previous obstetric outcome, 80 (90.9%) cases and 156

TABLE 2: Bivariate analysis of knowledge, attitude, and decision on place of delivery among cases and controls in Abobo Woreda, Gambella region, Southwest Ethiopia, 2019.

Variables	Category	Cases (88) No. %	Controls (176) No. %	COR (95% CI)	p value
Knowledge on danger sign of pregnancy	Poor	54 (61.4)	78 (44.3)	1.99 (1.18-3.36)	0.009*
	Good	34(38.6)	98(55.7)	1	
Knowledge on obstetric complications	Poor	62 (70.5)	58 (33.0)	4.85 (2.78-8.46)	<0.001 *
	Good	26 (29.5)	118 (67.0)	1	
Attitude towards delivery services	Negative	58 (65.9)	51 (29.0)	4.74 (2.74-8.19)	<0.001*
	Positive	30 (34.1)	125 (71.0)	1	
Decision on place of delivery	Self	26 (29.5)	49 (27.8)	0.97 (0.32-2.93)	0.961
	With husband	30 (34.1)	81 (46.0)	0.68 (0.23-1.99)	0.482
	Husband alone	26 (29.5)	35 (19.9)	1.36 (0.45-4.16)	0.588
	Others*	6 (6.8)	11 (6.3)	1	

Note: *significant at $p < 0.25$; others* (other family members like mothers). Abbreviations: COR: crude odds ratio; CI: confidence interval.

TABLE 3: Bivariate analysis of socioeconomic and health service-related factors of cases and controls in Abobo Woreda, Gambella region, Southwest Ethiopia, 2019.

Variables	Category	Cases (88) No. %	Controls (176) No. %	COR (95% CI)	p value
Media exposure	No	54 (61.4)	86 (48.9)	1.66 (0.99-2.8)	0.056*
	Yes	34 (38.6)	90 (51.1)	1	
Wealth index	Poor	41 (46.6)	46 (26.1)	3.12 (1.63-5.98)	<0.001*
	Medium	27 (30.7)	60 (34.1)	1.58 (0.80-3.09)	0.186*
	Rich	20 (22.7)	70 (39.8)	1	
Type of HF	Only HC	24 (27.6)	46 (26.6)	1	
	Both type	10 (11.5)	19 (11.0)	1.009 (0.4-2.51)	0.985
	Only HP	53 (60.9)	108 (62.4)	0.94 (0.52-1.70)	0.840
Accessibility of HF	≤5 km	78 (89.7)	169 (97.7)	1	
	>5 km	9 (10.3)	4 (2.3)	4.88 (1.46-16.32)	0.010*
Means of transportation	No	34 (38.6)	48 (27.3)	1.68 (0.98-2.89)	0.061*
	Yes	54 (61.4)	128 (72.7)	1	

Note: *significant at $p < 0.25$. Abbreviations: km: kilometer; COR: crude odds ratio; CI: confidence interval.

(88.6%) controls reported that they had not faced any obstetric problems during their last deliveries (Table 4).

5.1. Determinants of Home Delivery among Mothers. We found five variables significantly associated with home delivery: mothers who had no formal education (AOR: 5.07; 95% CI: 2.18-11.50), mothers who had poor knowledge on obstetric complication (AOR: 3.83; 95% CI: 1.98-7.40), mothers who had negative attitude towards delivery service (AOR: 3.25; 95% CI: 1.70-6.19), mothers who were in the poor wealth tertile (AOR: 4.55; 95% CI: 2.01-10.31), and mothers who had no ANC visit (AOR: 3.29; 95% CI: 1.63-6.63) (Table 5).

6. Discussion

This study, the first in the district, has identified factors that could predict home delivery among mothers in Abobo District of Gambella regional state. Our study has demonstrated results that are consistent with other studies in the literature. Accordingly, predisposing factors (educational status of mothers, knowledge about obstetric complications, and attitude of mothers towards delivery services), enabling factors (household wealth index), and need-based factors (ANC visit) were identified as predictors of home delivery.

Accordingly, those mothers who had no formal education had a significant association with home delivery than mothers who had secondary and above education. This finding is in line with other studies conducted in Bahirdar Ethiopia, South Tigray zone of Northern Ethiopia, Chandigarh of India, and Ghana [12, 13, 15, 16]. The observed difference could be level of awareness difference between the two groups. This highlights the need to educate mothers and the community as a crucial intervention step for substantial reduction of MMR.

Furthermore, the present study found that mothers' knowledge on obstetric complications had a significant

Table 4: Bivariate analysis of need-based factors of cases and controls in Abobo Woreda, Gambella region, Southwest Ethiopia, 2019.

Variable	Category	Cases (88) No. %	Controls (176) No. %	COR (95% CI)	p value
ANC visit	No	48 (54.5)	34 (19.3)	5.01 (2.86-8.79)	<0.001*
	Yes	40 (45.5)	142 (80.7)	1	
History of obstetric complication	No	80 (90.9)	156 (88.6)	1.28 (0.54-3.04)	0.573
	Yes	8 (9.1)	20 (11.4)	1	
Plan for last pregnancy	No	44 (50)	76 (43.2)	1.32 (0.79-2.19)	0.295
	Yes	44 (50)	100 (56.8)	1	

Note: *significant at p value <0.25. Abbreviations: COR: crude odds ratio; CI: confidence interval.

Table 5: Multivariable analysis for determinant factors of home delivery among mothers in Abobo District, Gambella region, Southwest Ethiopia, 2019.

Variable	Category	Cases No. %	Controls No. %	COR (95% CI)	AOR (95% CI)	p value
Mothers educational status	No formal education	42 (47.7)	29 (16.5)	4.94 (2.53-9.66)	5.07 (2.18-11.50)	<0.001*
	Primary (1–8)	24 (27.3)	72 (40.9)	1.14 (0.59-2.20)	1.39 (0.65-3.02)	0.394
	Secondary and above	22 (25.0)	75 (42.6)	1	1	
Knowledge on obstetric complications	Poor	62 (70.5)	58 (33.0)	4.85 (2.78-8.46)	3.83 (1.98-7.40)	<0.001 *
	Good	26 (29.5)	118 (67.0)	1	1	
Attitude towards delivery services	Negative	58 (65.9)	51 (29.0)	4.74 (2.74-8.19)	3.25 (1.70-6.19)	<0.001*
	Positive	30 (34.1)	125 (71.0)	1	1	
Wealth index	Poor	41 (46.6)	46 (26.1)	3.12 (1.63-5.98)	4.55 (2.01-10.31)	<0.001*
	Medium	27 (30.7)	60 (34.1)	1.58 (0.80-3.09)	1.78 (0.78-4.07)	0.172
	Rich	20 (22.7)	70 (39.8)	1	1	
ANC visit	No	48 (54.5)	34 (19.3)	5.01 (2.86-8.79)	3.29 (1.63-6.63)	0.001*
	Yes	40 (45.5)	142 (80.7)	1	1	

Note: *statically significant at p value <0.05. Abbreviations: AOR: adjusted odds ratio; COR: crude odds ratio; CI: confidence interval.

association with home delivery. Accordingly, mothers who had poor knowledge on obstetric complications showed higher odds on home delivery than their counter parts. It is supported by different studies [14, 17–19]. As knowledge of mothers on obstetric complication increases, they prefer to deliver at health facilities. Teaching mothers and the community on obstetric complication increases the need for professional care and preference of place of delivery, as this is likely to be more helpful in assisting decision-making.

Mothers who had negative attitude towards delivery service disclosed higher odds on home delivery than mothers with positive attitude. This finding is consistent with a study conducted in Zala District, Southern Ethiopia [20]. Negative attitudes affect positive practices. Improving the attitude of mothers on facility delivery services can play a significant role on the preference of delivery services. The district health office needs to play its role on increasing awareness of mothers and the community towards delivery service.

In the present study, mothers in the poor household wealth category were more likely to give birth at home than mothers in the rich category. This finding is similar with different studies conducted in Kenya and Ethiopia [5, 21, 22]. Even if maternal health services are free, there are different costs related to transportation. As different studies showed, financial capability of families and costs related to transportation may not be afforded by mothers from poor households [23, 24]. To improve health facility delivery, free transportation mechanisms and access to health facilities need to be considered.

Further, the odd of home delivery was higher among mothers with no ANC visit. This finding is in agreement with studies conducted in Istanbul Turkey, South Tigray zone, and Tanqua-Abergele district, Tigray Region, Ethiopia [14, 15, 25]. ANC package includes health education and promotion works related to pregnancy and its complication and recommended practices. Since the study area was rural setting, the communities including mothers' access to information on maternal and related health issues are limited to health facilities. If mothers miss their opportunity for ANC services during their pregnancy period, their decision on selection of place of delivery will be affected. Due to this, the area health office needs to boost ANC service utilization.

7. Strengths and Limitations

This study is the first to examine determinant factors for home delivery. It used a community-based case control approach among mothers who gave birth during the past one year.

The study considers only mothers who gave birth in the last one year preceding the current study; the evidence might not reflect the scenario of periods prior to this. Since data collectors were health workers, social desirability bias was the other limitations of this study and it could have effect on the report of mothers. However, helping mothers to remember the events, adequate training given to data collectors, and their supervision could minimize the effects of recall bias and social desirability bias.

8. Conclusion

This study provides evidence on the determinants of home delivery in Abobo District. It confirms that predisposing factors (mothers' educational status, knowledge on obstetric complications, and attitude towards delivery services), enabling factors (household wealth index), and need-based factors (ANC visit) were positively and significantly associated with home delivery among mothers in Abobo District, Southwest Ethiopia. From the identified determinants, majority were predisposing factors. Hence, the regional and district health office and other stakeholders need to tackle home delivery by focusing on mother's educational status, knowledge on obstetric complications, and attitude towards delivery services.

Abbreviations

ANC: Antenatal care
AOR: Adjusted odds ratio
CI: Confidence interval
COR: Crude odds ratio
EDHS: Ethiopian Demographic Health Survey
HC: Health center
HF: Health facility
HP: Health post
HSTP: Health sector transformation plan
km: Kilometer
MM: Maternal mortality
MMR: Maternal mortality ratio
PCA: Principal component analysis
SDG: Sustainable Development Goal
SPSS: Statistical Package for Social Science
VIF: Variance inflation factor.

Consent

"Not applicable" in this section.

Authors' Contributions

All authors made substantial contributions to conception and design, acquisition of data, or analysis and interpretation of data; took part in drafting the article or revising it critically for important intellectual content; gave final approval of the version to be published; and agree to be accountable for all aspects of the work.

Acknowledgments

We would like to thank Jimma University, Institute of Health, Faculty of Public Health, Department of Epidemiology, Abobo District health office and health facility staffs for their support from the beginning up to the end of the study. In addition, we would like to extend our thanks to supervisors, data collectors, and study participants for their unreserved participation during data collection period.

References

[1] World Health Organization, *World health statistics 2017: monitoring health for the SDGs, sustainable development goals*Licence CC BY-NC-SA 3.0 IGO. November 2018, http://www.who.int/gho/en/, 116–29.

[2] United Nations Economic Comissions, *Assessing progress in Africa towards the millennium development goals*, pp. 57–62, 2013.

[3] World Health Organization, *World health statistics 2018: monitoring health for the SDGs, sustainable development goals*, vol. -viii, World Health Organization, Geneva, 2018, Licence CC BY-NC-SA 3.0 IGO.

[4] WHO, UNICEF, UNFPA, World Bank Group and the United Nations Population Division, *Trends in maternal mortality: 1990 to 2015 Estimates by WHO, UNICEF, UNFPA, World Bank Group and the United Nations Population Division*, WHO Libr. Cat. Data, 2015.

[5] Centeral Stastical Agency(CSA)[Ethiopia] and ICF, *Ethiopia Demographic and Health Survey 2016*, CSA and ICF, Addis Ababa, Ethiopia, and Rockville, Maryland, USA, 2016.

[6] United nations newYork, "The millennium development goals report 2015," in *Time Glob. Action People Planet*, pp. 38–43, 2016.

[7] Federal Ministry Of Health, *HSTP I Annual Performance Report EFY 2008 (2015/2016)*, 2017.

[8] S. K. Chea, T. W. Mwangi, K. K. Ndirangu et al., "Prevalence and correlates of home delivery amongst HIV-infected women attending care at a rural public health facility in Coastal Kenya," *PLoS ONE*, vol. 13, no. 3, article e0194028, 2018.

[9] N. Diamond-smith and M. Sudhinaraset, "Drivers of facility deliveries in Africa and Asia: regional analyses using the demographic and health surveys," *Reproductive Health*, vol. 12, no. 1, 2015.

[10] Y. Tebekaw, Y. James Mashalla, and G. Thupayagale-Tshweneagae, "Factors Influencing Women's Preferences for Places to Give Birth in Addis Ababa, Ethiopia," *Obstetrics and Gynecology International*, vol. 2015, Article ID 439748, 7 pages, 2015.

[11] A. T. Gebrewold, E. M. Mwangi, L. Muiruri, and K. Bizuwork, "Factors influencing utilization of health facility delivery: a case of Abobo Woreda of Gambella Regional State, Ethiopia," *Health Systems Management Journal*, vol. 1, no. 1, pp. 1–10, 2018.

[12] M. L. Nanang and A. Atabila, "Factors predicting home delivery among women in Bosomtwe-Atwima-Kwanwoma district of Ghana: a case control study," *International Journal of Med-*

icine and Public Health, vol. 4, no. 3, article 137719, pp. 287–291, 2014.

[13] F. Abebe, Y. Berhane, and B. Girma, "Factors associated with home delivery in Bahirdar, Ethiopia: a case control study," *BMC Research Notes*, vol. 5, no. 1, p. 653, 2012.

[14] R. Tsegay, A. Aregay, K. Kidanu, M. Alemayehu, and G. Yohannes, "Determinant factors of home delivery among women in Northern Ethiopia: a case control study," *BMC Public Health*, vol. 17, no. 1, p. 289, 2017.

[15] H. Bayu, G. Fisseha, A. Mulat, G. Yitayih, and M. Wolday, "Missed opportunities for institutional delivery and associated factors among urban resident pregnant women in South Tigray Zone, Ethiopia: a community-based follow-up study," *Global Health Action*, vol. 8, no. 1, article 28082, 2015.

[16] K. Jeyashree, S. Kathirvel, K. Trusty, and A. Singh, "Socio-demographic factors affecting the choice of place of childbirth among migrant and native women - A case control study from Chandigarh, India," *Sexual & Reproductive Healthcare*, vol. 17, pp. 81–85, 2018.

[17] K. Asrese and M. E. Adamek, "Women's social networks and use of facility delivery services for uncomplicated births in North West Ethiopia: a community-based case-control study," *BMC Pregnancy Childbirth*, vol. 17, no. 1, p. 441, 2017.

[18] N. Tadele, "Utilization of institutional delivery service and associated factors in Bench Maji zone, Southwest Ethiopia: community based, cross sectional study," *BMC Health Services Research*, vol. 17, no. 1, p. 101, 2017.

[19] I. Temam and A. Banbeta, "Utilization of skilled birth attendant in Bonga Town, Kafa Zone, South West Ethiopia," *Gynecology & Obstetrics*, vol. 6, no. 9, 2016.

[20] K. Bedilu and M. Niguse, "Delivery at home and associated factors among women in child bearing age , who gave birth in the preceding two years in Zala Woreda, southern Ethiopia," *Journal of Public Health and Epidemiology*, vol. 9, no. 6, pp. 177–188, 2017.

[21] Jared Otieno Ogolla, "Factors associated with home delivery in West Pokot County of Kenya," *Advances in Public Health*, vol. 2015, Article ID 493184, 6 pages, 2015.

[22] M. Mekie and W. Taklual, "Delivery place preference and its associated factors among women who deliver in the last 12 months in Simada district of Amhara Region, Northwest Ethiopia: a community based cross sectional study," *BMC Research Notes*, vol. 12, no. 1, pp. 114-115, 2019.

[23] A. Gebeyehu, K. T. Dumga, and K. T. Cherie, "Home delivery practices and associated factors in Ethiopia," *Journal of Reproduction & Infertility*, vol. 20, pp. 102–108, 2019.

[24] S. Yaya, G. Bishwajit, and V. Shah, "Wealth, education and urban – rural inequality and maternal healthcare service usage in Malawi," *BMJ Global Health*, vol. 1, no. 2, article e000085, pp. 1–12, 2016.

[25] B. Catak and C. Oner, "Sociocultural factors affecting unplanned deliveries at home: a community-based case control study," *Social Work in Public Health*, vol. 30, no. 7, pp. 535–544, 2015.

25

Postabortion Contraception Acceptance and Associated Factors in Dessie Health Center and Marie Stopes International Clinics, South Wollo Northeast, Amhara Region, 2017

Ayele Mamo Abebe,[1] **Mesfin Wudu Kassaw**,[2] **and Nathan Estifanos Shewangashaw**[3]

[1]*Department of Nursing, Debre Birhan Health Sciences College, Debre Birhan 37, Amhara, Ethiopia*
[2]*Department of Nursing, College of Health Sciences, Woldia University, Amhara, Ethiopia*
[3]*Department of Nursing, College of Health Sciences, Wollo University, Amhara, Ethiopia*

Correspondence should be addressed to Ayele Mamo Abebe; ayelemamo12@gmail.com

Academic Editor: Daniel Vaiman

Introduction. Abortion is termination of pregnancy before the viability of the pregnancy. It is one of the major causes for maternal mortality in the world and in Ethiopia. Unintended pregnancies which end up in abortion occur due to contraception method nonuse or misuse. To limit unintended pregnancies and avoid repeated abortions promoting immediate postabortion contraception is crucial. *Objective.* To assess the proportion of postabortion contraception acceptance among women who got abortion care service and factors associated with it in Marie stopes international clinic and Dessie health center, Dessie, North eastern Amhara, 2017. *Methods.* An institutional based cross-sectional study design was conducted from May 1 to May 30, 2017, at Marie stopes international clinics and Dessie health center. A sample of 125 women were selected by means of systematic sampling techniques and 118 abortion clients were interviewed in Marie stopes international clinic and Dessie on the use/acceptance of postabortion family planning (PAFP). Data were collected through pretested structured questionnaire. Data was cleaned and checked. Chi-square test was done to assess the association between dependent and independent variables. Odds ratio was done to assess the strength of association. Frequency tables, pie chart, and graphs were used to present the finding of the study. *Results.* From a total of 125 participants recruited, 118 participated in the study while 7 were unwilling to participate in the study, yielding the response rate of 94.4%. Among the 118 study participants, 79 (66.9%) were within the age group 25-34. This study found a strong positive association between Postabortion contraception acceptance and age [P = *0.007* [X^2 test= *9.989*, COR=2.625)]. Study subjects aged 15–24 years were 3 times more likely to accept postabortion family planning as compared with those aged >35 years. *Conclusion and Recommendation.* This study revealed that the acceptance of postabortion family planning method was 84%. Age of women, marital status, ever use of history family planning, involvement of others in decision making, and family planning counseling were significantly associated with postabortion family planning acceptance. Therefore it is better to give emphasis on health education about family planning.

1. Introduction

1.1. Background. Abortion is the ending of pregnancy by removing a fetus or embryo before it can survive outside the uterus. The World Health Organization (WHO) and IFGO recommend that reproductive women who experience abortion should receive contraception assistance, so they can be pregnant in appropriate clinical conditions for the proper development of pregnancy. This requires a minimal interpregnancy interval of six months, mainly to minimize the risk of adverse health outcomes for women and children, such as maternal anemia, premature birth, and low birth weight. These outcomes are widely recognized as being associated with an interpregnancy interval lower than six months [1].

In 2011, the Ministry of Health (MOH) revised the Guidelines for Comprehensive Abortion Care, aiming at standardizing and qualifying women's health care. Aside from the abortion or miscarriage itself, qualified care to women who experience such an episode is considered a priority, primarily to minimize unfavorable outcomes such as maternal and neonatal death, a major challenge that persists in the current health care context [1].

The service includes postabortion care, emergency treatment of incomplete abortion, family planning counseling, STI evaluation and management, HIV testing, and counseling. The major cause for unintended pregnancy which ends up in abortion is nonuse or misuse of contraceptive methods [1].

Although the main aim of availing comprehensive abortion care service in recognized health institutions is to reduce maternal mortality through making abortion safer, the other important point is to introduce, initiate, and link the women with family planning methods after the abortion procedure through postabortion family planning counseling to prevent repeated unplanned pregnancy and abortion because fertility returns within ten days after abortion and the women can get pregnant again [2]. As a result of this, comprehensive postabortion care that includes treatments of incomplete and unsafe abortion, contraceptive, family planning counseling, reproductive and other health services, and abortion related counseling are crucial to prevent unintended pregnancy and repeated abortion

1.2. Statements of the Problem. Unsafe abortion is one of the leading causes for maternal mortality worldwide. About 80,000 (13%) maternal deaths per year are thought to be due to abortion complications, one in eight pregnancy-related deaths. An estimated 21.6 million unsafe abortions took place Worldwide in 2012; almost all were done in developing countries [2]. Numbers of unsafe abortions have increased from 19.7 million although the overall unsafe abortion rates remain unchanged at about 14 unsafe abortions per 1000 women aged 15-44 year [2]. This increase in number of unsafe abortions without a corresponding increase in the rate is mainly due to the growing population of women of reproductive age [3].

The national abortion rate is 23 abortions per 1,000 women of reproductive age.This reflects a high demand for abortion related services such as contraceptive methods [1, 4].

According to national family planning guidelines, the total Contraceptive acceptance rate in Ethiopia is 56.2% [2]. Studies done on unsafe abortion in selected health facilities in Ethiopia 2010 showed that fear of side-effects, perceived low risk of conception, inconvenience to use, and sociocultural factors are common reasons for the low use of contraceptives acceptance in general and postabortion family planning in particular [5–7]. However, the status of Postabortion contraception acceptance and factors associated with it in the Amhara region, Dessie health sectors, remains poorly understood.

Therefore, this study is expected to show the status of Postabortion contraception acceptance and associated factors in Dessie city, north eastern Amhara, so as to contribute to evidence based information that can be used by health program managers to design interventions aimed at promoting postabortion family planning among women.

1.3. Significance of the Study. Currently, Abortion is becoming a major public health problem in our country. Therefore, this study would be helpful to provide basic information for health care practitioners about Postabortion family planning acceptance. It also helps full for health care provider and other programmers to identify possible factors that affect postabortion family planning acceptance. It might be also helped heath care provider to establish strong postabortion and family planning service linkage based on the finding. It gives baseline information for local official about factors that hindered postabortion family planning acceptance. Additionally it could be contributed to a body of knowledge to further study and other researchers who might conduct a study on related topic and also for organizations working on Abortion and family planning services.

2. Literature Review

2.1. Introduction. Nearly 22 million unsafe abortions take place every year; these continue to contribute significantly to the global burden of maternal mortality and morbidity [7]. Considering abortion in Africa during 2010-2014, an estimated 8.3 million induced abortion occurred each year in Africa. The annual rate of abortion was estimated at 34 procedures per 1000 women of child bearing age. Abortion rate is roughly 26 for married women and 36 for unmarried women. The annual rate of abortion varies slightly by region, ranging from 38 per 1000 women of child bearing age in Northern Africa to 31 per 1000 in West Africa. In Eastern Middle and Southern Africa, rates are close to the regional average of 34 per 1000. The proportion of pregnancies ending in abortion ranges from 12% in West Africa to 23% and 24% in Northern Southern Africa, respectively. It is 13% and 14% in Middle and Eastern Africa, respectively [8].

2.2. Postabortion Contraception Acceptance. The prevalence of Postabortion contraception acceptance is varied. Study conducted in Brazil indicated that of all women enrolled in this study 97.4 percent accepted at least one contraceptive method. Most of them (73.4 percent) had no previous abortion history. From the women who had undergone a previous abortion, 47.5 percent reported undergoing unsafe abortion [2].

Following an intervention to strengthen FP as part of PAC services in rural health districts in Senegal, nearly twice as many PAC clients reported receiving FP counseling after an intervention as before the intervention. In addition, 20% of PAC clients left health care facility with modern contraceptive method compared with the baseline [9].

A nationwide hospital based survey of unsafe abortion, in 9 of the 11 administrative regions of Ethiopia that was conducted from June to December 2010, indicated that the majority of women (87%) were aware of contraceptive methods, but only about half of them ever used a family planning method. Of those pregnancies that ended in abortion, 60% were unplanned and 50% were unwanted. FP Method nonuse was responsible for 78% of pregnancies that occurred. Among those with induced abortion, the most common reason for termination of pregnancy was unmet contraceptive need [2].

Prevalence studies of postabortion contraception done in Ethiopia showed various results. More than 90% of all clients who received an abortion at MSI Clinic in Ethiopia by 2007 left with modern family planning methods [10], while the study done in Tigray from 2007 to 2009 to assess safe abortion care (SAC) monitoring framework showed that only 30% of all women who received abortion services left the facility with a contraceptive method [6].

The study conducted in Burayu, Oromia region, reported that Postabortion contraception acceptance was 88.5%. The usage of contraception is essential in reducing the number of unintended or unwanted pregnancies, which are causes for abortion. Two-thirds of unwanted pregnancies in the developing countries occur among women who are not using any method of contraception [3].

2.3. Associated Factor to Postabortion Contraception Acceptance. Despite wide spread adoption of family planning in the developing world, contraceptive use is still very low in sub-Saharan Africa including Ethiopia and other regions. The common cause for induced abortion is unintended or unwanted pregnancy due to varied reasons. Nonuse and misuse of contraception are the major reasons. Contraceptive prevalence rate (CPR) was 63.1%, 25.4%, and 14.7% worldwide, in Africa and in Ethiopia, respectively. This indicates that there was low utilization of contraception [11].

Studies revealed that various factors influence acceptance of postabortion family planning method. Age of women, educational status of women, occupational status, and marital status are among sociodemographic factors as identified by many studies. Family planning counseling by health care provider, previous history of abortion, and previous history use family planning are also indicated as reproductive abortion and related factors [2, 10, 12].

The study conducted in Pakistan revealed that majority of the PAC seekers aged between 25 and 34 years had 1 to 4 children (less educated and housewives). On the other hand, a study, done in Turkey, showed that postabortion contraception was influenced by age groups, educational levels, parity, future fertility plan, and previous induced abortion [4, 13].

Studies in Ethiopia indicated that women seeking induced abortion had a mean age of 23, and the majorities (57%) were single among women seeking induced abortion; only 24% of them reported contraceptive use before the current pregnancy. Furthermore, health care services factors play roles in promoting increased use of postabortion contraception. A cross-sectional survey, in two regions of Ethiopia (2002/3), showed that 53.4% of clients left health care facilities counseled about family planning and 44% with contraceptives [14].

From the study done to assess the future potential capacity and quality of PAC service delivery in public health facilities in three regions of Ethiopia, 23 percent health facilities reported they provide postabortion contraceptive service regularly. The rest of the facilities either rarely or never provide contraceptives. Postabortion counseling was reported to be a regular service provided by three fourths of the facilities but many of the health staffs (46%) who provide contraceptive method or counseling do not have special training in contraceptive counseling or provision [3].

From the study made in Addis Ababa on clients presented for abortion related services, only 57% were using contraceptive before presenting for abortion services. Among them, short-term method of contraception was common and almost one third reported one or more previous abortions. Women seeking safe termination are relatively young [8].

The study conducted in Burayu concluded that most of the women who seek abortion care service in the health centers were very young women. About 209 (53.5%) couples decide on Family planning together, whereas 165 (42.2%) women reported to decide by themselves. Most of women got counseling services more likely accepting PAFP than those who did not get counseling. Counseling, decision on family planning, abortion methods, and income of respondents were found to be determinant factors [15].

3. Objective

3.1. General Objective. The overall objective of the study is to assess the proportion of postabortion contraception acceptance among abortion care service clients and factors associated with it in Marie stopes international and Dessie health center, Dessie, Amhara, 2017.

3.2. Specific objectives

(1) The first is to determine the proportion of postabortion contraception acceptance in Marie stopes international and Dessie health center, Dessie, Amhara, 2017.

(2) The second is to identify factors associated with postabortion contraception acceptance in Dessie health in Marie stopes international and Dessie health center, Dessie, Amhara, 2017.

4. Methods

4.1. Study Area. The study was conducted in Marie stopes international clinics and Dessie health center, which provide postabortion service in Dessie Town. It is found at north direction of Amhara region about 480 km from Bahir Dar and 401 km from Addis Ababa, Capital City of Ethiopia. In Dessie town there are 2 general government hospitals, 3 private hospitals, 5 governmental health centers, and more than 4 private clinics. The health center has MVA service and medical abortion for early trimester abortions after which patients are counseled about different options of contraceptives and allowed to choose and use them.

4.2. Study Design and Period. Institutional based cross-sectional study was conducted from May 1 to May 30, 2017.

4.3. Source Population. All reproductive age women (15-49) got postabortion care service in Marie stopes international clinics and Dessie health centers.

Table 1

Health facility	Study participants	%
Marie stopes international clinic	101	80.8%
Dessie health center	24	19.2%

4.4. Study Population. The study population was all reproductive aged women who received abortion care service in Marie stopes international clinics and Dessie health centers during the study period.

4.5. Eligibility Criteria

4.5.1. Inclusion Criteria. These included women who attended abortion service.

4.5.2. Exclusion Criteria. These included those who were physically or mentally unable to make interview.

4.6. Sample Size and Sampling Techniques

4.6.1. Sample Size Determination. Sample size is calculated by using single population proportion formulas. Sample size was determined by taking p-value30% from related literature of postabortion contraceptive acceptance services in Tigray [16]. Confidence interval (95%) or Z=1.96 value of this formula N-sample size

Margin of error = 5%

$$n = \left(\frac{za}{2}\right)^2 \frac{p(1-p)}{d^2}$$
$$n = (1.96)^2 \frac{0.3(1-0.3)}{(0.05)^2} \quad (1)$$
$$n = 323$$

The final sample size will be made by correction formula nf=n/1+ (n/N)

$$nf = \frac{323}{1} + \frac{323}{176} = 114 \quad (2)$$

Adding 10% nonresponses

$$nf = 125 \quad (3)$$

4.6.2. Sampling Techniques. Sampling method was random, probability sampling because the study subjects are rare (abortion clients are rare) at the time of the data collection. All consecutive patients seeking postabortion care at sampling units at randomly selected days (i.e., Monday, Tuesday, Friday, and Saturday) during exit from abortion care service unit were included in the study. The study subjects were clients who received abortion care from Maria stopes international clinics and Dessie health centers from 1st of May till 30th of May, 2017. The total sample size was allocating to each health facilities based on the proportion of average clients served, allocated based on the previous three-month average clients' load.

4.7. Variables of the Study

4.7.1. Dependent Variable. This was postabortion contraceptive acceptance.

4.7.2. Independent Variable

Sociodemographic Characteristics. These were age, religion, marital status occupation, educational status, Residence, and Ethnicity.

Reproductive Health Related Variables. These were parity, history of family planning use, previous history of abortion, counseling by health care provider, decision making process, and reasons for not using family planning.

4.8. Operational Definition

Acceptance of FP. This is the use of contraceptive method among clients for abortion care in the health care facility.

Abortion. This is the termination of pregnancy before the viabilities of the fetus.

Postabortion Contraception. This is the use of contraceptives immediately after any abortion care procedure.

4.9. Method of Data Collection. Interviewer-administered structured questionnaires questions were developed based on review of literature. The questionnaire was prepared in English and then translated into Amharic keeping the content of the question using understandable words, as the study participants speak Amharic language. Before conducting the main study, pretest was carried out in Hayek health center which is not included in the main study. Pretest was done on 5% of the sample size before the data collection period. Based on the pretest result, the questionnaire was modified as necessary. The interview was filled by asking the women after they got the abortion care service. The filled interview was checked for their completeness and consistency (Table 1).

4.10. Data Entry and Analysis. Regarding descriptive statics means, proportion was done to see the distribution of sociodemographic characteristics. Chi-square was done to assess the association between postabortion family acceptance and independent variables. Odds ratio was done to assess the strength of association. Frequency tables, graphs, and pie charts were used to present the finding of the study.

4.11. Data Quality Assurance. We used pretested and structured questioners. The questionnaire was pretested among 5% of the sample size population in Haik. Investigators collected the data. Completed questionnaires were checked on a daily basis by investigators.

4.12. Ethical Considerations. Ethical clearance letter was obtained from Alkan Health Science, Business, and Technology College. A formal letter was given to Mario stopes international and Dessie health center. Informed consent was obtained from study participants before the interview. The participants of the study were told that they can refuse to continue or escape questions whenever they want, and confidentiality of the information they give was kept.

4.13. Dissemination of Result. The results of this study will be communicated to Zonal health department and other concerned bodies through reports. The study will be presented to Alkan Health, Business, and Technology College members

5. Result

5.1. Sociodemographic Characteristics. From a total of 125 participants recruited, 118 participated in the study while 7 were unwilling to participate in the study, yielding the response rate of 94.4%. Among the 118 study participants, 79 (66.9%) were within the age group 25-34. Half of the respondents, 63 (53.4%) were followers of Orthodox, 45 (38.1%) were Muslim, and 10 (8.5%) were protestants. The predominant ethnic group was Amhara 76 (64.4%). Majority of the respondents 69 (58.5%) were single; 73 (61.9%) of the study participants were unemployed (see Table 2).

Table 2: Distribution of sociodemographic characteristics among abortion care service clients in Marie stopes international and Dessie health center, Dessie, North eastern Ethiopia, 2017 (n=118).

Variables	Frequency (n=118)	%
Age		
18-24	24	20.4
25-34	79	66.9
>35	15	12.7
Ethnicity		
Amara	76	64.4
Tigray	13	11.0
Oromo	29	24.6
Religion		
Orthodox	63	53.4
Muslim	45	38.1
Protestant	10	8.5
Residence		
Dessie	83	70.3
Out of Dessie	35	29.7
Marital status		
Single	69	58.5
Married	49	41.5
Education		
Literate	91	77.1
Illiterate	27	22.9
Occupational status		
Employed	45	38.1
Unemployed	73	61.9

5.2. Reproductive Health, Family Planning, and Abortion Related Characteristics of Participants. Among the study participants, 44 (37.3%) of them had not a history giving birth and 109 (92.4%) of this study participants reported that they had no history of previous abortion (Table 3).

5.3. Reason for Not Using Family Planning. 33.9% of this study participants reported that they were not using family planning method because of fear of its side effect (Figure 1).

5.4. Respondents Age and Acceptance Family Planning. Among the 118 study participants, 79 (66.9%) were within the age group 25-34 which group had high acceptance of post abortion family planning (see Figure 2).

5.5. Acceptance of Postabortion Contraception. The overall acceptance of Postabortion contraception acceptance among abortion service clients in Marie stopes international and Dessie health center was 84.1 % (see Figure 3).

5.6. Factors Associated with Acceptance of Postabortion Contraceptive. This study found a strong positive association between Postabortion contraception acceptance and age [P = *0.007* [X^2 test= *9.989*, COR=2.625)]. Study subjects aged 15–24 years were 3 times more likely to accept postabortion family planning as compared with those aged >35 years and the odds ratios of accepting postabortion family planning among aborted women in the age group of 25-34 were 2 times higher than those aged >30 years.

Females who decide on family planning had significant association with Postabortion family planning acceptance. Females who made independent decision were two times more likely to accept PAFP compared with those decided by husband or both of them [P = *0.022*[X^2 test= *7.679*, COR=1.695)] (see Table 4).

6. Discussion

This study revealed that the magnitude of acceptance of postabortion contraception was 84%. Similar finding was reported in many studies [5, 15, 17]. On the other hand, the current study finding was higher than the finding of studies done in Pakistan (72.9%)[4] and lower than the studies done in Brazil (97.4%)[18]. This variation of findings across various studies might be due to cross-cultural limitations of diagnostic tools and reporting biases, differences in socioeconomic environments. Prevalence estimates also are likely to be influenced by stigma and discrimination.

Compared to general population, it can be assumed that acceptance of family planning is higher among clients who visit health facility for abortion, because of their condition. Comparing this study results with a Community based findings, we found our rates to be higher across the board: EDHS

TABLE 3: Reproductive health, family planning, and abortion related characteristics of participants, Dessie, Amhara, Ethiopia, 2017.

Variables	Frequency (n=118)	%
Have you ever given birth?		
Yes	44	37.3
No	74	62.7
Previous history of abortion		
Yes	9	7.6
No	109	92.4
Who give decision about use of FP?*		
Wife	61	51.7
Husband	36	30.5
Both	21	17.8
Have you ever been counseled by HP health about FP?		
Yes	70	59.3
No	48	40.7
Have you ever used FP?		
Yes	62	52.5
No	56	47.5

*FP**: family planning.

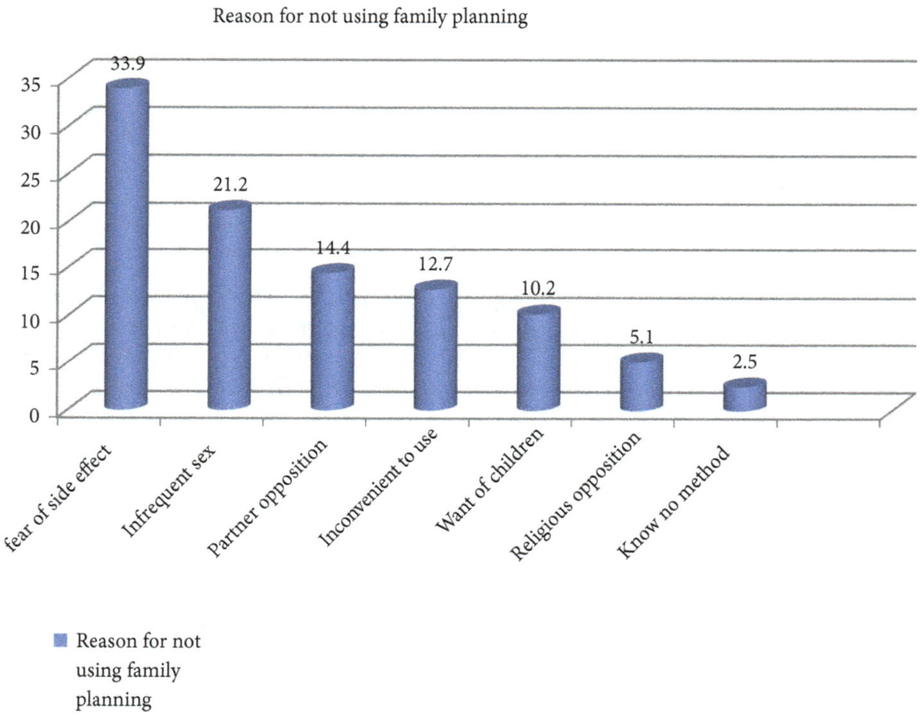

FIGURE 1: Study participants reason of not using family planning method among abortion service clients in Dessie, Amhara regional state, Ethiopia, 2017.

2000 (84.1% vs. 5.76%), EDHS 2005 (84.1% vs. 15.9%), EDHS 2011 (84.1% vs. 35.6%), and EDHS 2014 (84.1 % vs. 39.1%) [19]. Several factors can explain much higher acceptance of family planning among women who faced abortion. First, most of the women who came to get abortion care service had unintended/unplanned pregnancy; they all need to use contraception to avoid similar incidents. Second majority (80%) of these study participants were within the group 15-34; as a result they might not have stable relationships which make them at risk for unintended pregnancy which is unacceptable by the society.

This study found a strong positive association between Postabortion contraception acceptance and age [P = 0.007 [X^2 test= 9.989, COR=2.625)]. Study subjects aged 15–24

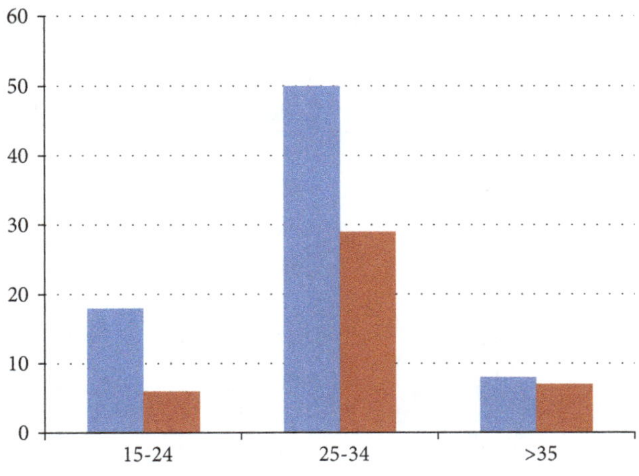

FIGURE 2: Age category and acceptance among postabortion service clients in Dessie, Amhara, Ethiopia, 2017.

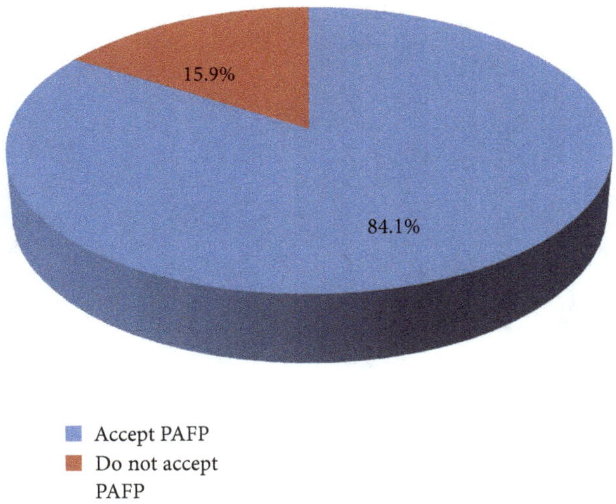

FIGURE 3: Acceptance of postabortion family planning among abortion service clients in Dessie, Amhara, Ethiopia, 2017.

years were 3 times more likely to accept postabortion family planning as compared with those aged >35 years and the odds ratios of accepting postabortion family planning among aborted women in the age group of 25-34 were 2 times higher than those aged >30 years. Similar relations were reported from the studies conducted in Ethiopia, Nepal, Vietnam, and Brazil [5, 15, 18, 20]. The possible reasons may be that young women have a greater probability of having unintended pregnancy which will end up with abortion.

In agreement with studies reported from 13 developing countries and Ethiopia in this study single women had high acceptance rate of postabortion family planning method [8, 15]. Participants who were single were 2 times more likely to accept postabortion family planning as compared with participants who were married [P = 0.0034 [X^2 test= 4.494, COR=2.398)]. The finding implies that females with unstable marital relationship increase acceptance of postabortion family planning. This may be due to first unmarried women may not use contraceptive as most of them have casual sex. Second those who are married are more likely to have settled and share the burden of increasing living cost which deceased fear of pregnancy and delivery; on the other hand single women have fear related with pregnancy because they do not have stable relationship and pregnancy without marital relationship is culturally unacceptable and discouraged.

This study result showed that females who decide on family planning had significant association with Postabortion family planning acceptance. Females who made independent decision were two times more likely to accept PAFP compared with those decided by husband or both of them [P = *0.022* [X^2 test= *7.679*, COR=1.695)]. This study finding is supported by studies done in Addis Ababa and Burayu [15, 21]. In addition, a study done in three regional states of Ethiopia, 2010, depicted that women make independent decision 46.5% regarding seeking postabortion care higher in magnitude than partner involvement decision making 42.4% [10]. The observed higher acceptance of postabortion family planning among females who passed independent decision might be explained as follows: since self-decision provides free space of choices females may tend to accept contraceptive.

Consistent with the study result in Burayu town which indicated that there is no significant association between participants family planning use history and acceptance of postabortion family planning, this study result showed that there is strong positive association between Postabortion contraception acceptance and family planning use history [15]. In this study females who had a use family planning had high acceptance postabortion family planning method when compared to those females who had not a history of family planning use [P= 0.000 [X^2 test= 63.621, COR=53.04)]. This might be due to the fact that those females who had a history of use family planning have better awareness on the method and side effect of family planning which facilitate choice of family planning, as supported by the result of this study which revealed that majority (56%) of this study participants reports fear of side effect which is the reason for why they did not accept postabortion family planning.

This study further depicts that women who did not get counseling were 4 [P = *0.03*[X^2 test= *4.333*, COR=2.369)] times less likely to accept postabortion family planning method compared with women who had counseled. This finding was supported by studies done in Ethiopia, Nepal, Brazil, and thirty countries [2, 5, 8, 15, 17, 22, 23]. This implies that family planning counseling is critical to raise acceptance of postabortion family planning method.

In this study occupational status, educational status, residence, place of abortion, those who ever give birth, and those who ever had abortion had no statistically significant association with acceptance postabortion family planning method as other studies found out [8, 22, 24, 25].

TABLE 4: Factors associated with Postabortion contraception acceptance among abortion service clients in Dessie, Amhara, Ethiopia, 2017.

Variables	Postabortion contraception acceptance		OR		
	Yes	No	COR	X^2 test	P-value
Age					
15-24	18	6	2.625	*9.989*	*0.007∗∗*
25-34	50	29	1.97		
35	8	7	1		
Education					
Literate	47	44	1.335	0.192	0.661
Illiterate	12	15	1		
Marital status					
Single	43	26	2.398	*4.494*	*0.034∗*
Married	20	29	1		
Occupational status					
Employed	24	21	1.385	.0.447	0.503
Unemployed	33	40	1		
Residence					
Dessie	44	39	1.065	0.002	0.964
Out of Dessie	18	17	1		
Place of abortion					
Marie stopes International	82	13	1.752	0.410	0.521
Dessie health centre	18	5			
Have you ever given birth?					
No	42	32	1.727	1.528	0.216
Yes	19	25	1		
Have you ever been counseled by HP about FP?					
Yes	44	26	2.369	*4.333*	*0.03∗*
No	20	28	1		
Have you ever used FP?					
Yes	52	10	53.040	*63.621*	*0.000∗∗∗*
No	5	51	1		
Who give decision about use of FP					
Wife	37	24	1.695	*7.679*	*0.022∗*
Husband	22	14	1.728		
Both	10	11	1		

∗∗∗0.000 ∗∗ <0.02 ∗ <0.05.

7. Strength and Limitation

7.1. Strength

(i) The first point is use of adopted, validated, and translated questionnaire.

(ii) The second point is the limited study in the area.

7.2. Limitations

(i) The first point is social desirability bias.

(ii) The second point is cross-sectional study design that established causal relationship impossible.

8. Conclusion and Recommendation

8.1. Conclusion. This study revealed that the acceptance of postabortion family planning method was 84%. Age of women, marital status, ever use of history family planning, involvement of others in decision making, and family planning counseling were significantly associated with postabortion family planning acceptance. Occupational status, educational status, residence, place of abortion, ever giving birth, and history of abortion had no statistically significant association with acceptance postabortion family planning method.

8.2. Recommendation. Based on this study finding the following recommendation was given.

(1) To Local Officials

(i) It is better to strengthen support health facility in establishing relation with school and community workers.

(2) Marie Stopes International Clinic and Dessie Health Center

(i) It is better to address young females through establishing link with schools.

(ii) It is better to strengthen family planning counseling services.

(iii) It is better to support females in decision making skills and process through establishing strong linkage with health extension and community workers.

(3) Health Educator and Researcher

(i) It is better for health educators to provide continuous health information about postabortion family planning methods and their side effects.

(ii) Researchers should further investigate other variable links with postabortion family planning and repeat the study with a comparison or control group to see the difference and the direction of relation.

Acronyms

DMPA: Depot-medroxyprogesterone acetate
FIGO: Federation of international gynecology and obstetrics
FP: Family planning
IUD: Intrauterine device
LARC: Long acting reversible contraceptives
MMR: Maternal mortality rate
MOH: Ministry of Health
MSIE: Marie stopes international clinic in Ethiopia
MVA: Manual vacuum aspiration
OR: Odd ratio
PAFP: Postabortion family planning.

Acknowledgments

Firstly, we would like to thank Alkan University Health Science and Business College, Department of Public Health, for giving this chance and financial support too. Secondly, we would like to say thanks to Marie stopes international and Dessie health center and for their cooperation. Last but not least we would deeply thank study participants.

References

[1] P. F. A. Van Look and J. Cottingham, "The World Health Organization's safe abortion guidance document," *American Journal of Public Health*, vol. 103, no. 4, pp. 593–596, 2013.

[2] A. Kesetebirhan, National Guideline for Family Planning Services in Ethiopia. Federal Democratic Republic of Ethiopia, Ministry of Health, 2011.

[3] A. Seid, A. Gebremariam, and M. Abera, "Integration of family planning services within post abortion care at health facilities in dessie –North East Ethiopia," *Science, Technology and Arts Research Journal*, vol. 1, no. 1, pp. 38–46, 2013.

[4] S. Khurram, Post abortion care family planning use in Pakistan, 2012.

[5] M. Puri et al., Post-abortion contraceptive use and continuation in Nepal, 2009.

[6] Central Stastical Agency, Ethiopia Demographic Health Servey, 2011.

[7] WHO and UNICEF, UNFPA AND theWorld Bank estimates maternal mortality; Geneva, 2012.

[8] S. Singh, "Hospital admissions resulting from unsafe abortion: estimates from 13 developing countries," *The Lancet*, vol. 368, no. 9550, pp. 1887–1892, 2006.

[9] S. L. Curtis, E. Evens, and W. Sambisa, "Contraceptive discontinuation and unintended pregnancy: an imperfect relationship," *International Perspectives on Sexual & Reproductive Health*, vol. 37, no. 2, pp. 58–66, 2011.

[10] Y. Melkamu, M. Betre, and S. Tesfaye, "Utilization of post-abortion care services in three regional states of Ethiopia," *Ethiopian Journal of Health Development*, vol. 24, no. 1, 2010.

[11] WHO Regional Office for Africa, I.o.O.B.f.P.o.M.-T.C.T.o.H., 2017.

[12] HIV/AIDS, J.U.N.P.o., AIDS scorecards: overview: UNAIDS report on the global AIDS epidemic 2010, UNAIDS, 2009.

[13] Post abortion family planning Tureky 2012.

[14] Federal Democratic Republic of Ethiopia, Ministry of health, (2006), National reproductive health strategy, 2006-2015.

[15] F. Andarge, Assessment of the Post abortion conteraception acceptanceand its assocatied factors in Burayu town ,Oromia region 2014.

[16] Monitering safe abortion care service provision in Tigray, Ethiopia, 2009.

[17] S. Worku and M. Fantahun, "Unintended pregnancy and induced abortion in a town with accessible family planning services: The case of Harar in eastern Ethiopia," *Ethiopian Journal of Health Development*, vol. 20, no. 2, pp. 79–83, 2007.

[18] A. L. Carneiro Gomes Ferreira, A. Impieri Souza, R. Evangelista Pessoa, and C. Braga, "The effectiveness of contraceptive counseling for women in the postabortion period: an intervention study," *Contraception*, vol. 84, no. 4, pp. 377–383, 2011.

[19] A. G. Worku, G. A. Tessema, A. A. Zeleke, and S. H. Räisänen, "Trends of modern contraceptive use among young married women based on the 2000, 2005, and 2011 ethiopian demographic and health surveys: a multivariate decomposition analysis," *PLoS ONE*, vol. 10, no. 1, Article ID e0116525, 2015.

[20] L. T. Vu, J. Oh, Q. T. Bui, and A. T. Le, "Use of modern contraceptives among married women in Vietnam: a multilevel analysis using the multiple indicator cluster survey (2011) and the Vietnam population and housing census (2009)," *Global Health Action*, vol. 9, no. 1, Article ID 29574, 2016.

[21] N. Prata, M. Holston, A. Fraser, and Y. Melkamu, "Contraceptive use among women seeking repeat abortion in Addis Ababa, Ethiopia," *African Journal of Reproductive Health*, vol. 17, no. 4, pp. 56–65, 2013.

[22] S. M. Tarekegn, L. S. Lieberman, and V. Giedraitis, "Determinants of maternal health service utilization in Ethiopia: analysis of the 2011 Ethiopian Demographic and Health Survey," *BMC Pregnancy and Childbirth*, vol. 14, no. 1, article 161, 2014.

[23] J. Benson, K. Andersen, D. Brahmi et al., "What contraception do women use after abortion? An analysis of 319,385 cases from eight countries," *Global Public Health*, vol. 13, no. 1, pp. 35–50, 2017.

[24] A. Sundaram, M. Vlassoff, A. Bankole, L. Remez, and Y. Gebrehiwot, "Benefits of meeting the contraceptive needs of Ethiopian women.," *Issues in brief (Alan Guttmacher Institute)*, no. 1, pp. 1–8, 2010.

[25] S. Singh et al., Adding It Up: The costs and Benefits of Investing in family Planning and maternal and new born health, Guttmacher Institute, 2009.

26

Adherence to Iron and Folic Acid Supplement and Its Associated Factors among Antenatal Care Attendant Mothers in Lay Armachiho Health Centers, Northwest, Ethiopia, 2017

Gashaw Agegnehu,[1] Azeb Atenafu,[2] Henok Dagne,[3] and Baye Dagnew[4]

[1] *Tikl Dingay Health Center, Ethiopia*
[2] *Department of Human Nutrition, Institute of Public Health, College of Medicine and Health Sciences, University of Gondar, Gondar 196, Ethiopia*
[3] *Department of Environmental and Occupational Health and Safety, Institute of Public Health, College of Medicine and Health Sciences, University of Gondar, Gondar 196, Ethiopia*
[4] *Department of Human Physiology, School of Medicine, University of Gondar, P.O. Box 196, Gondar, Ethiopia*

Correspondence should be addressed to Henok Dagne; enoch2313@gmail.com

Academic Editor: Stefania A. Nottola

Background. Iron deficiency is the leading nutrient deficiency globally affecting the lives of more than two billion people worldwide. Pregnant women are at higher risk of iron and folic acid deficiency due to lack of iron and folic acid or due to poor adherence. Adherence to iron and folic acid supplement is taking 65% or more of the recommended supplement, equivalent to taking the supplement at least 4 days a week during 3 months period using recording, reporting, and checking cards. *Objective.* The current study aimed at assessing adherence to iron and folic acid supplement during pregnancy and its associated factors among pregnant women attending antenatal care. *Methods.* Institution based cross-sectional study was conducted from February to March 2017. Systematic random sampling technique was used to select the study subjects. Data were collected using structured and pretested interviewer-administered questionnaire. Bivariable and multivariable logistic regression analysis were used to identify factors associated with adherence to iron and folic acid supplement among pregnant women. Adjusted odds ratio (AOR) with a 95% confidence interval (CI) was used to display the level of significance. Variables with a p-value less than 0.05 had been considered statistically significant. *Result.* Adherence to iron and folic acid in the current study was 28.7% with 95% CI (24.3, 33.6%). Educational status of mothers (AOR= 9.27 (95%CI: 2.47, 34.71)), educational status of husband (AOR= 0.31(95% CI: 0.11,0.88)), family size of four (AOR=3.70(95%CI: 1.08,12.76)), family size of five and above (AOR= 4.88(95% CI: 1.20, 19.85)), mothers who had 2500-3500 Ethiopian birr household average monthly income (AOR= 0.46(95% CI: 0.24,0.89)), mothers who had registered at 17-24 weeks of gestation (AOR=0.40(95% CI: 0.22-0.74)) and registered at 25-28 weeks (AOR=0.20(95% CI 0.10, 0.41)), and mothers who had collected their iron and folic acid starting at first visit at first month of pregnancy (AOR= 2.42(95% CI:1.05, 5.58)) had significant association with iron and folic acid adherence. *Conclusion and Recommendation.* Adherence of iron and folic acid was only 28.7% in the current study. Maternal and husband education status, family size, registration time, economic status, and first visit in the first month with duration of iron and folic acid taken were factors significantly associated with adherence to iron and folic acid supplement. Therefore, anaemia prevention strategy via improved iron and folic acid supplement adherence should comprise strategies of educating pregnant mothers, improving economic status, and early antenatal care (ANC) registration that can improve adherence to iron and folic acid supplement.

1. Introduction

Iron deficiency is the leading single most important nutrient deficiency globally which affects the lives of more than two billion people, accounting for over 30% of global population, the highest being in developing countries [1]. Pregnant women, postpartum women, and children aged 6-24 months are usually the most affected groups [2, 3].

Pregnant women are at high risk of iron and folic acid deficiency due to increased nutrient requirement during pregnancy [4, 5]. In Ethiopia, 17% women with reproductive age and 22% of pregnant women are estimated to be anaemic [6, 7]. According to the WHO and Ethiopia's national guidelines for control and prevention of micronutrient deficiencies, all pregnant women should receive and consume a standard dose of 60 mg iron and 400 μg folic acid daily for 6 months starting from first month of pregnancy or at the time of their first antenatal visit and three months of postnatal period. Iron and folic acid supplementation are required to balance increased physiological demand during puberty, pregnancy, and lactation [2, 3, 8, 9].

Iron is a trace mineral that is important for fetal growth and development. Iron is found in red blood cells to carry oxygen needed throughout the body. It is also essential for normal neuronal development. Folic acid is another important micronutrient used in the synthesis of neurotransmitters and particularly during early pregnancy. It has an essential role in synthesizing DNA during organogenesis [10].

The high physiological requirement for iron and folic acid in pregnancy is difficult to meet with the usual diet. Therefore, pregnant women should routinely receive iron and folic acid supplements. Adherence to a medication regimen is generally defined as the extent to which patients take medications as prescribed by their health care providers [11]. Adherence rates for individual patients are usually reported as the percentage of the prescribed doses of the medication actually taken by the patient over a specified period [12].

One in every three women had anaemia while one in every two had iron and folic acid deficiency, indicating that both folic acid and iron deficiencies constitute the major micronutrient deficiencies in Ethiopian women [4]. Iron and folic acid deficiency is a serious public health issue due to its high potential negative consequences. It can lead to several adverse outcomes including low birth weight, preterm delivery, stillbirth, and maternal and neonatal mortality. Infants are among the vulnerable groups of iron/folic acid deficiency. Since there is a link between maternal and neonatal iron status, interventions on infant alone are insufficient to decrease infant iron and folic acid status. Oral iron and folic acid supplementation is a feasible and cost-effective strategy in the prevention and control of iron and folic acid deficiency anaemia [13].

The risk of death decreases by 24% and 1.8 million deaths in children aged 28 days to 10 years will be avoided for each increase in 1 g/dl haemoglobin. Simple IFAS strategies are feasible ways to attain such increments in haemoglobin [13]. Early neonatal death was reduced by 57% in Nepal and 45% in Pakistan when more than 90 tablets are taken and started at or before fifth months of pregnancy. Similarly, the risk was decreased by more than half in those study participants who took IFAS during pregnancy [14]. Currently, iron and folic acid supplementation is the main strategy for anaemia control and prevention in Ethiopia [7, 9]. While many developing countries including Ethiopia are now implementing iron folic acid supplementation (IFAS) through antenatal care programs, only a few countries have reported significant improvement in IFAS adherence and control and prevention of anaemia [7, 15, 16].

This low achievement may be related to poor access and lower level of antenatal care service utilization, inadequate IFAS, poor counselling, poor knowledge about anaemia, and certain bad believes regarding IFAS [7]. However, many studies suggested that low level of maternal adherence to the regimen is the main reason for the ineffectiveness of the anemia prevention and control strategy [11, 15]. There is little feedback about the effectiveness of iron and folic acid supplement countrywide. Women may have low adherence to IFAS due to perceived side effects [17–19], forgetfulness [17, 18, 20, 21], and lack of access to IFAS supplement [11]. The factors associated with adherence to IFAS reported by various studies [18, 20–22] are not similar and there is a lack of information regarding the prevalence and associated factors of IFAS in the study area. In addition, previous studies mostly focused on adherence to IFAS and associated factors among pregnant women at community level where it lacks assessment of organizational related factors. Different sociodemographic, pregnancy and obstetric related, health service, and supplement related factors may contribute to adherence to IFAS (Figure 1). The level of education, the cultural practices, the strength of health service, and familial support vary from place to place. The current study focuses on assessment adherence and associated factors of IFAS among pregnant women in Lay Armachiho district health centers, Northwest, Ethiopia.

2. Methods

2.1. Study Design and Settings. An institution based cross-sectional study design was employed from February to March 2017 in Lay Armachiho district Health Centers. Lay Armachiho district is one of 22 districts in North Gondar administrative zone and is located at a distance of 769 *km* from Addis Ababa, 202 *km* from Bahirdar, and 22 *km* from Gondar administrative city. It encompasses about 129,272 km^2 area of land and is characterized by diverse climate and topography with a marked difference in the climate conditions. Most of the area is on the highland plateau and is characterized by rugged mountains, hills, and plateaus. Hence, the district has varied landscapes composed of steep fault escarpments and nearly mountainous and erodible landforms but draught did not occurr and no shortage of rain in a rainy season. It is located in Northwest of Gondar, Ethiopia and bordered by Wogera, Sanja, Chillga, Dembia, and North Gondar administrative city. According to figures from the Central Statistical Agency, 2007, the district had an estimated population of 140417, of whom 70911 are females. Estimated pregnant women are 5,616. There are 6 health centers, 26 health posts, 6 junior private clinics, 1 medium private clinic, and 2 private drug venders providing health services in the district [23].

2.2. Sample Size Determination. The sample size was calculated using single population proportion formula with the following assumptions: p (Proportion of Adherence to IFAS =

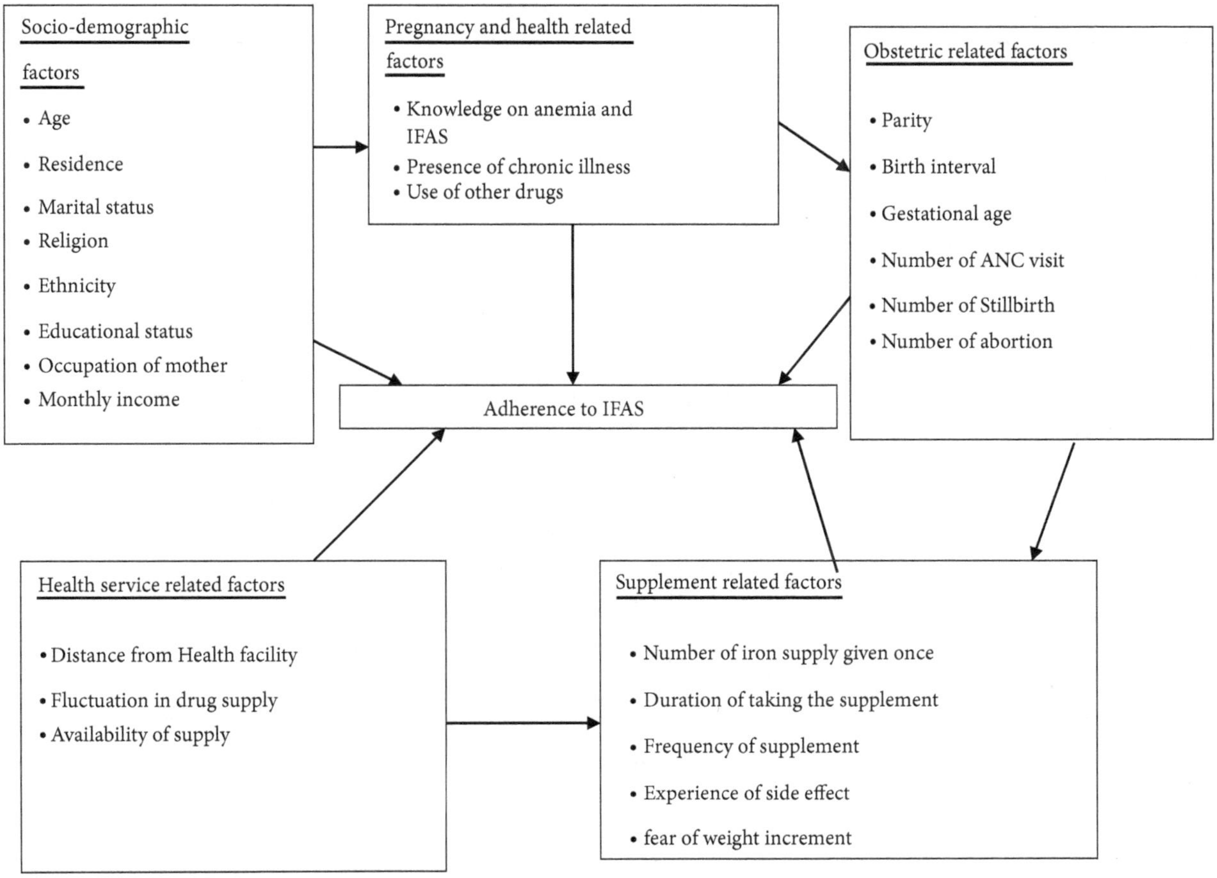

FIGURE 1: Conceptual framework adapted from different literature review [21, 24, 26].

55.5% [24], 95% confidence interval, and 5% margin of error (d)).

$$n = \frac{(z_{\alpha/2})^2 p(1-p)}{d^2} = \frac{(1.96)^2\, 0.555\,(1-0.555)}{0.05^2} = 380 \quad (1)$$

Considering, a 10% non-response rate, the final sample size was 418.

2.3. Sampling Procedures and Sampling Technique. There were a total of 838 pregnant women who fulfilled eligibility criteria (all pregnant mothers who were taking IFAS during their 2nd, 3rd, and 4th ANC follow-up were included in the study but mothers who were seriously ill at the time of data collection and pregnant mothers at the first trimester were excluded) during the study period in Lay Armachiho district, 2017. Using baseline information, a proportional number of study subjects were selected from each health center. The interval was determined as k = N/n, where k is the interval of sampling, N is total number of population, and n is the number of sample. With the total number of pregnant women N = 838 and the minimum sample size being n = 418, an interval of k = N/n = 838/418= 2. The first study participants were selected using lottery method and then every 2nd unit from ANC registration book was taken as study subject. Therefore, systematic random sampling technique was used to include a sample of 418 study participants.

2.4. Data Collection Procedures. A structured questionnaire was used to collect data. The questionnaire was pretested over 30 women out of the study area in an institution with similar characteristics prior to the actual data collection. Six BSc Nurses (worked as data collectors) and two BSc Public Health professionals (worked as supervisors) were involved in the data collection process. Training was given for the data collectors and supervisors. The overall interview process was supervised by supervisors. The collected data were checked by the data collectors immediately after finalizing the questionnaire before they left the health centers. Supervisors daily checked the completeness and consistency of information collected.

2.5. Operational Definition. Adherence to IFAS is the outcome variable in this study. Pregnant mothers are said to be "adherent " to IFAS if they took 65% or more of the recommended supplement, equivalent to taking the supplement at least 4 days a week during 3 months of period using recording, reporting, and checking their cards [25]. Early registration to ANC clinic was measured as those pregnant women who visit the ANC clinic before 16 weeks of gestation [26]. Knowledge of anaemia was measured by asking 6

Table 1: Sociodemographic factors of respondents, Lay Armachiho district Health Centers, Northwest Ethiopia, 2017 (n=418).

Variable	Categories	Frequency (n)	Percent (%)
Age	17- 25	211	50.5
	26- 35	155	37.1
	36- 45	52	12.4
Residence	Rural	312	74.6
	Urban	106	24.4
Religion	Orthodox	415	99.3
	Muslim	3	0.7
Ethnicity	Kemant	380	90.9
	Amhara	38	9.1
Educational status of mother	Cannot read and write	148	35.4
	Can read and write	188	45
	Completed primary and above	82	19.6
Educational status of husband	Cannot read and write	152	36.4
	Can read and write	118	24.6
	Completed primary and above	148	35.4
Occupation of mother	Housewife	347	83
	Employed	71	17
Occupation of husband	Employed	66	15.8
	Farmers	352	84.4
Family size	Two	101	24.2
	Three	77	18.4
	Four	64	15.3
	Five and above	176	42.1
Monthly income (ETB*)	500- 2500	165	39.5
	2501- 3500	161	38.5
	>3500	92	22
**Knowledge about IFAS and anaemia	Knowledgeable	57	13.6
	Non-knowledgeable	361	86.4

* ETB: Ethiopian birr; ETB = 24 USD; ** knowledgeable means those who have correctly answered above the mean of knowledge questions regarding anemia and IFAS.

knowledge questions whether respondents know the illness called anemia, causes of anemia, and consequences of anemia during pregnancy and identify who is more susceptible to anemia and whether they know methods of anemia prevention during pregnancy. Mothers who score median and more questions on anaemia are said to be knowledgeable [21]. Knowledge about IFAS was measured by asking 8 knowledge questions about IFAS (regarding knowledge of Iron/folate drug, health benefit of IFAS for the fetus and child, whether they believe taking IFAS has risks, and whether they know for how long they should take the IFAS). Those who score median and above on questions prepared to assess comprehensive knowledge of IFAS of the respondents were considered as having "good knowledge" and those who scored below the median were having "poor knowledge" [26]. Total knowledge for both variables together was computed and respondents who score mean and above mean of the knowledge questions were considered as knowledgeable.

2.6. Data Management and Statistical Analysis. Data were entered using EPI-INFO version 3.5.1 and exported into SPSS version 20 for analysis. For most variables, data were presented by frequencies and percentages. Bivariable logistic regression analysis was used to explore candidate variables for the multivariable logistic regression analysis and variables with p-value less than 0.2 during the bivariable analysis were then analyzed by multivariable logistic regression for controlling the possible effect of confounders and finally variables which had significant association with IFAS adherence were identified on the basis of AOR with 95% CI and $p < 0.05$. Hosmer and Lemeshow goodness of fit test was used to check model fitness. Variance inflation factor (VIF) was also used to test interactions between variables.

3. Results

3.1. Sociodemographic Information. A total of 418 study participants were included in this study with 100% response rate. The mean age of respondents was 27.2 (SD±6.3) years. Majority of respondents 312 (74.6%) were rural dwellers. Four hundred fifteen (99.3%) of the study subjects were followers of Orthodox Christianity. The majority (83%) of the study subjects were housewives (Table 1).

TABLE 2: Pregnancy, obstetric, and health-related factors of respondents, Lay Armachiho district Health Centers, Northwest Ethiopia, 2017 (n=418).

Variable	Categories	Frequency (n)	Percent (%)
Gravidity	One	114	27.3
	Two- Five	219	52.4
	Six- Ten	85	20.3
Parity	Zero	117	28
	One- five	257	61.5
	Six- Eight	44	10.5
History of stillbirth	Yes	22	5.3
	No	396	94.3
Number of stillbirth	One	18	4.3
	Two or more	4	0 .96
History of abortion	Yes	39	9.3
	No	379	90.7
Number of abortion	One	29	6.9
	Two or more	10	2.4
ANC follow up	Yes	415	99.3
	No	3	0.7
Time of ANC registration	0- 16 weeks	124	29.7
	17- 24weeks	160	38.3
	25- 28 weeks	134	32.1

3.2. Pregnancy, Obstetric, and Health-Related Factors of Respondents. Majority of respondents (72.2%) had less than three times ANC visit. Among the respondents, 124 (29.7%) had started ANC during the first trimester (before 16 weeks of gestation) (Table 2).

3.3. Respondents Knowledge of Anaemia and Benefit of IFAS. Less than one-fifth of respondents 57 (13.6%) were knowledgeable about anaemia and IFAS, while 361 (86.4%) of respondents were not knowledgeable about anaemia and IFAS (Table 3).

3.4. Health Service-Related Factors of Respondents. Only 4 study participants have used iron and folic acid for greater than three months (90 tablets). Among the respondents, 80% were provided health education about IFAS (Table 4).

3.5. The Adherence to IFAS. From a total of 418 participants included in this study, only 120 (28.7%) 95% CI (24.3, 33.6%) participants adhered to IFAS. The reason that most mothers reported for not adhering to IFAS were forgetfulness 167 (40%), pill burden 21 (5%), side effects of the drugs 207 (49.5%), epigastric burning sensation (gastritis) 206 (49.3%), unpleasant taste of IFAS 101 (24.2%), and vomiting 166 (39.7%).

3.6. Factors Associated with Adherence to IFAS. Bivariable logistic regression was used to choose variables for the final model on the basis of p-value less than 0.2. Place of residence, educational status of mothers, educational status of husband, number of pregnancy, number of delivery, knowledge on anaemia and IFAS, occupation of mother, occupation of husband, family size, early registration, average household monthly income, disease confirmed by physician like gastritis, treatment of disease, and first visit at first month were variables selected for the final model. Variance inflation factor (VIF) was calculated considering one independent variable as the dependent variable turn by turn to test interactions between variables to minimize effect of multicollinearity. The test result showed that VIF for all variables was below 3, the threshold for collinearity diagnostics. This showed that there is no multicollinearity effect between independent variables.

Table 5 shows variables associated with adherence to IFAS. Adherence to IFAS was significantly associated with the educational status of participants. The probability of adherence to IFAS was 9.27 times higher among participants whose educational status was primary education and above [AOR= 9.27, 95%CI= (2.47, 34.71)] as compared to study participants who cannot read and write.

About 69% of study participants whose husbands have an educational status above primary education were less likely adhered to IFAS as compared to those study subjects whose husbands cannot read and write [AOR= 0.31, 95% CI = (0.11, 0.89)]. The probability of IFAS adherence was 3.7 times higher among participants who have a family size of four as compared to those having only two family members [AOR=3.70, 95% CI = (1.08,12.76)]. Adherence of IFAS among study participants with five and above family members was 4.88 times higher than those only with 2 family members [AOR=4.88, 95% CI = (1.20, 19.85].

TABLE 3: Respondents' knowledge of anaemia and benefit of IFAS in Lay Armachiho district Health Centers, Northwest Ethiopia, 2017 (n=418).

Variables		Frequency (n)	Percent (%)
Knowledge on anaemia and IFAS	Good	57	13.6
	Poor	361	86.4
The source of information	Health professionals	310	74.2
	Mass media	41	9.8
	Friends	21	5
Iron/and folic acid currently taking	Yes	403	96.4
	No	15	3.6
Duration of iron and folic acid used	1 month (30 Tablets)	162	38.8
	2 month (60 Tablets)	140	33.5
	3 month (90 Tablets)	116	27.8

TABLE 4: Health service-related factors of respondents, Lay Armachiho district health centers, Northwest, Ethiopia, 2017 (n=418).

Variable	Categories	Frequency (n)	Percent (%)
Health education delivered during collection of drugs about	Use of drugs	335	80
	Methods used	221	52.9
	Side effects	181	43.3
	Appointment	261	62.4
Tablets collected in each follow up	30 tablets	396	94.7
	60 tablets	7	1.7
*Problem faced in health centre during health care delivery	Yes	24	5.7
	No	377	90.4

* Respondents were asked if they encountered problems such as shortage of IFAS, long waiting time, poor communication that hindered them from taking the IFAS.

As revealed by this study, adherence to IFAS was associated with average monthly household income. The study participants whose average monthly income is 2501 to 3500 ETB were less likely adhered to IFAS compared to those who earned 500 to 2500 ETB [AOR= 0.46, 95% CI = (0.24,0.90)]. Participants who had registered 17-24 weeks of gestation [AOR=0.40, 95% CI (0.22-0.74)] and participants who had registered at 25-28 weeks [AOR=0.20, 95% CI (0.10, 0.41)] were less likely to adhere to IFAS. The probability of adherence to IFAS was 2.42 times higher among study participants collecting their pill at first visit at first month of pregnancy with duration of pill used [AOR= 2.42, 95% CI (1.05, 5.58)].

4. Discussion

Pregnant women are prone to iron deficiency anemia. Iron and folic acid supplementation has been a major strategy to reduce iron/folic acid deficiency anemia. However, issues of poor adherence remain a challenge. Adherence to IFAS found in this study was 28.7% which is lower than studies conducted in Cambodia [14], Indonesia [13], studies done among pregnant women in Eritrean refugee camps, Northern Ethiopia [19], among pregnant women attending ANC at University of Gondar hospital [18], Governmental Health Centers in Akaki Kality Sub City [22], among pastoralist pregnant women in Burji districts, Southern Ethiopia [17], among pregnant woman in west Dembia [27], and among pregnant women attending antenatal care follow up at Debre Tabor General hospital, Ethiopia [28]. It was similar to the adherence reported for rural women by Gebre et al. [26]. But the adherence in the current study is higher than results from studies conducted in Kenya [29], Goba, Ethiopia [24], a study done in 8 rural districts of Ethiopia [21], and a study conducted in Mecha district in Amhara region [30].

This difference could be due to the differences in the socioeconomic status of the study populations and the time of the study, the data collection tool used, and the difference in the study setting. This also might be due to differences in training level of health care professionals regarding IFAS and the professional skill of teaching mothers regarding the health benefit of IFAS and standard of the health care institution in the different level of health care facilities as this study was conducted on health centers. This rationale is supported by several studies as in well-organized set-ups adequate counselling and sustainable product availability is better [27].

This study depicted that the educational status of the mother was significantly associated with adherence to IFAS. The adherence was higher among mothers who have completed primary education and above.

This finding is in line with the findings of other studies in Ethiopia [17, 22, 30] and India [31]. Education is more likely to enhance female awareness of micronutrient deficiency and ways to overcome these deficiencies. Overall, educated women have a greater ability to stick to health care inputs

TABLE 5: Factor associated with adherence Lay Armachiho district Health Centers, Northwest Ethiopia, 2017 (n=418).

Variables	Category	Adherence status of respondents		COR(95% CI)	AOR(95% CI)
		Adhered	Non-adhered		
Residence	Rural	80(19.1)	232(55.5)	1	1
	Urban	40(9.6)	66(15.8)	0.57(0.36, 0.91)	0.60(0.27, 1.30)
Educational status of mother	cannot read and write	27(6.5)	121(28.95)	1	1
	Read and write	43(10.3)	145(34.7)	0.57(0.44, 1.29)	1.34(0.64, 3.05)
	Completed primary and above	50(12)	32(7.7)	5.27(3.01,9.22)	9.27(2.47,34.71) *
Educational status of husband	Cannot read and write	36(8.6)	116(27.8)	1	1
	Read and write	28(6.7)	90(21.5)	0.10(0.57, 1.76)	0.78(0.38, 1.61)
	Completed primary and above	56(13.4)	92(22)	1.96(1.14, 3.35)	0.31(0.11-0.88) *
Family size	Two	19(4.5)	82(19.6)	1	1
	Three	49(11.7)	127(30.4)	2.33(1.18,4.62)	2.33(0.86, 6.32)
	Four	27(6.5)	50(12)	2.77(1.36,5.62)	3.70(1.08, 12.76) *
	Five and above	25(6)	39(9.3)	1.67(0.92, 3.03)	4.88(0.90, 4.80)
Occupation of mother	House wife	81(19.4)	266(63.6)	1	1
	Employed	39(9.3)	32(7.7)	4.00(2.36,6.80)	1.13(0.46,2.79)
Occupation of husband	Employed	39(9.3)	27(6.5)	1	1
	Farmer	81(19.4)	271(64.8)	0.63(0.24, 1.67)	0.66(0.25, 1.72)
Monthly income	500-2500 birr	28(6.7)	133(31.8)	1	1
	2501-3500 birr	40(9.6)	125(29.9)	0.66(0.38,1.13)	0.46(0.24,0.89) *
	>3500 birr	52(12.4)	40(9.6)	4.06(2.34,7.00)	2.08(0.90,4.79)
Gravidity	One	28(6.7)	86(20.6)	1	1
	Two	46(11)	126(30.1)	1.76(0.95,3.26)	0.86(0.06,12.49)
	Three	15(3.6)	32(7.7)	1.44(0.86,3.04)	1.29(0.06,28.35)
	Four and above	31(7.4)	54(12.9)	1.12(0.65,1.93)	2.58(0.11,61.09)
Parity	Zero	28(6.7)	88(21.1)	1	1
	One	45(10.8)	124(29.7)	1.94(1.06, 3.55)	0.86(0.07, 11.32)
	Two	13(3.1)	55(13.2)	1.32(0.07,2.86)	0.61(0.03,12.78)
	Four and above	34(7.1)	31(7.4)	1.14(0.66,1.97)	0.22(0.01, 4.46)
Early registration	0-16weeks	55(13.2)	69(16.5)	1	1
	17- 24 weeks	44(10.5)	116(27.8)	0.48(0.29, 0.78)	0.40(0.22, 0.74) *
	25- 28 weeks	21(5)	113(27)	0.66(0.13, 0.51)	0.20(0.10,0.41) **
Duration of pill taken	3months	100(23.9)	283(67.7)	1	1
	>3months	20(4.8)	15(3.4)	3.77(1.86, 7.66)	2.42(1.05, 5.58) *
Health problem	Yes	3	26	1	1
	No	117	272	3.73(1.12,12.56)	1.32(0.12,14.64)
Treatment for health problem	Yes	2	22	1	1
	No	118	276	4.70(1.09, 20.32)	1.86(0.11, 33.18)
Knowledge on anemia and IFAS	Good	12(2.9)	45(10.8)	1	1
	Poor	108(25.8)	253(60,5)	0.63(0.32, 1.23)	0.77(0.36, 1.64)

Note. ** significant at P-value < 0.001; * significant at P-value <0.05; Hosmer and Lemeshow test = 0.434 showed that the model fit well.

such as IFA which offer better care for both the infant and the mother. A husband who completed primary education and above was less likely to promote adherence of IFAS. This result is inconsistent with a study conducted in Indonesia where both mothers and husbands had promoted and enhanced adherence status of pregnant women equally [32]. This might be due to low autonomy of mothers on their own health care in Indonesia [32]. In the current study mothers are autonomous on utilization of IFAS without the consent of their husbands.

Household average monthly income was associated with IFAS. The current study has revealed that those participants with lower family income are less likely to adhere to IFAS compared to those with higher family income. This was consistent with a study conducted in Kenya [29]. Family size was significantly associated with adherence of IFAS. This might be because those participants who had multiparity would have medical advice, health education, counselling, and access to more information about the benefits of IFAS during pregnancy and early pregnancy than nulliparous participants.

Early time of registration was significantly associated with IFAS adherence. This finding is consistent with a study done in Kenya [29].

Finally, this study is not without limitation. The gold standard method of measuring adherence like electronic and pills counting method was not used. The cross-sectional nature of the study does not allow establishing a strong cause-effect relationship. The use of larger sample size and pretested questionnaire made this study generalizable and the reliability was checked and found to be good.

5. Conclusion/Recommendations

The adherence of IFAS among antenatal care attendant women in Lay Armachiho district health centers was low and significant proportion of women do not adhere to IFAS. Educational status of participants, educational status of husband, family size, household average monthly income, registration time, and tablet collection time were identified as factors associated with adherence to IFAS. Educating pregnant mothers, improving economic status, and early ANC registration can improve adherence to IFAS. Professionals at the health centers should strive a lot to increase the adherence of pregnant women on IFAS. There are many barriers that hinder the pregnant women from adherence to IFAS including forgetfulness and fear of side effects of the drugs. To minimize or prevent forgetfulness to take the drug, health professionals should counsel the women with strategies such as correlating taking the drugs with natural events. Regarding fear of side effects, health professionals should deliver counseling and make the pregnant women aware that side effects are minor as compared with the advantage of taking IFAS, and if major side effects occurred, they should go to health facilities for better management.

List of Abbreviations

ANC: Antenatal care
AOR: Adjusted Odds Ratio
CI: Confidence interval
COR: Crude Odds Ratio
IFAS: Iron folic acid supplementation
Km: Kilometer
Km^2: Square kilometers
mg: Milligram
SPSS: Statistical Package for Social Sciences
VIF: Variance inflation factor
WHO: World Health Organization
μg: Microgram.

Consent

This manuscript does not contain any individual person's data. Verbal informed consent was obtained from the study participants.

Disclosure

There were no risks due to participation in this research project. The collected data were used for this research purpose only and kept with complete confidentiality. Researchers provided health education for the study subjects about the importance of IFAS.

Authors' Contributions

All the authors actively participated during the conception of the research issue, development of a research proposal, analysis and interpretation, and writing of various parts of the research report. Gashaw Agegnehu designed the protocol; participated in data collection; entered data into Epi-Info epidemiological software; analyzed the data; and supervised the overall research process. Azeb Atenafu designed the protocol and supervised the overall research process. Henok Dagne designed the protocol, supervised the overall research process, and prepared the manuscript. Baye Dagnew undertook data analysis, commented on the manuscript, and revised accordingly. All the authors read and approved the final manuscript.

Acknowledgments

The authors are pleased to acknowledge data collectors, field supervisors, study participants, the University of Gondar, and the managers and staff members of Lay Armachiho District Health Centers for their unreserved contributions to the success of this study. The authors of this study did not receive funds from any funding institution. However, the University of Gondar covered questionnaire duplication and data collection fees.

References

[1] L. N. Gathigi, *Factors Influencing Utilization of Iron and Folic Acid Supplementation Services among Women Attending Antenatal Clinic at Nyeri Provincial Hospital Kenya*, 2013.

[2] WHO. Guideline, *Guideline: Daily Iron and Folic Acid Supplementation in Pregnant Women*, 2006.

[3] K. Mahomed, "Iron supplementation in pregnancy (Cochrane Review)," *The Cochrane Library*, p. 2, 2000.

[4] M. Y. Yakoob and Z. A. Bhutta, "Effect of routine iron supplementation with or without folic acid on anemia during pregnancy," *BMC Public Health*, vol. 11, no. 3, article no. S21, 2011.

[5] J. A. Haidar and R. S. Pobocik, "Iron deficiency anemia is not a rare problem among women of reproductive ages in Ethiopia: a community based cross sectional study," *BMC Hematology*, vol. 9, no. 1, 2009.

[6] Ethiopia Central Statistical Agency and ICF International, *2011 Ethiopia Demographic and Health Survey: Key Findings*, ICF International, Calverton, Maryland, USA, 2012.

[7] FMOH, *A Rapid, Initial Assessment of the Distribution and Consumption of Iron-Folic Acid Tab-lets through Antenatal Care in Ethiopia in Selected Four Regions*, SPRING, 2013.

[8] W. D. o. M. P. S. (MPS), *Iron and Folic acid Supplementation. Standards for Maternal & Neonatal Care. Integrated Management of Pregnancy and Childbirth (IMPAC)*, Geneva, Switzerland, 2006.

[9] FMOH, *Programme Implementation Manual of National Nutrition Programme*, Ethiopia, Addis Ababa, Ethiopia, 2013.

[10] O. Ogundipe, C. Hoyo, T. Østbye et al., "Factors associated with prenatal folic acid and iron supplementation among 21,889 pregnant women in Northern Tanzania: A cross-sectional hospital-based study," *BMC Public Health*, vol. 12, no. 1, 2012.

[11] R. Galloway and J. McGuire, "Determinants of compliance with iron supplementation: supplies, side effects, or psychology?" *Social Science & Medicine*, vol. 39, no. 3, pp. 381–390, 1994.

[12] Z. M. Ibrahim et al., "Assessment of adherence to iron and folic acid supplementation and prevalence of anemia in pregnant women," *The Medical Journal of Cairo University*, vol. 79, no. 2, 2011.

[13] C. R. Titaley and M. J. Dibley, *Factors associated with not using antenatal iron/folic acid supplements in Indonesia: the 2002/2003 and 2007 Indonesia Demographic and Health Survey*, Federation of American Societies for Experimental Biology, 2013.

[14] P. Lacerte, M. Pradipasen, P. Temcharoen, N. Imamee, and T. Vorapongsathorn, "Determinants of adherence to iron/folate supplementation during pregnancy in two provinces in Cambodia," *Asia-Pacific Journal of Public Health*, vol. 23, no. 3, pp. 315–323, 2011.

[15] M. Zakia et al., "Assessment of Adherence to Iron and Folic Acid Supplementation and Prevalence of Anemia in Pregnant Women Ismailia governorate," *The Medical Journal of Cairo University*, vol. 79, no. 2, 2011.

[16] B. Kulkarni, P. Christian, S. C. LeClerq, and S. K. Khatry, "Determinants of compliance to antenatal micronutrient supplementation and women's perceptions of supplement use in rural Nepal," *Public Health Nutrition*, vol. 13, no. 1, pp. 82–90, 2010.

[17] N. Boti, T. Bekele, W. Godana et al., "Adherence to Iron-Folate Supplementation and Associated Factors among Pastoralist's Pregnant Women in Burji Districts, Segen Area People's Zone, Southern Ethiopia: Community-Based Cross-Sectional Study," *International Journal of Reproductive Medicine*, vol. 2018, pp. 1–8, 2018.

[18] T. M. Birhanu, M. K. Birarra, and F. A. Mekonnen, "Compliance to iron and folic acid supplementation in pregnancy, Northwest Ethiopia," *BMC Research Notes*, vol. 11, no. 1, p. 345, 2018.

[19] M. Getachew, M. Abay, H. Zelalem, T. Gebremedhin, T. Grum, and A. Bayray, "Magnitude and factors associated with adherence to Iron-folic acid supplementation among pregnant women in Eritrean refugee camps, northern Ethiopia," *BMC Pregnancy and Childbirth*, vol. 18, no. 1, p. 83, 2018.

[20] W. Niguse and R. Murugan, "Determinants of adherence to iron folic acid supplementation among pregnant women attending antenatal clinic in Asella town, Ethiopia," *International Journal of Therapeutic Applications*, vol. 35, pp. 60–67, 2018.

[21] S. Gebremedhin, A. Samuel, G. Mamo, T. Moges, and T. Assefa, "Coverage, compliance and factors associated with utilization of iron supplementation during pregnancy in eight rural districts of Ethiopia: a cross-sectional study," *BMC Public Health*, vol. 14, no. 1, article 607, 2014.

[22] B. Gebreamlak, A. F. Dadi, and A. Atnafu, "High adherence to iron/folic acid supplementation during pregnancy time among antenatal and postnatal care attendant mothers in Governmental Health Centers in Akaki Kality Sub City, Addis Ababa, Ethiopia: Hierarchical negative binomial poisson regression," *PLoS ONE*, vol. 12, no. 1, Article ID e0169415, 2017.

[23] Annual health report 2016, Lay Armachiho Woreda Health office.

[24] Birhanu, *Adherence to prenatal iron/folic acid supplements and associated factors among ANC attendant mothers of Debere markos town, south East Ethiopia, in Haramaya University*, Harar, Ethiopia, 2016.

[25] A. Lynette, *Factors Associated with Adherence to Iron/Folate Supplementation among Pregnant Women Attending Antenatal Clinic at Thika District Hospital in Kiambu County, Kenya*, University of Kenyata, 2013.

[26] A. Gebre, A. Mulugeta, and B. Etana, "Assessment of factors associated with adherence to iron-folic acid supplementation among urban and rural pregnant women in north western zone of Tigray, Ethiopia: Comparative Study," *International Journal of Nutrition and Food Sciences*, vol. 4, no. 2, pp. 161–168, 2015.

[27] T. Molla, T. Guadu, E. A. Muhammad, and M. T. Hunegnaw, "Factors associated with adherence to iron folate supplementation among pregnant women in West Dembia district, northwest Ethiopia: a cross sectional study," *BMC Research Notes*, vol. 12, no. 1, 2019.

[28] A. D. Gebremariam, S. A. Tiruneh, B. A. Abate, M. T. Engidaw, D. T. Asnakew, and S. S. Budhathoki, "Adherence to iron with folic acid supplementation and its associated factors among pregnant women attending antenatal care follow up at Debre Tabor General Hospital, Ethiopia, 2017," *PLoS ONE*, vol. 14, no. 1, p. e0210086, 2019.

[29] L. A. Dinga, A. Mwangi, and G. Abong, *Factors Associated with Adherence to Iron/Folate Supplementation among Pregnant Women Attending Antenatal Clinic at Thika District Hospital in Kiambu County*, University of Nairobi, Food Science, Nutrition and Technology, Faculty of Agriculture, Nairobi, Kenya, 2013.

[30] B. Taye, G. Abeje, and A. Mekonen, "Factors associated with compliance of prenatal iron folate supplementation among women in Mecha district, Western Amhara: a cross-sectional study," *Pan African Medical Journal*, vol. 20, article 43, 2015.

[31] P. Mithra, B. Unnikrishnan, T. Rekha et al., "Compliance with iron-folic acid (IFA) therapy among pregnant women in an urban area of south India," *African Health Sciences*, vol. 13, no. 4, pp. 880–885, 2013.

[32] C. R. Titaley and M. J. Dibley, "Factors associated with not using antenatal iron/folic acid supplements in Indonesia," *Asia Pacific Journal of Clinical Nutrition*, vol. 23, no. 4, 2014.

Permissions

All chapters in this book were first published by Hindawi Publishing Corporation; hereby published with permission under the Creative Commons Attribution License or equivalent. Every chapter published in this book has been scrutinized by our experts. Their significance has been extensively debated. The topics covered herein carry significant findings which will fuel the growth of the discipline. They may even be implemented as practical applications or may be referred to as a beginning point for another development.

The contributors of this book come from diverse backgrounds, making this book a truly international effort. This book will bring forth new frontiers with its revolutionizing research information and detailed analysis of the nascent developments around the world.

We would like to thank all the contributing authors for lending their expertise to make the book truly unique. They have played a crucial role in the development of this book. Without their invaluable contributions this book wouldn't have been possible. They have made vital efforts to compile up to date information on the varied aspects of this subject to make this book a valuable addition to the collection of many professionals and students.

This book was conceptualized with the vision of imparting up-to-date information and advanced data in this field. To ensure the same, a matchless editorial board was set up. Every individual on the board went through rigorous rounds of assessment to prove their worth. After which they invested a large part of their time researching and compiling the most relevant data for our readers.

The editorial board has been involved in producing this book since its inception. They have spent rigorous hours researching and exploring the diverse topics which have resulted in the successful publishing of this book. They have passed on their knowledge of decades through this book. To expedite this challenging task, the publisher supported the team at every step. A small team of assistant editors was also appointed to further simplify the editing procedure and attain best results for the readers.

Apart from the editorial board, the designing team has also invested a significant amount of their time in understanding the subject and creating the most relevant covers. They scrutinized every image to scout for the most suitable representation of the subject and create an appropriate cover for the book.

The publishing team has been an ardent support to the editorial, designing and production team. Their endless efforts to recruit the best for this project, has resulted in the accomplishment of this book. They are a veteran in the field of academics and their pool of knowledge is as vast as their experience in printing. Their expertise and guidance has proved useful at every step. Their uncompromising quality standards have made this book an exceptional effort. Their encouragement from time to time has been an inspiration for everyone.

The publisher and the editorial board hope that this book will prove to be a valuable piece of knowledge for researchers, students, practitioners and scholars across the globe.

List of Contributors

Modou M. Mbaye
Laboratory of Physiopathology, Genetics Molecular and Biotechnology (PGMB), Faculty of Sciences Ain Chock, Research Center Health and Biotechnology, University Hassan II of Casablanca, Morocco
In Vitro Fertilization Center IRIFIV, IRIS Clinic, Casablanca, Morocco

Bouchra El Khalfi, Saida Ouzamode and Abdelaziz Soukri
Laboratory of Physiopathology, Genetics Molecular and Biotechnology (PGMB), Faculty of Sciences Ain Chock, Research Center Health and Biotechnology, University Hassan II of Casablanca, Morocco

Noureddine Louanjli
In Vitro Fertilization Center IRIFIV, IRIS Clinic, Casablanca, Morocco

Brahim Saadani
Laboratory of Medical Analyses, Reproductive Biology, Labomac, Casablanca, Morocco

Dagmawit Birhanu Kebede, Yeshitila Belay Belachew, Desta Workneh Selbana and Admasu Belay Gizaw
Jimma University School of Nursing and Midwifery, Ethiopia

Faisel Dula Sema
Department of Clinical Pharmacy, School of Pharmacy, College of Medicine and Health Sciences, University of Gondar, Ethiopia

Deres Gezahegn Addis, Eshetie Azezew Melese and Demeke Dana Nassa
School of Pharmacy, College of Medicine and Health Sciences, University of Gondar, Ethiopia

Zemene Demelash Kifle
Department of Pharmacology, School of Pharmacy, College of Medicine and Health Sciences, University of Gondar, Ethiopia

Giani Silvana Schwengber Cezimbra and Dioclécio Campos Junior
Department of Pediatrics, Faculty of Medical Sciences-University of Brasília (UnB), Brasília-DF 70.910-900, Brazil

Edward Araujo Júnior and Cristina Aparecida Falbo Guazzelli
Department of Obstetrics, Paulista School of Medicine-Federal University of São Paulo (EPM-UNIFESP), São Paulo-SP 04021-001, Brazil

Álvaro Nagib Atallah
Discipline of Evidence-Based Medicine, Paulista School of Medicine-Federal University of São Paulo (EPM-UNIFESP), São Paulo-SP 04024-002, Brazil

Shamsudeen Mohammed
Department of Population, Family and Reproductive Health, School of Public Health, Kwame Nkrumah University of Science and Technology, Kumasi, Ghana

Roderick Emil Larsen-Reindorf
Department of Obstetrics & Gynaecology, School of Medical Science, Kwame Nkrumah University of Science and Technology, Kumasi, Ghana

Issahaku Awal
Department of Medicine, Renal Dialysis Unit, Tamale Teaching Hospital, Tamale, Ghana

Haile Zewdu Tsegaw
Maternity Ward, Gondar University Comprehensive and Specialized Referal Hospital, Ethiopia

Endeshaw Admassu Cherkos, Marta Berta Badi and Muhabaw Shumye Mihret
Department of Midwifery, College of Medicine and Health Sciences, University of Gondar, Ethiopia

Haileyesus Gedamu, Adane Tsegaw and Etsubdink Debebe
School of Nursing, Bahir Dar University, Bahir Dar, Ethiopia

Mirwais Saheem
Master of Public Health Program, Faculty of Medicine, Kandahar University, Kandahar, Afghanistan

Muhammad Haroon Stanikzai
Public Health Department, Faculty of Medicine, Kandahar University, Kandahar, Afghanistan

Ghulam Mohydin Mudasir and Najeeb Rahimy
Para Clinic Department, Faculty of Medicine, Kandahar University, Kandahar, Afghanistan

Najibullah Fazli
Internal Medicine Department, Faculty of Medicine, Kandahar University, Kandahar, Afghanistan

Hadia Sayam
Para-clinic Department, Malalay Institute of Higher Education, Kandahar, Afghanistan

Negussie Boti, Tezera Bekele, Wanzahun Godana, Eskeziyaw Getahun and Feleke Gebremeskel
Department of Public Health, College of Medicine and Health Sciences, Arba Minch University, Arba Minch, Ethiopia

Behailu Tsegaye
Department of Biomedical Sciences, College of Medicine and Health Sciences, Arba Minch University, Arba Minch, Ethiopia

Bilcha Oumer
Department of Midwifery, College of Health Sciences, Arba Minch, Ethiopia

Tchoula Mamiafo Corinne
Department of Biochemistry, Faculty of Sciences, University of Yaoundé I, PB 812 Yaoundé, Cameroon

Pieme Constant Anatole and Ngogang Yonkeu Jeanne
Department of Biochemistry, Faculty of Medicine and Biomedical Sciences, University of Yaoundé I, PB 1364 Yaoundé, Cameroon

Farrukh Ishaque Saah
Department of Epidemiology and Biostatistics, School of Public Health, University of Health and Allied Sciences, Hohoe, Ghana

Elvis Enowbeyang Tarkang, Joyce Komesuor, Eric Osei and Hubert Amu
Department of Population and Behavioural Sciences, School of Public Health, University of Health and Allied Sciences,Hohoe, Ghana

Evelyn Acquah
Institute of Health Research, University of Health and Allied Sciences, Ho, Ghana

C. C. Ifemelumma, C. C. Anikwe, F. A. Onu, J. A. Obuna, B. N. Ejikeme and O. P. Ezeonu
Department of Obstetrics and Gynaecology, Federal Teaching Hospital Abakaliki Ebonyi State, PMB 102 Abakaliki, Ebonyi State, Nigeria

B. C. Okorochukwu
Department of Obstetrics and Gynaecology, Federal Medical Centre Owerri, Owerri, Imo State, Nigeria

Sita Chhetri
Charak Hospital Nursing College, Pokhara, Kaski, Nepal

Rajani Shah
Nepal Public Health Foundation, Kathmandu, Nepal

Laxmi Rajbanshi
Teaching Hospital, Chitwan Medical College, Bharatpur, Nepal

Júlia Kefalás Troncon
MSc in Obstetrics and Gynecology, Department of Obstetrics and Gynecology, Ribeirão Preto Medical School, University of São Paulo, Ribeirão Preto, SP, Brazil

Júlio César Rosa-e-Silva and Francisco José Candido-dos-Reis
Associate Professor, Department of Obstetrics and Gynecology, Ribeirão Preto Medical School, University of São Paulo, Ribeirão Preto (SP), Brazil

Rayssa Miranda
Undergraduate student, Ribeirão Preto Medical School, University of São Paulo, Ribeirão Preto, SP, Brazil

Omero Benedicto Poli-Neto
Associate Professor, Department of Obstetrics and Gynecology, Ribeirão Preto Medical School, University of São Paulo, Ribeirão Preto, SP, Brazil

Antônio Alberto Nogueira
PhD, Professor, Department of Obstetrics and Gynecology, Ribeirão Preto Medical School, University of São Paulo, Ribeirão Preto, SP, Brazil

Prince Kubi Appiah
Department of Family and Community Health, School of Public Health, University of Health and Allied Sciences, Ho, Ghana
Department of Medical Law and Ethics, Asian Institute for Bioethics and Health Law, College of Medicine, Yonsei University, Seoul, Republic of Korea

Blaise Bagyliku Kuubabongnaa and Mohammed Bukari
Health Information Unit, District Health Administration, Ghana Health Service, Wa East District, Upper West Region, Ghana

Simon Nidoolah Yiri-Erong
Department of Public Health and Community Medicine, Institute of Medicine, University of Gothenburg, Sweden

Kwabena Owusu
Health Information Unit, District Health Administration, Ghana Health Service, Wa West District, Upper West Region, Ghana

George Borogyante Atanga
Health Information Unit, District Health Administration, Ghana Health Service, Sissaala West District, Upper West Region, Ghana

Stephen Nimirkpen
Health Information Unit, Municipal Health Administration, Ghana Health Service, Lawra Municipal, Upper West Region, Ghana

Martin Adjuik
Department of Epidemiology and Biostatistics, School of Public Health, University of Health and Allied Sciences, Ho, Ghana

Negash Wakgari
Department of Midwifery, Ambo University, Ambo, Ethiopia

Terefe Woyo, Emnet Kebede and Hirut Gemeda
Department of Midwifery, Hawassa University, Hawassa, Ethiopia

Wakgari Binu
School of Public Health, Wolaita Soddo University, Wolaita, Ethiopia

Gonfa Moti
Ambo University Referral Hospital, Ambo, Ethiopia

Kefena Etita Bedada
Ambo Town Health Office, Ambo, Ethiopia

Tufa Kolola Huluka
Department of Public Health, College of Medicine and Health Silences, Ambo University, Ambo, Ethiopia

Gizachew Abdissa Bulto and Ephrem Yohannes Roga
Department of Midwifery, College of Medicine and Health Sciences, Ambo University, Ambo, Ethiopia

Nick A. Bersinger, Markus Eisenhut, Petra Stute and Michael von Wolff
University Women's Hospital, Division of Gynaecological Endocrinology and Reproductive Medicine, University of Berne, Switzerland

Yohannes Kelifa Emiru, Betelhem Anteneh Adamu and Abyot Endale Gurmu
Department of Pharmacognosy, School of Pharmacy, College of Medicine and Health Sciences, University of Gondar, Gondar, Ethiopia

Melak Erara
Department of Clinical Pharmacy, School of Pharmacy, College of Medicine and Health Sciences, University of Gondar, Gondar, Ethiopia

Tigist Chanie
University of Gondar Compressive Specialized Hospital, University of Gondar, Gondar, Ethiopia

Mengstu Melkamu Asaye, Tewodros Syoum Nigussie and Worku Mequannt Ambaw
Midwifery Department, College of Medicine and Health Sciences, University of Gondar, Gondar, Ethiopia

Christine Nimwesiga
Institute of Public Health and Management, Clarke International University, Kampala, Uganda

Mereth Murezi
Uganda Nursing School, Bwindi-UCU Affiliate, Uganda

Ivan Mugisha Taremwa
Institute of Allied Health Sciences, Clarke International University, Kampala, Uganda

Manish Banker, Parul Arora and Sandeep Shah
Nova IVF Fertility, Ahmedabad, India

Jwal Banker
IVI RMA, Madrid, Spain

Oloruntoba Ayodele Ekun, Oluwatumininu Mary Olawumi and Nkeiruka Ogochukwu Ogidi
Department of Medical Laboratory Science, College of Medicine, University of Lagos, Nigeria

Christian Chigozie Makwe
Department of Obstetrics and Gynaecology, College of Medicine, University of Lagos, Nigeria

Asmelash Abera Mitiku
Gambella Regional Health Bureau, Gambella Region, Ethiopia

Abraham Lomboro Dimore and Solomon Berhanu Mogas
Department of Epidemiology, Jimma University, Jimma, Oromia, Ethiopia

Ayele Mamo Abebe
Department of Nursing, Debre Birhan Health Sciences College, Debre Birhan 37, Amhara, Ethiopia

Mesfin Wudu Kassaw
Department of Nursing, College of Health Sciences, Woldia University, Amhara, Ethiopia

Nathan Estifanos Shewangashaw
Department of Nursing, College of Health Sciences, Wollo University, Amhara, Ethiopia

Gashaw Agegnehu
Tikl Dingay Health Center, Ethiopia

Azeb Atenafu
Department of Human Nutrition, Institute of Public Health, College of Medicine and Health Sciences, University of Gondar, Gondar 196, Ethiopia

Henok Dagne
Department of Environmental and Occupational Health and Safety, Institute of Public Health, College of Medicine and Health Sciences, University of Gondar, Gondar 196, Ethiopia

Baye Dagnew
Department of Human Physiology, School of Medicine, University of Gondar, Gondar, Ethiopia

Index

www.ingramcontent.com/pod-product-compliance
Lightning Source LLC
LaVergne TN
LVHW082221200926
848484LV00008B/2284
* 9 7 9 8 8 8 7 4 0 4 3 3 2 *